4/18 Wrinkled pages, last page slightly skied TC

The Mississippi Valley's
Great Yellow Fever Epidemic
of 1878

Khaled J. Bloom

THE MISSISSIPPI VALLEY'S GREAT YELLOW FEVER EPIDEMIC OF 1878

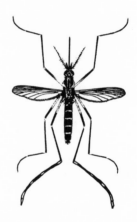

LOUISIANA STATE UNIVERSITY PRESS   Baton Rouge and London

Copyright © 1993 by Louisiana State University Press
All rights reserved
Manufactured in the United States of America
First printing
02 01 00 99 98 97 96 95 94 93   5 4 3 2 1

Designer: Glynnis Phoebe
Typeface: Galliard
Typesetter: G&S Typesetters, Inc.
Printer and binder: Thomson-Shore, Inc.

Library of Congress Cataloging-in-Publication Data

Bloom, Khaled J., 1954–
    The Mississippi Valley's great yellow fever epidemic of 1878 /
Khaled J. Bloom.
        p.   cm.
    Includes index.
    ISBN 0-8071-1824-9 (cloth : alk. paper)
    1. Yellow fever—Mississippi River Valley—History—19th century.
    2. Yellow fever—Mississippi River Valley—Epidemiology.   I. Title.
    [DNLM: 1. Yellow Fever—history—United States.   2. Disease
Outbreaks—history—United States.   3. History of Medicine, 19th
Cent.—United States.   WC 532 B655m 1993]
    RA644.Y4B56   1993
614.5′41′097709034—dc20
DNLM/DLC
for Library of Congress   93-2965
                                                                CIP

To the memory of my father,
Cedric Parnell Bloom

CONTENTS

ACKNOWLEDGMENTS

Perhaps more than most monographs, this work fed, grew, and matured on the favors of others. I can do no better than quote my good cousin, Stephen Jaeger, in his preface to one of his fine books: "Rather than pay them back piecemeal and unevenly here, I should take recourse to whatever is the author's equivalent of bankruptcy and give up all my collected assets in the form of this book. Such as they are, they are much richer for the help of many donors."

The reference and interlibrary loan departments of the Health Sciences Library, University of California, Davis, were eyes and hands to me in the early stages of research. The university's Northern Regional Library Facility and various branch libraries on the Berkeley, San Francisco, and Los Angeles campuses also supplied important materials and services. I owe a particular debt of gratitude to the Lane Medical Library, Stanford University, for access to its wonderful collection of nineteenth-century medical books and journals. I thank the Civil Reference Branch of the National Archives for prompt replies to all my inquiries. I am likewise beholden to many public and academic libraries in the southern states, notably the Memphis and Shelby County Public Library in Memphis, the Tennessee State Library and Archives in Nashville, and the Division of Libraries of the Louisiana State University Medical Center in New Orleans.

To Frederick Simoons, a scholar in the best sense of the term, I am grateful for both precept and example. I am indebted to my friends Kenneth Thompson and Calvin Schwabe for their criticisms of the original draft. I am privileged to acknowledge a review of the final manuscript by John Duffy, whose work in the field of American medical history I have long admired. Some finishing touches were advised by Gabriele Ludwig, a woman of uncommon discernment.

I thank Helen, Kevin, and Elisabeth Switzer-Patterson, the valiant little Davis family whose hospitality and patience were so valuable when much of the research and writing were under way. I thank my mother, Jeanne, and Mr. Carl Zarcone for the same. I thank the faculty, staff, and students of the Geography Department, University of California, Davis, for their indulgence.

I am under the greatest obligation to Louisiana State University Press and everyone connected with it. I thank Margaret Fisher Dalrymple for her encouragement of the work early on. I thank Catherine Landry and Julie Schorfheide for their good services in steering things along. And the luck of the draw was certainly mine when Jane Taylor was engaged as my copy editor; my most lavish and sincere thanks to her.

The Mississippi Valley's
Great Yellow Fever Epidemic
of 1878

ONE

Yellow Fever: A Sketch of Its Natural and Human History

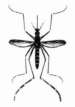

"The King of Terrors continues to snatch victims with fearful rapidity," the Memphis *Avalanche* reported dolefully, as epidemic yellow fever tightened its grip on the city in the summer of 1878. "One by one those who remain in the city and are liable to the monster malady are taken down. . . . Our streets are deserted, our stores and residences empty. . . . But three weeks have passed since the fever broke out among us, and from six to eight weeks must elapse before relief can be extended and the fever checked by the appearance of frost."[1] The King of Terrors had not yet visited its full fury on Memphis. When the anticipated frost finally arrived seven weeks later to check the disease, the death toll in the Tennessee city exceeded five thousand. Memphis, which formerly boasted a population of fifty thousand, thus found itself literally decimated, after passing through an ordeal much worse than decimation if we consider the city's mostly deserted condition at the time. "The grandest misfortune that ever marked an American city," the *Avalanche* called it, while journals across the country exclaimed that for sheer desolation by pestilence, the Memphis of 1878 had its parallel only in the plague-ravaged Florence of 1348. We may discount the historical accuracy of the latter assertion, but the Memphis epidemic indeed stands out as one of the very worst catastrophes in American urban history, its toll in human life surpassing that of the Chicago fire, San Francisco earthquake, and Johnstown flood combined.

1. Memphis *Avalanche,* September 1, 1878.

The yellow fever calamity of 1878 was not confined to Memphis, how-ever: more than four thousand lives were swept away by the pestilence at New Orleans, more than one thousand at Vicksburg, and at least another five thousand in over two hundred towns and villages in nine states of the Mississippi Valley.[2] And while the toll in sickness and death was terrible enough, it was perhaps the lesser part of the story. As the New York *Bulletin* observed, the epidemic was "more than a local misfortune, it is a positive national calamity. . . . The whole valley of the Mississippi is pre-cipitated into a fright. Railway and steamboat communication between cities is suspended, the mails even are turned back, and all the ordinary operations of commerce and trade are paralyzed. The paralysis has ex-tended to the cities of the Atlantic seaboard, and we doubt if millions of dollars would today repair the losses which have already resulted." In its aftermath a Louisville medical editor warned: "The importance of the yel-low fever question can not be exaggerated. No question comparable in im-portance has been presented to the people of America since the civil war. The entire country is interested in it pecuniarily if not vitally. The pecu-niary losses entailed by the late scourge are estimated at $200,000,000, and the lives destroyed at from fifteen to twenty thousand."[3]

It is fair to assert that in the Americas at least, yellow fever was the most dreaded epidemic malady of the eighteenth and nineteenth centuries, and yet its prevalence was almost entirely limited to those two centuries. There is no mention whatever of yellow fever in early European or Ori-ental writings, ancient or medieval. The disease came to the attention of the Old World only after discovery of the New. The initial consensus among historians of yellow fever was that the infection was native to tropi-cal America—it was known to the Carib and Maya Indians, had plagued Columbus' first colony on Hispaniola, and was encountered in Darien by the Spanish when they first landed there. This view was being maintained

2. Enumerations of the dead as well as listings of the places visited by the fever were, of course, quite inexact. What appear to be the two most complete summaries are found in John M. Keating, *The Yellow Fever Epidemic of 1878 in Memphis, Tenn.* (Memphis, 1879), 92–97, and J. P. Dromgoole, *Yellow Fever Heroes, Honors, and Horrors of 1878* (Louisville, 1879), 107–25.

3. L. P. Yandell, "The Late Yellow Fever Outbreak in Louisville," *Louisville Medical News,* VI (1878), 277.

by Leland Howard, for example, as late as 1912.[4] In the last great work of his career, Henry Rose Carter, one of yellow fever's most sedulous and productive students, carefully examined early records of sickness and mortality in the pioneer settlements of Mexico, Panama, and the Spanish Main. Carter demonstrated that none of the many plagues described in the old histories truly satisfied the symptomological and etiological conditions of yellow fever; he determined that the first definite accounts of epidemic yellow fever in America record it in Yucatán in 1648 and Cuba in 1649. Carter argued that the disease had originated in West Africa and was probably introduced to the Caribbean by way of the slave trade, which had gotten into full swing earlier in the 1600s. Since 1931, when Carter's book was published, biological evidence has accumulated confirming the African origin of yellow fever.[5]

Yellow fever appears to have become thoroughly seeded and naturalized around the Caribbean Basin by 1700, established there on an endemic basis in the tropical climate, and it was the Caribbean, with its close maritime ties to northern ports, that came to be regarded as the great nidus and distribution center of the disease. It was unquestionably from Havana, Veracruz, and other permanently infected ports around the "Mexique Bay" that yellow fever made its deadly summer excursions to higher latitudes in the following century. By 1800 it had been recorded at least once at most of the tidewater cities of the east coast of North America—the story of the terrible epidemic at Philadelphia in 1793 is fairly well known—and had also crossed the Atlantic to visit some of the southern ports of Iberia. Desolating epidemics occurred at Cádiz and Seville in 1800, and at Gibraltar and Málaga in 1804. In 1821 it raged at Barcelona, as well as at Palma on the island of Mallorca. There was a severe epidemic at Lisbon in 1857, evidently introduced by ships from Rio de Janeiro. At Rio, just inside the Tropic of Capricorn, the disease did not appear until 1849, but thereafter established itself as a notorious endemic plague, some years claiming thousands of victims. Before long the Brazilian capital had a reputation

4. Leland O. Howard, Harrison G. Dyar, and Frederick Knab, *The Mosquitoes of North and Central America and the West Indies* (4 vols.; Washington, D.C., 1912), I, 294–98. See also George Augustin, *History of Yellow Fever* (New Orleans, 1909), 639–49.

5. Henry Rose Carter, *Yellow Fever: An Historical and Epidemiological Study of Its Place of Origin* (Baltimore, 1931), 81–197.

for insalubrity rivaling that of Havana.[6] In areas favored by short summers and cool winters, yellow fever was known only as an occasional scourge, one which could be severe in an unusually warm season, but which, like the seed falling in stony places in the parable, would not take permanent root and showed little or no tendency to spread from the coastal cities to the interior. Among major port cities outside the tropics, it was only at New Orleans that yellow fever became entrenched as a recurrent (though not truly endemic) public health problem, and only in New Orleans' hinterland, the lower Mississippi Valley, with its long subtropical summer, that epidemic outbreaks of the disease began to involve an increasingly wider territory. This development in the geographic distribution of yellow fever was clearly seen later on in the nineteenth century. The epidemic of 1878 was the most fatal and extensive diffusion of the disease.

Well into the twentieth century, even after the disease's mode of transmission had been established and quite thoroughly analyzed, such unspecific terms as *the infective principle* and *the parasite* were being used in the medical literature to designate the causative agent of yellow fever. The discovery of a number of susceptible laboratory animals in the late 1920s brought about a flourish of productive virological and immunological research, and within a few years the long-sought yellow fever "germ" was finally isolated, its physical and chemical properties described, and its cellular pathology studied. A practicable vaccine was available by 1938. We know today that yellow fever is caused by a mosquito-borne virus that invades through the lymphatic system and rapidly proliferates in visceral tissue cells. The liver, kidneys, and heart are principally involved, and the degenerative changes in those organs are responsible for most of the clinical symptoms. The general progress of organ damage in yellow fever is described as cloudy swelling and icteric staining of the organ tissue, continuing through degenerative fatty infiltration, and culminating in local necrosis; the prospect of recovery or of collapse and death depends on the degree of injury. Although details of the toxic process and the physiological damage involved were not understood until the present century, the gross pathological appearances in yellow fever were quite well recognized

6. Augustin, *History of Yellow Fever,* 356–635, 767–1024; E. Cleary, "Report upon the History of Yellow Fever in Rio de Janeiro since 1849," in U.S. Marine Hospital Service, *Report for Fiscal 1896,* 380–81.

by 1878, and autopsies were often performed to establish a diagnosis in questionable cases.[7]

As to its outward symptoms, yellow fever is apt to be sudden in its onset, ushered in with malaise, headache, chills, and generalized aches and pains in muscles and joints. In mild cases the symptoms end there, and might pass off in as little as forty-eight hours. An unusually observant doctor in a small town outside Memphis in 1878 noted: "Many persons who kept on their feet throughout the epidemic gave unmistakable evidence of the effects of the poison in their systems. . . . From examinations made at the time, I found a red and dry tongue and yellowish scanty urine very common, attended by head and backache, a feverish condition, and insomnia. I suffered thus myself, as did the other physicians of the place."[8] Such cases were liable to go entirely unnoticed, and if detected at all were very easily mistaken for flu, dengue, or one or another of the ordinary "bilious" or malarial fevers. As James Carroll advised in 1903: "Genuine yellow fever may be so mild in character that no one, no matter how extensive his experience may have been, would dare diagnose it as such unless he knew the disease to be prevailing at the time."[9] As a result, early cases of the fever more often than not went unrecognized and undeclared until the infection had already gotten a substantial foothold in the community. The mild cases were, to be sure, the most insidious carriers and spreaders of the disease and not only posed an insurmountable challenge to practical sanitarians and quarantine enforcers, but had the effect of inspiring much misconceived theorizing about the "spontaneous" origin of yellow fever in "local causes," or about its transmission via "fomites." In fact most nineteenth-century physicians did not recognize the contagiousness of yellow fever even in its most frank and malignant form, and very

7. John C. Bugher, "The Pathology of Yellow Fever," in *Yellow Fever*, ed. George K. Strode (New York, 1951), 142–59. Compare Joseph Jones, "Yellow Fever," in *A Dictionary of Medicine*, ed. Richard Quain (New York, 1883), 1800–1803. See also "In the Dead House," Louisville *Courier-Journal*, September 30, 1878.

8. John F. Cochran, "Observations on Yellow Fever at Bartlett, Tenn.," *Richmond and Louisville Medical Journal*, XXVII (1879), 13.

9. James Carroll, "Remarks on the History, Cause, and Mode of Transmission of Yellow Fever," *Journal of the Association of Military Surgeons*, XIII (1903), 193. On the problem of differential diagnosis, see J. Austin Kerr, "The Clinical Aspects and Diagnosis of Yellow Fever," in *Yellow Fever*, ed. Strode, 400–416; Rubert W. Boyce, *Yellow Fever and Its Prevention* (New York, 1911), 197–207.

few were as perceptive as S. O. Vanderpoel, who warned in 1873: "Those half-sick often deceive the most rigid scrutiny, yet they possess the same specific element as the graver cases, and in point of contagion, the same danger."[10]

In more serious cases the symptoms, extending over three to seven days, advance and intensify. Frontal headache and pains in the lower back and limbs become severe, even violent. Nausea, stomach cramps, constipation, and urinary suppression are distressing symptoms. Fever remains high, while the pulse falls. There is general congestion, with a horrible tendency to hemorrhage in many places, even from the urethra and ears. The eyes are red and glistening at first, becoming deeply bloodshot and even seeping blood. The face becomes flushed; the lips and tongue puff, crack, and bleed; the gums in particular swell painfully and ooze blood; and there is a tendency to heavy and persistent nosebleeds. Often the skin becomes blotched with purpuric spots; old bruises exude blood spontaneously. Uterine bleeding, sometimes heavy, is common in women, and pregnant women usually miscarry. In the most malignant cases appears what is perhaps the most ghastly symptom of the disease, the throwing up of greater or lesser amounts of "black vomit." This grumous, "coffee-grounds" matter represents the partially digested blood, blackened by gastric juices, that seeps into the gut through capillary hemorrhages in the mucous lining of the stomach and duodenum.

Nervous irritability and restlessness are often significant premonitory symptoms, abiding and often worsening as the attack progresses. In the past this effect of the disease was widely mistaken for a predisposing cause. Several times in the course of the 1878 epidemic the New Orleans *Picayune* editorialized on "Damaging Emotions" and the imperative to maintain perfect tranquillity, and to that end the mayor of the city repeatedly ordered the police to suppress all unnecessary and disturbing noisemaking in the city, from whistle blowing by tugs on the river to yelling and bell ringing by hucksters on the streets. The belief also tended to encourage

10. S. Oakley Vanderpoel, "General Principles Affecting the Organization and Practice of Quarantines," *Reports and Papers, American Public Health Association*, I (1873), 412. Contrast Vanderpoel's insight with A. N. Bell, "Some Observations on Yellow Fever and Its Habitudes, as Opposed to the Fallacies and Dangers of Personal Quarantine," *Reports and Papers, American Public Health Association*, XIV (1888), 55–61.

the misuse of alcohol and opiates as prophylactics by nervous individuals. Delirium, ranging in degree from mild confusion to active maniacal raving, often appears in the last stage of malignant yellow fever. In the worst cases it is awful to behold; clinically it was and is considered to be of very grave import; and in the violent epidemics of the past, this dreaded symptom was undoubtedly the inspiration of much of the distress and panic sparked by the appearance of Yellow Jack. "Men, delirious, rush from their rooms into the street," was the terse headline of the Memphis *Avalanche* on August 31, 1878, summing up for all who read it the awful desolation and helplessness of the stricken city. The agitation is thought to be the result of congestion and swelling of the minute capillaries of the brain. Coma due to hepatic collapse, or toxic convulsions from kidney failure, usually supervene in fatal cases. "The death is a horror—as bad as confluent smallpox or hydrophobia," wrote H. R. Carter, whose personal acquaintance with epidemics of this disease extended from Memphis in 1879 to Guayaquil in 1916. Climaxing the ugly symptom complex of malignant yellow fever, and adding much to its mystery and horror in the past, is the hideous skin discoloration appearing just before and after death, a deep jaundice caused by necrosis of the liver, and from which the disease takes its name. "Like a rotten pumpkin" was a simile frequently used by reporters both medical and journalistic. In very bad cases the hue is bronze or mahogany yellow.[11]

A good description of a fatal case of yellow fever, displaying most of the symptoms characteristic of the disease in its most malignant form, survives in an account of the 1878 epidemic at Bartlett, Tennessee, a small town on the railroad eleven miles outside Memphis. The victim was a Captain LaFevre, described as "a robust farmer about forty years of age," who died on September 14. It was said he had been into Memphis about a month before, but in the meantime he had frequently been in Bartlett

11. Kerr, "Clinical Aspects," in *Yellow Fever,* ed. Strode, 389–400; Boyce, *Yellow Fever,* 127–96; H. R. Carter, "Yellow Fever," in *The Practice of Medicine in the Tropics,* ed. William Byam and R. G. Archibald (2 vols.; London, 1922), II, 1235–43; René LaRoche, *Yellow Fever, Considered in Its Historical, Pathological, Etiological, and Therapeutical Relations* (2 vols.; Philadelphia, 1855), I, 129–42. For firsthand clinical accounts from the 1878 epidemic, see A. Hausmann, "Observations on Yellow Fever," *St. Louis Medical and Surgical Journal,* XXXVI (1879), 19–28; J. B. Marvin, "Yellow Fever," *American Practitioner,* XVIII (1878), 295–307.

and the nearby town of Raleigh, both of which had cases of yellow fever. At Raleigh he had visited one house where a person had died. LaFevre died at his establishment in the country two miles outside Bartlett. It was noted that his family and servants, five persons in all, were in constant attendance on him during his sickness, but none of them came down with the fever. The case history also presents a good description of the medical treatment of yellow fever typical at that time:

> He had suffered twice during the summer from intermittent fever. On September 9th, 7 A.M., he had a slight chill, or rather chilly sensations, followed by violent febrile reaction, with unusual pain in the head (frontal) and backache, sore throat, irritability of the bladder, and difficulty in emptying it. He spent a very disagreeable night. Next day, at 1 P.M., the fever having failed to pass off as usual, I was called to see him. He had already taken, at his own option, "McLean's pills" and eighteen grains of quinine. Pulse 100, temperature 104°F, skin pungently hot, and had not been moist at all. Urine sufficient, but passed with straining and pain. Frontal headache, pain in lumbar region, and aching of limbs and shoulders. The restlessness of the patient was striking; he could not be kept still, nor covered; had not slept a moment. Countenance flushed; eyes injected; brilliant and intolerant of light; tongue had a little white coating, with red edges, and plain indentations of the teeth; thirst decided; stomach quiet; bowels had acted scantily, and there was slight cinchonism. I suspected yellow fever, and, contrary to my better judgment, gave grs. x calomel and grs. xx quinine. I requested a consultation, and Dr. Duncan of Raleigh saw him with me at 5 P.M. There was no material change in his condition, except that cinchonism was now profound. Diagnosis, unquestionable yellow fever. Mustard footbaths, sage tea, and frequent sponging of the surface with tepid water and whiskey, were ordered with a view to their quieting and sudorific effect.
>
> September 11th, 11:30 A.M.—Pulse 90, temperature 102°F. Has spent another restless night, without any sleep or perspiration. Countenance bears an expression of anxiety; tongue has thick white coating in the center; papillae enlarged and red; edges quite red, presenting very much the appearance of the tongue of scarlet fever. Mouth dry; thirst great; gums ragged and inclined to bleed; lips scarlet; nasal passages dry; urine scanty, and of an orange color, and evidently laden with the epithelial coating of the bladder. Calomel had acted freely; dejecta black and wa-

tery. Stomach quiet; very restless. Sponging and baths, which had a momentarily quieting effect, continued. Watermelon-seed tea to be given freely.

5 P.M.—Pulse 90, temperature 103°F. Condition about the same, and treatment continued.

September 12th, 8 A.M.—Pulse 84, temperature 102°F. Another restless night. Urine almost suspended, without deposit, except a little bright red material, which drifted into lines in the bottom of the vessel when decanted. The patient now presented a degree of mental and bodily excitement I had not witnessed before; his whole frame was in a tremor; his mind was clear and painfully alive to impressions from what he saw or heard; he was bleeding from the nose, gums, and lips; dejections from the bowels black, watery, and frequent; stomach uneasy, but no vomiting; thirst intense; he said he was "burning up inside"; respiration sighing and irregular. Acetate potass. was added to the watermelon-seed tea, and turpentine stupes were used to back and abdomen.

3:30 P.M.—Pulse 76, temperature 101°F. Champagne was added to the morning directions. No encouragement from the kidneys; patient more quiet.

September 13th, 10:30 A.M.—Pulse 84, temperature 101°F; kidneys secreting a little better; about three ounces passed during the night. Has slept in snatches; vomited several times mucus and water containing dark flocculi. Nothing allowed now by stomach but a little water and ice.

4:30 P.M.—Pulse 84, temperature 100°F. He rested quietly two hours during the morning. Passed about one ounce of urine. Stomach would retain nothing; had vomited a quantity of blood. Delirium had set in; he was unmanageable, except by force. The extremities were getting cold. He died early next morning.[12]

Secondary infections may account for a few late deaths, but recovery from yellow fever is ordinarily rapid and complete, with no significant complications or sequelae. It is very important to note that one attack of the disease confers lifelong immunity. It was an old observation that a sweeping epidemic of yellow fever had the effect of rendering most of those who lived through it resistant to future attacks, even many who had not been recognizably sick; and at New Orleans, as well as at Havana and

12. Cochran, "Yellow Fever at Bartlett," 8–10.

Rio de Janeiro, it was proverbial that mortality from the fever corresponded directly with the pulse of fresh immigration to the city. In the eighteenth and early nineteenth centuries, when the fever was generally thought to be produced by poison in the atmosphere, this acquired resistance was explained as an adjustment or hardening of the individual system to the causative miasm, and was termed "acclimation." As late as 1875 the president of the Louisiana Board of Health could wonder: "How, is the question, is toleration to yellow fever produced by continuous exposure to its poisonous cause, or by being accustomed to high temperatures, to be answered? It is probably better to use the expression of resistance to the poison, as such resistance to other zymotic poisons is frequently seen." It was only as the germ theory gained ground that physicians began to understand the phenomenon of "acclimation" to yellow fever in terms of the modern concept of acquired immunity.[13]

The awful mortality attributed to yellow fever would of course explain most of the terror with which its epidemic visitations were regarded in the past. The modern literature, however, has progressively downplayed this feature of the disease. Current medical textbooks place the normal case fatality rate in yellow fever at just 5 to 10 percent, while admitting death rates of up to 50 percent in severe outbreaks. The tendency is to presume that the high ratio of deaths to cases reported in past epidemics can be explained by the likelihood that a great many mild infections simply escaped recognition in times before diagnostic procedures were refined. Laboratory studies, however, have established marked differences in the pathogenic properties of different strains of yellow fever virus, and the mortality statistics of 1878 certainly indicate that a strain of peculiar virulence and deadliness was going the rounds that year. Its severity is exhibited in the fact that of an estimated 6,000 to 9,000 whites who lingered in and around Memphis through the whole course of the epidemic, 4,204 died; of not more than 500 whites who stayed in Grenada, Mississippi, 260 died; and of a similar number in Holly Springs, Mississippi, 210 died.

The whole human family is equally susceptible to infection by the

13. Jo Ann Carrigan, "The Saffron Scourge: A History of Yellow Fever in Louisiana, 1796–1905" (Ph.D. dissertation, Louisiana State University, 1961), 364–98; Louisiana Board of Health, *Report for 1875* (New Orleans, 1876), 35; Stanford E. Chaillé, "Acclimatisation, or Acquisition of Immunity from Yellow Fever," *New Orleans Medical and Surgical Journal,* n.s., VIII (1880), 141–59.

yellow fever virus, but the severity of the disease varies considerably according to race; blacks, at least those of West African extraction, suffer much less than Caucasians. Of the 4,046 yellow fever deaths officially recorded at New Orleans in 1878, only 183 were among the blacks, who made up one-third of the city's population, and even that was considered an unusually high figure. It was said not a single Negro or mulatto was among the 226 who died in the city in the lesser epidemic of 1873. Of the 5,150 deaths tallied at Memphis, only 946 were among "the colored population," although blacks were thought to comprise at least 14,000 of the estimated 20,000 who remained in the city through the epidemic. Now that the geographic origin of yellow fever has been established, it is clear that this comparative resistance is only to be expected in a race exposed to the disease for countless generations in its African homeland.[14]

The disease also tends to be quite mild, often practically undiagnosable, in young children of any race. A doctor at Hernando, Mississippi, thought he saw a connection: he conjectured that since Negroes and children were alike characterized by simple minds, "being incapable of taking a comprehensive view of the situation," they were "not depressed with so much anxiety" as white adults, therefore less given to the mental stress that predisposed a body to yellow fever. The native whites of New Orleans in the last century congratulated themselves on possessing a so-called creole immunity to yellow fever, due not as they thought to some occult process of acclimation, but to having had an unrecognized case of the disease as infants in one or another of the epidemics that swept the city on an almost yearly basis. But an unusually large number of children perished in the 1878 epidemic—at New Orleans, children under ten made up fully half the list of dead many days. That sad deviation from the norm, along with the relatively high mortality suffered by blacks, is another indication of an unusually malignant strain of yellow fever in 1878.[15]

By 1878, indeed well before 1878, it was generally recognized that yellow fever was not a contact disease—that it was not directly communi-

14. Louisiana Board of Health, *Report for 1878* (New Orleans, 1879), 171; Keating, *Epidemic of 1878 in Memphis,* 116; Mississippi Board of Health, *Report for 1878–79* (Jackson, 1879), 45, 61–62.

15. Mississippi Board of Health, *Report for 1878–79,* 74; "Yellow Fever," New Orleans *Picayune,* August 13, 1878; S. M. Bemiss, "Report upon Yellow Fever in Louisiana in 1878, and Subsequently," *New Orleans Medical and Surgical Journal,* n.s., XI (1883), 92–93, 110.

cated from the sick to the well, but was somehow propagated through the medium of a "poisoned" or "infected" environment. "Extrinsic" and "extra-organismal" were among the adjectives applied to this puzzling characteristic of the infection, and over the years a vast amount of speculation was spawned about the peculiar combination of localized atmospheric and telluric influences that could account for it. Two interesting papers submitted to the Medical Society of Tennessee in 1879 considered this matter at some length, drawing illustrations from the epidemic at Chattanooga in 1878. Chattanooga, in the highlands of east Tennessee, had never experienced an outbreak of yellow fever before that unusual summer, and never would again. Though locally quite virulent, causing at least 140 deaths, the disease seemed to have met with a shortage of those unknown "influences" favoring its wider propagation and dissemination and it spread unsteadily or not at all outside a certain "infected district" embracing two slum wards in the center of town. Numerous instances were cited of fever victims who were removed outside (sometimes not very far outside) the infected district but failed to spread the disease behind them; of doctors, nurses, and friends intimately exposed to the transported sick and their exhalations and discharges who did not contract the fever, provided they themselves had not made the mistake of straying into the infected district. "Other conditions are always necessary, aside from simple personal contact with yellow fever patients, to transmit the disease from one to another," was the conclusion. "Other ways of dissemination must account for the spread of yellow fever than that of personal intermingling." Another mysterious property of the infection was the way it clung to buildings even after they had been deserted by their occupants: "Houses, after once being infected, retained their infection for some considerable period of time. This was made known to us by the return of refugees, several of whom, whose houses were in the infected district, were stricken down." [16]

Similar observations were made elsewhere that year and on many

16. W. T. Hope, "Facts on the Introduction and Dissemination of Yellow Fever by Persons," in *Transactions of the Medical Society of the State of Tennessee, 1879* (Nashville, 1879), 155–57, and G. A. Baxter, "Atmospheric Dissemination of Yellow Fever at Chattanooga," *ibid.*, 158–60. See also George M. Sternberg, "Yellow Fever at Pensacola, Fla., in 1873, 1874, and 1875," *Reports and Papers, American Public Health Association*, II (1875), 468–78; U.S. Navy, Bureau of Medicine and Surgery, *Report on Yellow Fever in the* U.S.S. *Plymouth in 1878–9* (1880), 29–33.

other occasions in epidemics both before and after 1878. Dr. Jerome Cochran of the Alabama Board of Health expressed the common view in an 1888 article: "Its growth in the environment seems hardly to admit of question. Upon no other hypothesis can we explain the infection of localities. . . . While the disease spreads from the patient it is not, perhaps at all, and certainly not to any considerable extent, contagious from person to person like smallpox. It seems to take root in the locality—in the soil, as it were—and to be contracted from the environment of the patient rather than from the patient himself; and the locality remains infected after the patient has been removed—remains infected for weeks, and even months."[17] Clearly, the "extrinsic" or extracorporeal character of the yellow fever infection was well recognized by nineteenth-century doctors, but medical theory would twist and turn for many years before finally connecting it to a thing so obscure as the mosquito.

Medical thinkers earlier in the century considered the frequent failure of infection to spread from cases taken out of an infected place to be sufficient evidence for the spontaneous origin and essentially noncontagious character of yellow fever, concluding that the disease was produced by unwholesome conditions in the local atmosphere and nothing else. This school of opinion, dominant well into the 1850s, regarded the disease as a simple intoxication or poisoning engendered by a miasm or vapor in the corrupt air of unclean towns and cities in warm climates.[18] Writing in 1850, Dr. Daniel Drake favored the generally accepted view that yellow fever was the result of a peculiar "civic malaria" catalyzed when a city atmosphere vitiated by "animal exuvia and impure exhalations and secretions from a dense population" was acted on by abnormal weather conditions. Drake insisted that any new theory of yellow fever's etiology was bound to take into account "the necessary, though indirect, agency of a particular local condition of the atmosphere."[19] In a treatise published five years later, Dr. René LaRoche also emphasized the agency of some "peculiar alteration in the surrounding air." In outlining the necessary measures of "public prophylaxis," LaRoche stressed that "streets, alleys, gutters, sinks,

17. Jerome Cochran, "Problems in Regard to Yellow Fever and the Prevention of Yellow Fever Epidemics," *Reports and Papers, American Public Health Association,* XIV (1888), 42–43.
18. LaRoche, *Yellow Fever,* II, 329–68; Carrigan, "Saffron Scourge," 301–17.
19. Daniel Drake, *A Systematic Treatise, Historical, Etiological, and Practical, on the Principal Diseases of the Interior Valley of North America* (2 vols.; Philadelphia, 1854), II, 286–98.

and sewers must be cleaned and expurgated, all sources of noxious effluvia must be removed." In an 1854 report, the Sanitary Commission of New Orleans endorsed the same general idea of an "epidemic constitution of the atmosphere" and offered the same sanitary prescription, taking the view that various gases arising from the organic waste of cities played a role in yellow fever "congenerous" or analogous to that of marsh exhalations in producing the malaria of rural districts. If certain conditions of atmospheric heat and humidity, combined with the various "filthy deposits" inevitably found in towns and cities, were the ever-present concomitants of yellow fever epidemics, it seemed to the Sanitary Commission that "the fact is clearly inferable, that being the sine qua non, they form them."[20]

The attribution of epidemic disease to peculiar changes and conditions in the air—to "miasma" or to an "epidemic constitution of the atmosphere"—was one of medicine's most enduring traditions, with venerable precedents from Sir Humphry Davy to Hippocrates, and there were many things about yellow fever that made the doctrine seem especially applicable. It is not, after all, a "catching" disease in the absence of the mosquito that transmits it, and if we consider the general character of the mosquito vector, the basic perception of a "poisonous" local atmosphere was really not illogical, or even inaccurate. Continued experience with yellow fever gradually made evident a number of contradictions and inadequacies in the miasmatist doctrine, however. Chiefly, there was the fact that the disease occurred only some years, although there was no significant year-to-year difference in weather conditions, and the supposed precursory condition of "noxious effluvia" was likewise always present. There was also the fact that the disease was almost always confined to lines of travel, to communities located on railroads and navigable rivers, and was always at least indirectly associated with human movement and communication with previously infected places. The notion of an infectious "ferment" or "germ," not contagious from person to person, perhaps, but transplantable from place to place, and endowed with the capability of propagating itself outside the human body under the right conditions of warmth, moisture, and decomposition, began to seem a more consistent

20. LaRoche, *Yellow Fever*, II, 624, 751; *Report of the Sanitary Commission of New Orleans on the Epidemic Yellow Fever of 1853* (New Orleans, 1854), 493–97.

and adaptable explanation for these peculiarities of yellow fever, while still respecting the obvious fact that the appearance of this mystifying disease was somehow contingent on "a particular local condition of the atmosphere."[21]

The ideas of noncontagion and local causation, or at least the more inflexible versions of those ideas, were largely discarded by 1878, but the secret of the extrinsic propagation and indirect transmission of yellow fever's hypothetical "germ" remained to tease and baffle medical decipherers. Physicians, of course, could only speculate about the ultimate character of the germ. The New Orleans Board of Health gradually adopted the view that it was animalcular, while many doctors, with as much reason, took the position that it was fungal. The mode of infection was also a subject of interminable conjecture. Most theorists assumed that the germ invaded the human body in active form after passing a certain stage of maturity in outer nature, but some contended that the disease actually resulted from a toxin generated as a by-product of the germ's development in the environment, the way alcohol was generated by yeast proliferating in must or wort. Inasmuch as it recognized a "living cause" of yellow fever afloat in the environment, and shifted understanding of the disease's operation from an inorganic to a biological basis, the germ theory represented a considerable advancement in etiological thinking, yet it did not entail any radical recasting of views as far as practical control measures

21. It should not be supposed that the doctrine of spontaneous origin was completely extinguished by the 1870s. The published proceedings of local medical societies show that even as late as 1879 a considerable number of physicians had not yet settled their views on the germ theory versus local causation. See "Yellow Fever: Discussion, Medical Section, Polytechnic Institute of Kentucky," *Medical Herald* (Louisville), I (1879), 147–56. And at least one professional journal in the region was still vigorously upholding the local-origin position. See "Yellow Fever Commission," *Atlanta Medical and Surgical Journal*, XVI (1878), 558–64. "Hundreds of non-malarious places have been made the test of personal infection by having yellow fever cases brought to them, and the disease did not spread," said the latter. "No 'spark' is necessary to ignite the 'tinder.' When malaria is in sufficient quantity and of sufficient virulence, malignant fever in the form of congestive, yellow, or haemeturial will be found." But most physicians by that time fully recognized the infectious character of yellow fever and would have agreed with Samuel Bemiss when he answered that citing the nonspread of infection in nonsusceptible places as an argument against it was exactly like asking, "If females are impregnated by connection with males, why are not all females impregnated who expose themselves by this act?" ("Yellow Fever Commission—Note on the Review by Dr. Burroughs," *Virginia Medical Monthly*, VI [1879], 56).

were concerned. "Filth," in the ordinary sense of the word, was still regarded as the sine qua non of yellow fever, no longer operating directly, as
a source of poisonous vapors, but supportively, as the "culture medium"
in which the germ of the disease would develop and fructify when introduced. The idea of a free-living saprophytic germ, maturing in sources of
filth and decomposition and diffusing itself into the miasmatic air, seemed
at last to provide a logical and consistent explanation for the extrinsic nature of the yellow fever infection, and took such a hold on medical thought
as to completely overshadow other views, diverting efforts against the disease into completely false channels for the balance of the century. It should
be acknowledged that the backward sanitary condition of the southern and
tropical cities most subject to yellow fever furnished ample credit for the
filth theory of the disease's origin, as this sickening description of the privy
system of New Orleans, written in 1879 by one of the city's sanitary inspectors, testifies:

> During wet weather these vaults or sinks quickly fill with water and over-
> flow, flooding yards and gutters with ordure. Under a sun almost tropical
> one half the year, this ferments and emits a most abominable stench,
> which of all others must be a fruitful source of disease, operating directly
> in its production, and indirectly in lowering the vital stamina of the
> inhabitants.
>
> While in wet seasons these vaults are flooded, in dry weather they
> are largely emptied by their fluid contents soaking into the ground, thus
> saturating the soil upon which we live with human excrement. In this
> respect it may be properly stated that the people have a huge privy in
> common, and that the inhabitants of New Orleans live upon a dung-
> heap.
>
> Is it possible to imagine a sanitary condition more deplorably
> bad? . . . However, so long as this flagrant disobedience of sanitary law
> exists, so long must we surely pay the price, as we paid it last summer.[22]

In the wake of the 1878 epidemic, the editor of the country's leading
public health journal quoted Sir John Simon on cholera being "equally
applicable to yellow fever": "Through the unpolluted atmosphere of
cleanly districts it migrates slowly, without a blow; that which it can kindle

22. Louisiana Board of Health, *Report for 1878*, 87.

into poison lies not there. To the foul, damp breath of low-lying cities it comes like a spark to powder. Here is contained that which it can quickly make destructive—soaked into soil, stagnant in water, griming the pavement, tainting the air—the slow rottenness of unremoved excrement, to which the first contact of this foreign ferment brings the occasion of changing into more and more deadly combinations."[23]

While the germ theory of yellow fever retained many elements of miasmatism, experience made it clear that air currents were not significant factors in disseminating the disease over any considerable distance, even within an infected city. Enormous emphasis came to be placed on the supposed role of "fomites"—mail, merchandise, any items that had been contaminated by the sick or exposed to the exhalations of an infected place. Such articles were thought to absorb and retain the infectious principle, usually conceived in terms of a microscopic seed or spore, which would subsequently germinate and begin multiplying and spreading wherever the fomites were carried, provided the right atmospheric and telluric conditions were present. "Some of these carriers of infection have exhibited an almost marvelous intensity of the poison when considered in connection with the small compass of the material containing it," wrote Dr. Samuel Bemiss, a prominent medical editor of New Orleans, in 1882. "There is trustworthy evidence that a cotton bandana communicated yellow fever to five persons who were all within range of its infection when first opened, and who were all attacked within five days after the exposure."[24] Such reports were thought to buttress rather than discredit the fomites theory. The mysterious phenomenon, frequently recorded in widespread epidemics, of yellow fever erupting in places where there had been no known exposure to a prior case from outside the locality, made the explanation of "infection from fomites" very attractive and plausible, just as it had been cited to support earlier ideas about local miasms and the spontaneous origin of yellow fever. We know in retrospect that such

23. A. N. Bell, "Quarantine," *Sanitarian*, VII (1879), 81.

24. S. M. Bemiss, "Chapters from the Report of Yellow Fever Commission of 1878," *New Orleans Medical and Surgical Journal*, n.s., X (1882), 334. A classic example of supposed fomites infection, perhaps the very one Bemiss was referring to, is described in W. W. Moore, "The Yellow Fever at Mr. Y. R. Griffin's, Four Miles East of Summit," in Bemiss, "Yellow Fever in Louisiana," 172–74. See also "The Cause of the Recent Yellow Fever Outbreak at Pensacola—Findings of the Court of Inquiry," *Medical News*, XLII (1883), 528.

seemingly mysterious instances can be explained very simply as introduction of infection via missed or inapparent cases. It was, of course, only inevitable that mail, merchandise, people, and pestilence should turn up together at the same places during an epidemic season, as natural correlates of necessary commerce and communication. If the spontaneous generation of infection from local causes was no longer a credible explanation for the disease's appearance, and if an infecting case from outside the community was impossible to identify (as it usually was), it seemed logical to trace the introduction of the disease to a germ that had ridden in secretly on papers, fabrics, or other goods. Time and again in the 1878 epidemic we shall see with what facility the fomites doctrine could be stretched and adapted to cover almost any anomaly in the spread of yellow fever from place to place.[25]

"Yellow fever is so feebly contagious from the persons of the sick," Dr. Bemiss declared, "that it is questionable, in instances where it is supposed to have been communicated directly from the exhalation of the body, if the clothing or other things about the patient were not really the fomites to spread the disease." Dr. John M. Woodworth, surgeon general of the U.S. Marine Hospital Service, stated it even more positively: "Evidence warrants the assertion that yellow fever poison is transported by *things,* and not by persons considered apart from their clothing."[26] Of course a few doctors were alert to the contradictions inherent in the fomites doctrine, such as Ezra Hunt of the New Jersey Board of Health, who asked: "Has not the person a relation to the surcharging of articles called fomitic? If the disease cannot be communicated from one person to another, then how is it possible for the sick man to infect his clothing so that it may be the means of spreading the disease?"[27] Nevertheless, most

25. It should be pointed out that the fomites theory was not limited to yellow fever but was applied to many other infectious diseases, notably cholera and smallpox. See "Report of the Special Committee on the Disinfection of Rags," *Reports and Papers, American Public Health Association,* XII (1886), 170–97, and Charles V. Chapin, *The Sources and Modes of Infection* (2nd ed.; New York, 1916), 212–58.

26. Bemiss, "Chapters from the Report," 325; John M. Woodworth, "Internal Quarantine for Yellow Fever," *Medical Record,* XIV (1878), 238. See also Henry Fraser Campbell, "The Yellow Fever Quarantine of the Future, Based upon the Portability of Atmospheric Germs, and the Non-Contagiousness of the Disease," *Reports and Papers, American Public Health Association,* V (1879), 131–44.

27. "Proceedings and Discussions," *Reports and Papers, American Public Health Association,* V (1879), 219.

physicians right up to the turn of the century were deeply engrossed with the fomites idea, often even in the face of clear and direct evidence of infection from persons. The doctor who reported to Bemiss on the epidemic at Labadieville, Louisiana, in 1878 identified the initial case there as a woman who had gone into infected New Orleans to nurse her sick brother, falling ill with yellow fever herself a few days after returning home. The disease later appeared in others of her household and spread through the whole village, killing fifty of its two hundred inhabitants. The reporting doctor unblinkingly referred the origin of the Labadieville epidemic not to the person of the sick woman, but to the baggage she brought back with her from New Orleans.[28] The obsession with fomites infection was if anything even more prevalent and compelling at the popular level. The newspapers in 1878 were full of reports of shipments of supposedly infectious merchandise being seized, condemned, and destroyed by fire at rigidly quarantined towns around the region. In more than a few instances, whole railroad cars were burned, and river barges sunk, by nervous quarantine enforcers.

A scientifically correct picture of that "peculiar alteration in the surrounding air" postulated by earlier observers slowly began to emerge after 1878. The association of mosquitoes with a sickly atmosphere had frequently been observed by the old miasmatists, but the relationship was regarded as symptomatic, not causative, and usually was mixed together uncritically with other observations of a perfectly irrelevant character. The atmospheric "prodromes" of yellow fever at Lake Providence, Louisiana, in 1853 were summarized this way by the Sanitary Commission of New Orleans: "Fruits had dark and unhealthy spots; animals more sickly, and many had swellings; musquetoes tenfold more numerous; mould more than common; toadstools vastly more plentiful; a peculiar smell pervaded the atmosphere." The epidemic of 1853 was widespread as well as malignant, and a superabundance of mosquitoes was also observed that year at Biloxi, Centerville, Donaldsonville, Clinton, and Natchez.[29] In a long es-

28. T. B. Pugh, "Yellow Fever in Assumption," in Bemiss, "Yellow Fever in Louisiana," 183–85. Noncontagionists earlier in the century had soundly rejected fomites transmission. Discussing alleged cases of infection from fomites, LaRoche astutely commented in 1855, "We may well infer that some error has crept in, something has been omitted or overlooked, and production of the disease was really due to some other agency than the one contended for" (LaRoche, *Yellow Fever*, II, 522).

29. *Report of the Sanitary Commission of New Orleans*, 265–66.

say on the mosquito nuisance published in the *New Orleans Medical and Surgical Journal* in 1856, Dr. Bennett Dowler of New Orleans remarked that many people had come to regard "any increase in the number of mosquitoes as a precursor or prelude to yellow fever." He dismissed the whole line of conjecture rather summarily, though: "These are opinions which, however untenable, many persons believe firmly. It is evident on taking an enlarged view of the climatic range, habits, and stations of the mosquito, that its appearance cannot be a reliable sentinel or precursor of yellow fever, as for example in the Polar Regions."[30] As far as any scientific discussion or investigation was concerned, the matter slumbered soundly for at least twenty years thereafter.

A "living cause" of yellow fever—one that existed independently of its manifestation among human beings, which grew and multiplied in its season, then drooped and died out as the season declined—certainly suggested parallels in insect life. Respected physicians like Josiah Nott and Greensville Dowell repeatedly called attention to those parallels, but neither they nor any of their students made the direct connection. The unusual prevalence of mosquitoes when yellow fever raged seems to have been recognized by a great many people, nevertheless, and it even appears that the guilty species of mosquito had been correctly singled out in public judgment. In 1878 an item in the Louisville *Courier-Journal* mentioned "the gray-back mosquito," considered by the old inhabitants of Mississippi to be "a certain forerunner of the yellow fever."[31] We shall come across a number of other contemporary references to this insect in the course of our story. In all the formal medical literature issuing from the experience of 1878, however, nothing at all was said about the mosquito. In 1881 the eccentric Dr. Carlos Finlay of Havana, Cuba, published a paper implicating a particular species of mosquito, the one we know today as *Aedes aegypti*, as the transmitter of yellow fever. *A. aegypti*, it turns out, is indeed the small, gray-backed "cistern mosquito" familiar to the Caribbean countries and to our southern states. Finlay's idea was almost totally ignored by leading scientists at the time, however; a number of attempts by him to prove it experimentally were clumsy and unresultful.[32]

30. Bennett Dowler, "Researches into the Natural History of the Mosquito," *New Orleans Medical and Surgical Journal*, XII (1856), 187.

31. "The Insect Theory," Louisville *Courier-Journal*, September 17, 1878.

32. George M. Sternberg, "Dr. Finlay's Mosquito Inoculations," *American Journal of the Medical Sciences*, n.s., CII (1891), 627–30.

An empirical breakthrough came in 1899, when H. R. Carter developed his classic study of the spread of infection in houses and the interval between infecting and secondary cases in yellow fever. Carter secured the case records of a government doctor who had ministered to the people of an isolated group of farms in north-central Mississippi during a minor yellow fever outbreak the previous summer. Carefully piecing together and correlating the sequence of cases, he determined that there had been a fairly regular interval of time, never fewer than twelve and usually more than fifteen days, between the first "infecting case" from the outside and the appearance of the first "secondary cases" among the people dwelling there. This time lag he called "the period of extrinsic incubation of yellow fever infection." He also noted that once a house had become infected, it could impart sickness to a nonimmune newcomer after as little as three days of exposure. Carter's observations pointed intriguingly to the presence of some kind of intermediate host and, taken in light of the then-recent (1898) discovery of the mosquito transmission of malaria, served to stimulate reconsideration of the mosquito as a possible vector of yellow fever. The subsequent work of the U.S. Army Yellow Fever Commission in Cuba, under the direction of Dr. Walter Reed, formed one of modern experimental medicine's most brilliant chapters.[33]

Reed's group confirmed, in the first place, that yellow fever is indeed transmitted by *A. aegypti* and only by that mosquito. Fomites infection was tested and retested and shown to be a false doctrine entirely. Later developments would show that the central conclusion of the army commission was not absolutely true. Tropical yellow fever research in the 1930s revealed a previously unsuspected "forest cycle" in the jungles of South America and Central Africa involving a variety of arboreal primates and certain species of mosquitoes other than *A. aegypti,* and in which man is not a necessary component, though he might be an occasional victim. The forest cycle of yellow fever, maintaining the infection permanently in wild reservoirs too vast for control, is of crucial importance in the present epidemiology of the disease, but it was never of any direct consequence in North America, where neither the monkeys nor the mosquitoes concerned in it exist. And while laboratory investigations have shown that the yellow

33. H. R. Carter, "Contributed Articles," in U.S. Marine Hospital Service, *Report for Fiscal 1900,* 230–52; "Board for the Study of the Etiology and Prevention of Yellow Fever," in U.S. Secretary of War, *Report for Fiscal 1901* (3 vols.), I, 714–40; Aristides Agramonte, "The Inside History of a Great Medical Discovery," *Scientific Monthly,* I (1915), 209–37.

fever virus can be retained for brief periods by a variety of peridomestic blood-sucking insects, including bedbugs, fleas, and stable flies, all attempts at transmitting the infection with those species have failed. So far as the devastating urban epidemics of the last century are concerned, therefore, blame is still laid solely to the *A. aegypti* mosquito. Fomites, it should be emphasized, play no role whatsoever in the spread of yellow fever.[34]

In an extensive series of experiments, the U.S. Army Yellow Fever Commission showed that the transmission of yellow fever was not a simple bite-to-bite transfer of infected blood, but involved a certain period of incubation in the mosquito, tentatively determined to be twelve to eighteen days, a term amazingly close to the "period of extrinsic incubation" that had been posited by Carter. We know today that the so-called extrinsic incubation of yellow fever represents the time it takes for the imbibed virus to develop in the body of the mosquito and travel to its salivary glands, whence it can be injected into human victims in subsequent blood meals. Later research has shown that under favorable conditions, extrinsic incubation may be as short as ten days, perhaps only eight days. Once mosquitoes become infectious, they remain so all their breeding, biting life, which might be as long as two or even three months. It was also determined that, after being bitten by an infected mosquito, three to six days were required for symptoms of the disease to develop in the human victim—again a remarkable correspondence with Carter's earlier observations of house infection. One other important fact emerged from the army commission investigations: the mosquito can pick up infection from the human host only during the first three days of a person's illness. This is when free virus overflowing from the infected viscera is found circulating in the blood, before a stage of stasis and remission sets in. These undreamed-of complexities and contingencies in the transmission of yellow fever were among the factors that contributed to the confusion among early investigators over whether or not it was a transmissible disease.[35]

"Cisterns are engendering places of yellow fever," the Memphis *Ava-*

34. On the forest cycle of yellow fever, see Richard M. Taylor, "Epidemiology," in *Yellow Fever*, ed. Strode, 442–538; John Duffy, ed., *Ventures in World Health: The Memoirs of Fred Lowe Soper* (New York, 1977), 168–200.

35. "The Publications of Walter Reed and his Associates on the Commission in Regard to Yellow Fever," in *Yellow Fever: A Compilation of Various Publications* (Washington, D.C., 1911), 53–174.

lanche advised on August 4, 1878. The observation, in retrospect so aston- ishing, continued: "Cisterns are the homes of the larvae of insects—the mosquito particularly." The unknown journalist came remarkably close to making an important statement, but instead veered off into an explanation of how the dead insect larvae, along with accumulated "fungus" and "in- fusoria," putrefied in the warm water of the tanks to "render noxious the element" and release "mephitic vapors," all of which could be neutralized, he said, by sprinkling the water with potassium permanganate or some other precipitating agent. That newspaper item nevertheless serves to in- troduce some important points about the life history and bionomics of *A. aegypti.* This species is preeminently peridomestic in its habits, found only in and about the habitations of man. While it is occasionally found living and breeding in tree holes and rock pools in the wild, it is not, as a rule, a mosquito of the marshes, woods, or fields. And *A. aegypti*-borne yellow fever, accordingly, is not a paludal, sylvan, or campestral malady, but is distinctly a plague of developed human environments. In the past, residents of places liable to yellow fever demonstrated a sound practical understanding of this fact of the disease's etiology when they immediately took off for the forests and swamps on first rumor of Yellow Jack in the towns. "Yellow fever is essentially a disease of towns and cities," as Dr. Daniel Drake recognized. "The inhabitants of the country, even within a few miles of a town where the disease is epidemic, generally escape it, unless they venture within its sphere of prevalence."[36]

A. aegypti manifests no liking for standing water on the open ground, but has the peculiar characteristic of living and breeding only in shaded containers with solid sides to which it can cement its eggs. House cisterns undoubtedly were the principal "engendering places" of the yellow fever mosquito at most localities in the past. Cistern storage of water was a universal practice in the rainy tropical and subtropical countries around the Gulf and the Caribbean, even in large cities—at New Orleans, for example, a sanitary survey in 1879 revealed that over 35,000 houses were watered from cisterns, while fewer than 5,000 were served with piped mu- nicipal water. The people, of course, always saw to it that their cisterns

36. S. R. Christophers, *Aedes aegypti (L.), the Yellow Fever Mosquito: Its Life History, Bionomics, and Structure* (Cambridge, Eng., 1960), 54, 57–59; Howard, Dyar, and Knab, *Mos- quitoes of North and Central America,* I, 283–86; Carter, *Yellow Fever,* 10–14; Boyce, *Yellow Fever,* 269–72; Drake, *Diseases of the Interior Valley,* II, 188.

contained water, and the large, covered vats were necessarily closely attached to dwellings, affording eggs and larvae much better protection from adverse temperatures than any smaller and more exposed receptacles scattered around the yards. Yellow fever sanitarians of the mosquito era did not take long to recognize that the house cisterns served as the "mother-foci" of *A. aegypti* infestation at virtually every southern town liable to yellow fever, and concentrated their clean-up efforts on them accordingly. Nonetheless, every conceivable domestic collection of water, no matter how small, can serve as an acceptable seasonal breeding-place. This includes rain barrels and horse troughs alongside buildings, fire buckets and flower vases inside houses, discarded cans and jars in backyards, even fonts for holy water in churches.[37]

A. aegypti prefers clear though not necessarily clean water and tends to shun muddy water and water polluted by urine and feces. In 1878 and the years following, a vast expenditure of labor and material was directed at cleansing and sanitizing house privies and street gutters, then regarded as the main niduses of the "germ" of yellow fever, all of which was of virtually no coincidental benefit as affecting *A. aegypti*. As H. R. Carter emphasized: "The progress of civic improvement tends to remove or lessen *aegypti* infestation in towns, and by that factor to render them noninfectible; but it is piped water doing away with its domestic storage, not sewerage, drainage, or general cleanliness, which has this effect." This mosquito is strictly a pot-breeder and it does not haunt cesspools and street ditches, though occasionally it can be discovered sheltering in stagnant sections under culverts in lined gutters, conditions that sufficiently resemble its preferred habitat. The street ditches and drains of New Orleans in 1878 were indeed extensive, quite stagnant, and very foul, but nearly all were open and unlined. The "innumerable insect life" found teeming in the gutters that summer by a St. Louis visitor must therefore have referred to flies and to mosquitoes of the *Culex* genus but not to *A. aegypti*. A recommendation made in 1854 by the Sanitary Commission of New Orleans, advising that all the city's gutters be curbed with brick or

37. George E. Waring, *Report on the Social Statistics of Cities* (2 vols.; Washington, D.C., 1887), II, 282–84; William R. Horsfall, *Mosquitoes: Their Bionomics and Relation to Disease* (New York, 1955), 481–83; Asa C. Chandler, "Factors Affecting the Uneven Distribution of *Aedes aegypti* in Texas Cities," *American Journal of Tropical Medicine*, XXV (1945), 145–49.

stone, and covered over where possible, would, ironically, only have aggravated the situation with regard to the yellow fever mosquito.[38]

In the quotation that opened this chapter we saw how the coming of frost was anxiously awaited in fever-stricken Memphis. One of the early established characteristics of yellow fever was its close correspondence with the level of the thermometer and the turn of the season. It was repeatedly seen how epidemics became entrenched in warm, humid, stagnant weather and then declined with the advent of cool weather, ceasing abruptly after the occurrence of a hard frost. Miasmatists once pointed to the controlling influence of air temperature on yellow fever as one of the main proofs of their doctrine, compelling evidence that the sickness was essentially due to a physical disorder of the atmosphere—to the presence of some unknown gas presumably congealed, like water vapor, by cold temperatures. The same evidence was later invoked to support the germ theory, freezing supposedly destroying the life of the invisible pathogenic animalcules. Today, of course, it is plain that the phenomenon had everything to do with the activity of the yellow fever mosquito. *A. aegypti* is, fortunately, rather limited in its temperature tolerance: it is most active between 70° and 90° F; its activity gradually diminishes below 70°; it grows sluggish and will not feed below 60°, and is quite inert below 50°. "Without knowing with certainty what its particulate cause may be," Dr. John Rauch of the Illinois Board of Health wrote in 1888, "we do know that a temperature below 32° F destroys the vitality of the cause, and that a continuous temperature of not less than 70° is necessary for its origin and spread."[39] It is interesting, and a little distressing, to see how many of the conditions for yellow fever were recognized, and even quite precisely defined, while all the time its ultimate cause remained painfully elusive.

It was common knowledge in the past that the "poison" or "germ" of yellow fever could not survive a northern winter and that even in Louisiana the disease was probably not "indigenous," or as we would express

38. Carter, *Yellow Fever*, 13, 28; Rubert W. Boyce, *Report to the Government of British Honduras upon the Outbreak of Yellow Fever in that Colony in 1905* (London, 1906), 25–37; "A Howard Visitor," New Orleans *Picayune*, October 26, 1878.

39. John H. Rauch, "Yellow Fever Panics and Useless Quarantines—Limitation by Temperature and Altitude," *Reports and Papers, American Public Health Association,* XIV (1888), 139; Christophers, *Aedes aegypti,* 263–65, 474–75, 550–51; Carter, *Yellow Fever,* 14–17.

it, endemic. Concerning the supposed "poison-germ" of yellow fever, Dr. Woodworth of the U.S. Marine Hospital Service observed in an 1878 circular: "It cannot be said to be indigenous in the United States. It appears to have about as much resistance of cold as the banana plant. When the banana stalk is killed down by the frost, the yellow fever does not recur until again imported." Although cold weather effectively kills off adult mosquitoes and suppresses the larvae, the eggs of *A. aegypti* are fairly hardy and, laid in and around human shelters, were normally able to overwinter in appreciable numbers everywhere in the lower Mississippi Valley. The effect of the region's cold season on the abundance of the following summer's mosquitoes, and hence on the potential intensity of yellow fever infection, was by way of limiting the length of time they had to actively multiply. The development of *A. aegypti* from egg to imago normally takes fifteen to forty days, depending on temperature conditions. An extra month of suitably warm weather at the beginning of summer therefore would have meant an extra round or two of mosquito breeding—and every extra generation meant, of course, an exponential increase in mosquito numbers.[40]

The winter of 1877–1878 was by all accounts extraordinarily mild in the Mississippi Valley—New Orleans had experienced freezing temperatures but a single night in December. The spring came warm and early, and the early summer was disagreeably hot. "The climatic lines were virtually carried a thousand miles north of their ordinary position," the *Annual Cyclopaedia* claimed. "An unacclimated people as far north as the Ohio were exposed to the ordinary temperatures of the Gulf States, while the Gulf States were tropical." According to Signal Service observations, mean monthly temperatures in the period from December, 1877, through April, 1878, ranged from eight to fifteen degrees above normal in the lower Missouri Valley, and from three to eleven degrees above normal in the Ohio Valley and Tennessee. In Tennessee it was said the violets had bloomed all winter, and the hyacinths were out in January. At Memphis even light frosts had disappeared by the end of February, and temperatures as high as 80° F were recorded in March. Vegetation around the city was said to be "much advanced" by then, with the peach and plum trees and

40. "Instructions to the Marine Hospital Service," New York *Herald*, August 17, 1878; Christophers, *Aedes aegypti*, 38–40, 55–56, 150–51; Carter, *Yellow Fever*, 40–45.

most ornamentals in full flower. The month of July, leading up to the explosion of yellow fever, brought unusually hot weather to the region. St. Louis registered 163 deaths from sunstroke in July. Memphis also reported considerable "heat sickness" in the last half of the month, enough to cause "a partial suspension of business" (we can only wonder how much of this was actually yellow fever). It was, however, the prolongation rather than the intensity of heat that favored mosquito activity. The queer procession of seasons, which a Philadelphia professor believed had "dropped a strange climate upon an unacclimated people," had in fact given a running start to the swarms of *A. aegypti* that were on hand to disseminate the yellow fever virus when it was brought up from the endemic zone that spring.[41]

Other "atmospheric peculiarities" of yellow fever observed in the nineteenth century can also be readily explained in terms of the mosquito vector. The disease often displayed the property of spreading outward from an initial "focus of infection" in short extensions, proceeding quite steadily from house to house even when there had been no communication between the inhabitants. "When a wharf or a house becomes infected, the poison at once commences to spread, creeping slowly in all directions," observed Surgeon General Woodworth. It was this feature of epidemics that led doctors in the 1870s to visualize an extrinsic infection spreading over localities like mold on leather or ringworm on skin, and persuaded them to launch expensive "disinfection" campaigns, treating the surrounding ground with strong antiseptic chemicals in an effort to encircle, confine, and kill the unseeable "germs."[42] In other instances the infection seemed mysteriously heavy and inert, unable to cross a wide avenue or even a high board fence. Dr. Samuel Bemiss wrote: "It seems probable that certain qualities belonging to yellow fever germs, perhaps ponderability and that unknown quality which causes it to adhere to surfaces, are sufficient to prevent atmospheric accumulations, except in close contiguity with the surface of the earth. It has been properly spoken of as a lowlaying poison, creeping, as it were, near the surface of the ground." Mod-

41. *Appelton's Annual Cyclopaedia and Register of Important Events*, n.s., III (1878), 315; *Monthly Weather Review*, V–VI (December, 1877–July, 1878); "On Yellow Fever," New Orleans *Picayune*, September 18, 1878.

42. S. S. Herrick, "Review of Yellow Fever in New Orleans, 1869–74," *New Orleans Medical and Surgical Journal*, n.s., II (1875), 645–52.

ern entomologists tell us that *A. aegypti,* a rather weak flier, is generally disinclined to leave the house in which it hatches out, and when it does fly off, normal dispersal is something less than fifty yards, usually just going far enough to make it to the closest shelter.[43]

That the spread of infection was slowed by windy or stormy weather, and promoted or intensified by calm, dry spells, was another old truism that can be referred to the behavior of this mosquito, which indeed tends to lie low in unsettled weather. An outbreak at New Orleans in 1871 was thought to have been completely abated when the city was struck by an October hurricane bringing violent rains and winds. The long-lived belief that the germ or poison of yellow fever was somehow suppressed by the "ozone" generated in the atmosphere by storms probably stemmed from such observations. Other bygone legends concerning the relation of yellow fever to atmospheric conditions are more difficult to evaluate. In New Orleans it was firmly believed that rainstorms, while slowing the spread of infection, also had the unwelcome effect of increasing mortality among existing cases. The same was said about north winds. Another old idea was that sleeping in an upper-story room lessened one's liability to contract the disease. And nineteenth-century observers all insisted that a distinctive odor enveloped places infected by yellow fever. "You can easily distinguish it," said the New York *Herald*'s correspondent at Grenada, Mississippi, in 1878: "There is a peculiarity about it which, once discovered, never can be forgotten." It was said to be a sweetish smell; some writers described it as "cadaveric," others likened it more to rotting hay.[44]

One of the persistent mysteries of yellow fever, so confounding to scientists in the past but perfectly understandable in light of present knowledge, was its seeming propensity to detour some towns completely, while nearby communities were violently scourged. Memphis, Tennessee, and Grenada, Mississippi, were devastated by the fever in 1878, while Sardis, Mississippi, midway between them, had not a case. In a similar way, Huntsville, Alabama, was bypassed, although Decatur, Alabama, to the west, and Chattanooga, Tennessee, to the east, became seriously infected. In remarks before the American Public Health Association that fall, a Huntsville doctor could only attribute his town's reprieve to its "scrupu-

43. Bemiss, "Yellow Fever in Louisiana," 99; Christophers, *Aedes aegypti,* 516.

44. Louisiana Board of Health, *Report for 1871* (New Orleans, 1872), 25; New Orleans *Picayune,* September 15, 19, 1878; New York *Herald,* September 7, 1878.

lous cleanliness," as contrasted with the sanitary condition of its neighbors. Other places in similar situations credited their escape to the fancied "perfection" of their local quarantine measures. The backward town of Pope, Mississippi, not only failed to clean up and disinfect during this epidemic but had a faulty quarantine as well, and ended up being exposed to several imported cases of yellow fever, but aside from a few local cases of questionable identity, the town never became infected. A Pope physician came nearest of all to the truth of the matter when he admitted: "I can give no reason satisfactory to myself why we did not have the fever in its violence; I can only suppose the atmosphere not to have been in a proper condition to receive the poison." Of course the underlying reason for the different fortunes of these towns hinged on the simple question of whether *A. aegypti* was present or absent.[45]

In 1905, when quarantine officials were contending with what was to be Yellow Jack's last serious invasion of this country, the U.S. Public Health Service issued a circular that defined the "infectible territory" of the United States to be "broadly stated, that part of the United States south of a line drawn from the Atlantic coast through Washington to St. Louis, Missouri, and thence to El Paso, Texas." That statement merely delimited the general climate region where average temperatures suitable for the year-to-year propagation of the yellow fever mosquito prevailed. *A. aegypti* is a species exotic to North America—biologists consider it to be, like the virus it transmits, a native of Central Africa—and historical evidence indicates that its diffusion and establishment over its rather extensive potential range on this continent was in fact a very gradual and irregu-

---

45. "Abstract of Discussions," *Reports and Papers, American Public Health Association,* IV (1878), 383–85; Mississippi Board of Health, *Report for 1878–79,* 32, 116–17, 128. The latter document contained seventy-two pages of reports from ninety-four towns and thirty-two counties, nearly all vouching for the great effectiveness of their rigid quarantines in 1878. In November, the American Public Health Association overwhelmingly endorsed the following proposition: "Quarantine established with such rigor and precision as to produce absolute non-intercourse will prevent the importation of the specific cause of yellow fever." Not many were as skeptical as the Houston doctor who pointed out: "All history teaches that no General or Commandant of a post, with all the power and machinery of war, has been able to establish perfect non-intercourse. . . . Almost every place that had yellow fever in 1878 had quarantines" (J. J. Burroughs, "Origin and Nature of the Late Yellow Fever Epidemic—Report of the Yellow Fever Commission Partially Reviewed," *Virginia Medical Monthly,* V [1879], 950).

lar process. Its increase and dispersal within a town or city after being introduced therein tended to be steady, but not necessarily rapid or uniform, hence Dr. Daniel Drake's observation that yellow fever tended to be "less prevalent in the infancy of cities than in their more advanced and populous condition." The mosquito was obviously well established at New Orleans when the first confirmed yellow fever epidemic occurred there in 1796, but at Vicksburg, for example, three hundred miles up the Mississippi, the first occurrence of yellow fever in epidemic form was not recorded until 1839. In the severe epidemic of 1853, several score of yellow fever cases appeared among Louisiana refugees at Memphis, five hundred miles upriver from New Orleans, but no instances of communication of the disease to local people were reported. A similar situation seems to have obtained in 1878 at Nashville, which remained uninfected despite the arrival of numerous refugee cases from Memphis and elsewhere. In 1905, however, health officials found the mosquito in considerable numbers at Nashville, and the city, formerly considered secure from yellow fever, was declared "infectible." By the 1930s entomologists could find *A. aegypti* breeding and overwintering as far north as Carbondale, Illinois, and as far west as Stillwater, Oklahoma.[46]

The yellow fever mosquito did not spread by independently winging its way from place to place. Rather, its diffusion depended on the transportation people unwittingly gave it. There can be no doubt that ocean-going ships—and, later on, river steamers—were the primary means of carrying *A. aegypti* to new territory and establishing new points of infestation. In terms of furnishing habitat for this insect, a freshwater cask on shipboard was precisely like a cistern in a house on land, and, once infested by egg-laying mosquitoes, qualified the vessel as a perfect mobile breeding colony. The association of yellow fever outbreaks on land with the arrival of ships from the tropics, and the fact that the disease for a long time appeared to be confined in its range to seaports and river cities, gave rise to persistent speculation that yellow fever was essentially a "nautical" disease. "Its spread from one city to another is chiefly accomplished by ves-

46. Geo. A. Smith and W. J. Tuck, "Letters on Yellow Fever at Memphis, Tennessee, in 1853," *New Orleans Medical and Surgical Journal*, X (1854), 662–67; J. Berrian Lindsley, "Report on the Yellow Fever in Nashville, Tennessee, September and October, 1878," *Reports and Papers, American Public Health Association*, IV (1878), 241–42; *Public Health Reports*, XX (1905), 1752, 1882. On the distribution of *A. aegypti* in North America see Carter, *Yellow Fever*, 28–33, 40–45; Christophers, *Aedes aegypti*, 36–37.

sels—their damp, filthy holds and bilge water being its favorite lurking places," advised Surgeon General Woodworth in 1878. "In some instances it has been carried inland with the people flying from infected localities, but it has never shown a disposition to spread epidemically to points removed from the continuous water-roads of commerce, or to lodge in high, salubrious places." Discussions at the 1879 meeting of the American Public Health Association revealed that in the minds of some doctors it was still an open question, whether the infection of yellow fever might not be spontaneously generated in the hot, foul, dank holds of ships cruising tropical waters. As late as 1893, experts of the U.S. Marine Hospital Service attempted to trace an epidemic at Brunswick on the Georgia coast to "germs" diffused from a pile of filthy ballast dumped by a ship from Havana.[47]

Dr. Daniel Drake, writing around 1850, could find no instance on record of yellow fever occurring epidemically away from navigable water and supposed this represented a fixed characteristic of the disease's etiology and geography. Even as he wrote, however, the construction of railroad lines throughout the Mississippi Valley was preparing the way for a dramatic expansion of the territory susceptible to yellow fever. Adult mosquitoes straying from nearby buildings could easily be closed up in the cars and coaches of trains halted at an infested place and so be transported many miles inland in short order, to fly off at stops along the line and begin breeding in places where conditions were right. In some instances, perhaps, the mosquitoes might even have begun breeding in the water vessels carried for various purposes on board the trains. The explosive outbreaks of yellow fever at dozens of railroad towns in Mississippi and Tennessee in 1878 forcefully demonstrated that trains had been scarcely less efficient than boats as conveyors and distributors of *A. aegypti*. We must admire the reasoning of Dr. Stanford Chaillé, who in 1880 observed:

> While yellow fever never did and never will originate spontaneously on ships, yet it continued, throughout the long period during which ships

47. Howard, Dyar, and Knab, *Mosquitoes of North and Central America*, I, 298–303; Carter, *Yellow Fever*, 24–27, 34–38; Boyce, *Yellow Fever*, 42–47; "Proceedings and Discussions," *Reports and Papers, American Public Health Association*, V (1879), 185–93, 211–13, 221–22; U.S. Marine Hospital Service, *Report for Fiscal 1893*, II, 32–34. The transfer of *A. aegypti* by boat is still witnessed today; see Dave D. Chadee, "*Aedes aegypti* Aboard Boats at Port-of-Spain, Trinidad, West Indies," *Mosquito News*, XLIV (1984), 1–3.

were the chief vehicles of transportation from infected places, to be, in a certain sense, a "nautical," "oceanic," and "sea-port" disease; but with the invention of steamboats, it in the same sense became a disease of towns on navigable streams, and with the invention of railroads, it became a disease of inland railroad depots. Hence, though ships continue for obvious reasons to be the best carriers of yellow fever, this is no more a "ship disease" than it is a steamboat or railroad disease, and no more an "oceanic disease" than it is a fluvial, riparian, or inland disease.[48]

More pedestrian means of transportation for the mosquito were available as well. Although water is in most respects as crucial to the existence of this insect as it is to a fish, research has shown that *A. aegypti* is capable of surviving for rather long periods under waterless conditions. Experiments performed early in this century by the U.S. Marine Hospital Service in connection with certain questions of quarantine procedure established that adult yellow fever mosquitoes can live for as long as forty-eight hours when packed away among dry fabrics, and if the material is just slightly damp, survival time is increased to six to eight days. Close observers have witnessed this mosquito's fondness for secreting itself in pockets and folds of clothing, especially when the weather is cool. It is not difficult to imagine an occasional female mosquito getting imprisoned in a trunk or suitcase and then being carried overland to a place remote from both railroads and navigable water, at which place she escapes, finds water, and lays her eggs. In addition, the eggs of *A. aegypti* are fairly resistant to temporary drying and, clinging to the inside of an occasional crock or barrel, could have been carried away from an infested place to mature and hatch when the container arrived at its new location and was again filled with water.[49]

Such modes of diffusion could not have been very probable or frequent, but that they had occurred often enough over the years was evident in 1878, when yellow fever appeared at more than a few isolated farms and hamlets in the delta country, places whose only link to the outside world were dirt roads. The Mississippi State Board of Health published an inter-

48. Stanford E. Chaillé, "The Alleged Spontaneous Origin of Yellow Fever on Ships," *New Orleans Medical and Surgical Journal*, n.s., VIII (1880), 426. On the conveyance of *A. aegypti* by train, see Howard, Dyar, and Knab, *Mosquitoes of North and Central America*, I, 299–301.

49. S. B. Grubbs, *A Note on Mosquitoes in Baggage*, (Washington, D.C., 1902); Christophers, *Aedes aegypti*, 147–49; Boyce, *Yellow Fever*, 283–85.

esting account of an outbreak at a Tallahatchie County plantation, twenty-seven miles from the nearest town, Grenada. Thirty-six out of the forty people living there were stricken and seventeen died, though all the other farms in the neighborhood were completely untouched by the pestilence. "Yet the fever was carried by persons who visited Dr. Payne's to other places in the neighborhood, where they died, but did not communicate the fever to other members of their families." The physician making the report ruminated: "Exclude local causes and the fever will not be epidemic. What these local causes are I don't know. Who does? Yet we see the fever prevail fearfully at some places and in some years, and not at others. Some factor, as yet unknown, must exist at the one place and not at the others to account for this difference. . . . There is," he noted, "nothing at the Doctor's place more than at others in the neighborhood to cause the fever, unless it be the cistern"—which, he observed, "was not cleansed properly last year."[50] Here was another example (we shall come across a good many more) of how a vagrant speculation could get so close, and yet be so far off, when it came to divining the ultimate mystery of yellow fever.

The yellow fever mosquito was not present everywhere in 1878. It was not even established at a majority of places, otherwise the epidemic would have been even more destructive than it was. It is nevertheless clear that a century of settlement and traffic in the region had prepared a sufficiently wide and fertile circuit for the King of Terrors when it made its grand sweep in the summer of 1878.

50. J. M. Calhoun, "The Epidemic at Valley Home, 1878," in Mississippi Board of Health, *Report for 1878–79*, 85–89.

Two

The Burden of Yellow Fever
in the Mississippi Valley

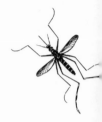

The Mississippi Valley's consternation over yellow fever in 1878 was all with regard to the extraordinary scope and intensity of the epidemic—the disease itself was nothing new to the region. The European colonization of Louisiana began in 1718, when the settlement of New Orleans was laid out on a bend of the Mississippi River nearly one hundred miles upstream from the Gulf of Mexico. For at least the first thirty or forty years of its existence, the isolated French outpost was not troubled by yellow fever to any notable extent. Of course, occasions for the disease's introduction would have been infrequent in a "backwater of empire," having only a modest commerce in pelts and the produce of a few plantations. The first probable references to the disease at New Orleans show up in the 1760s. Those references are somewhat ambiguous; they are unclear from a clinical standpoint, but suspicious in view of the fact that the town had been garrisoned with Cuban troops, and much more frequent contacts with Havana had been initiated after the takeover of Louisiana by Spain in 1762.[1]

Colonial records do contain the first definite accounts of a yellow fever outbreak at New Orleans. The year was 1796. The unusual amount of descriptive writing, sprinkled with references to the terrible "black vomit of Philadelphia" three years before, suggests that local officials were unusually worried by this appearance of the disease. The colony's attorney gen-

---

1. Jo Ann Carrigan, "The Saffron Scourge: A History of Yellow Fever in Louisiana, 1796–1905" (Ph.D. dissertation, Louisiana State University, 1961), 13–20.

eral estimated that 250 of New Orleans' 8,000-odd people had died, not counting "strangers." The mayor of the town ascribed the origin of the plague to a combination of fetid exhalations from the marshes on the opposite side of the river, stagnant waters in the town's street ditches, and dead animals and putrid offal carelessly dumped on the riverbank. Those basic etiological conclusions would be elaborated on very little over the next 100 years. It is also well to note how the various goings-on described in 1796 previewed the public reaction to Yellow Jack that would be exhibited in all subsequent epidemics. Normal daily business was abruptly suspended as all who could fled to the plantations outside town. Various nostrums and prophylactic measures, including the chewing of cinchona, drinking of herb teas, and sprinkling of camphor and vinegar around dwellings, were optimistically tried by those who stayed, but really seemed to be of little avail. Pine tar was burned in the streets, a measure that was still considered useful in 1878, but the medieval expedient of burning of animal hides, horns, and hoofs would not be repeated in the nineteenth century. It was observed that the epidemic was finally terminated by frost, and that the Negroes and creoles had fared relatively well, while the plague had been especially hard on "strangers to the country"—in this case mostly "Englishmen and Protestants"—the general category of resident that would later be known as "the unacclimated." The latter observation suggests this was really not the first time yellow fever had gone the rounds in New Orleans.[2]

The United States acquired Louisiana in 1803. In a matter of months the population of New Orleans more than doubled, and in the summer of 1804 yellow fever flared up violently in the city, mainly affecting this horde of new "unacclimated" subjects. Governor William Claiborne, who lost his wife, daughter, and personal secretary to the disease that year, estimated in a report to Washington that as many as one-third of the recent immigrants had been swept away by yellow fever. In the wake of the epidemic, Claiborne read to the first territorial legislature a letter from his friend, Thomas Jefferson, expressing concern that yellow fever might prove to be a serious handicap to the settlement of the region and to the city's prosperity. As a possible ameliorative measure, Jefferson recommended that New Orleans' future growth be arranged on a checkerboard

2. *Ibid.*, 26–34.

plan, leaving the alternate squares thickly planted with trees to shade the ground and absorb miasms. The imaginative president explained the larger theory behind his suggestion:

> In the middle and northern parts of Europe, where the sun rarely shines, they may safely build cities in solid blocks without generating disease; but under the cloudless skies of America, where there is so constant an accumulation of heat, men cannot be piled one on another with impunity. Accordingly, we find this disease confined to the solid-built parts of the towns and the parts on the water side, where there is the most matter for putrefaction, but rarely extending into the thin-built parts of the towns, and never into the country. In these latter places it cannot be communicated. In order to catch it you must go into the local atmosphere where it prevails. Is not this then a strong indication that we ought not to contend with the laws of nature, but should decide at once that all our cities should be thinly built? [3]

"For beauty, pleasure, and commerce it would certainly be eminent," Jefferson said of his plan, and he hoped that "those more interested should think as favorably of it as I do." Whatever its medical merits, however, the scheme obviously would have idled too much valuable real estate and was therefore completely ignored in New Orleans' subsequent expansion. Yellow fever came again and again to afflict the young city. It is estimated that at least five hundred died in the epidemic of 1811, and eight hundred in the visitation of 1817. Confirmed annual mortality from yellow fever at New Orleans exceeded one thousand for the first time in 1819. And the malady started gradually finding its way into the interior after the inauguration of steamboat traffic on the rivers in 1812. It appeared at Baton Rouge and at Natchez, both on the Mississippi River, in 1817, and at Alexandria on the lower Red River in 1819. By the end of the 1820s it had reached out to perhaps a dozen country towns in Louisiana, including Opelousas on Bayou Teche and Thibodaux on Bayou Lafourche. By this time yellow fever was becoming a serious embarrassment to New Orleans, commercially and politically as well as medically. Perceiving their own liability to the transported scourge, communities in the interior started imposing their own seasonal quarantines against the metropolis, the pre-

---

3. Quoted in Joseph Jones, "Comparative Pathology of Malarial and Yellow Fevers," in *Proceedings of the Louisiana State Medical Association, 1879* (New Orleans, 1879), 92.

sumed source of infection, and also brought pressure on the state legislature in 1821 to organize a general maritime quarantine of the state. The merchants of the Crescent City naturally chafed at the inconveniences of quarantine—a public resolution in 1823 called it "not only useless but in the highest degree oppressive and injurious to the commerce of this city." When the device failed to avert a major epidemic there in 1822 (eight hundred deaths) and a moderately severe outbreak in 1824 (over one hundred deaths), it seemed to be discredited in theory as well as in practice and was discontinued in 1825. New Orleans lost over nine hundred people to yellow fever in 1829.[4]

Local thinking tended to focus on the probability that yellow fever was the product of an atmospheric "poison" or "miasm" generated *de novo* by certain local conditions. In an 1824 message, Mayor Raffignac of New Orleans offered this explanation for the seasonal prevalence of yellow fever in the city, which was supposed to represent the consensus of the local medical faculty at that time:

> The internal causes are 1st, the filth daily created in a populous city; 2dly, the low grounds and pools where stagnant water lies, and the wooden gutters, constantly wet and fermenting under the rays of the torrid sun; 3dly, the want of privies in most of the populous districts, which renders it necessary to resort to the disgusting and dangerous use of tubs.
>
> The external causes are 1st, the marshes lying north and west of the city, uncovered but undrained, and deprived, by the cutting down of trees, of the shelter formerly afforded to them by the shade of a luxuriant vegetation for which the many miasms which now spread disease and desolation among us was a source of life and vigor; 2dly, to the south and east, the Mississippi, which in its periodical retreat, at the hottest season of the year, leaves on its banks a great portion of the filth which has been thrown into the current, but is brought back by eddies; 3dly, the winds, which at the moment we feel most secure, may, as was the case in 1822, convey to us the deadly effluvia of the dangerous spots which they sweep in their course.[5]

Continued experience with yellow fever gradually sharpened and refined the atmospheric theory, and some things formerly supposed to be contributing causes were gradually ruled out as factors in the disease's

---

4. Carrigan, "Saffron Scourge," 40–66.
5. Quoted in Jones, "Comparative Pathology," 106.

etiology. It became clear that the poison of yellow fever had nothing to do with the ordinary marsh-malaria of the countryside when unacclimated persons were observed residing in perfect health just a few miles off in the midst of the swamps while the city was ravaged by the pestilence. In 1847, Dr. John Harrison, professor of physiology at the University of Louisiana, ventured an explanation for this in a long and elaborate article in the *New Orleans Medical and Surgical Journal*. He observed that the physical environment of New Orleans differed from the surrounding country not in soil, elevation, drainage, or any element of topography, but rather "in the want of vegetation; in masses of mankind being crowded together; in the want of free ventilation; in the accumulation of vast quantities, from year to year, of human excrement, both urine and night soil." He offered that the putrid "animal matters" which abounded in the city contained more nitrogen and sulfur than the decomposing plant materials that characterized the swamps, and thought this might be a clue to the secret condition of the atmosphere that produced yellow fever in the city but not the country. Harrison described recent experiments in which he had injected liquid strained from an assortment of putrefying "animal matters" into the veins of dogs and violent poisoning resulted. On autopsy he found the dogs' livers affected with fatty infiltration not unlike that seen in yellow fever in man. He claimed similar effects were produced by confining dogs in cages over open cases in which similar materials were rotting: "The theory, then, of the etiology of yellow fever may be thus stated: From the accumulation of filth in large cities (chiefly night soil and the animal matters of urine), putrefaction must necessarily take place, and from this putrefaction, under certain meteorological conditions, there is generated a poison, which either in the form of a volatile oil, or other organic essence, held in solution by ammonia, floats in the atmosphere, is inhaled during the respiratory movements, is taken into the circulation and poisons the system." Like miasmatists before and after him, Harrison failed to identify the specific poison that induced the symptoms of yellow fever, saying that in the putrefaction of organic materials, as in the smelting of metals, an infinite variety of "peculiar volatile substances" were given off in an enormous range of states and combinations. He was nevertheless sure that it existed somewhere in the complex mix of "ammoniacal, phosphorescent, sulphurous, hydrocyanic, etc., emanations which are discharged into the air from our privies and sewers, and from everyone who breathes and gives back to our atmosphere a disoxygenated air impregnated with all the vapours which the respiratory surfaces exhale." And he believed his demonstration of the effects of "putrid miasms" was enough to point the lesson: "Keep the city clean—remove all filth as soon as it is discovered, and let it be cast into the river."[6]

Yellow fever death tolls of 400 in 1832 and 1,000 in 1833, coupled with a cholera mortality of 5,300, made those two years the most terrible in the medical history of New Orleans, whose population then was estimated at 55,000. Cholera tended to fade away and return after long intervals, but yellow fever was now an almost yearly visitor, and for the next two decades it accounted for ever-increasing losses at New Orleans. Over 1,300 died in the epidemic of 1837, at least 1,300 again in 1841, and more than 2,800 in 1847.[7] This was the great period of "Cotton Prosperity" in the antebellum Mississippi Valley; jobs and money were to be had, and the region's chief port city was thronged with immigrants. An estimated 20,000 newcomers, mostly Germans and Irish, landed at New Orleans in the winter of 1852–1853, an influx of unacclimated fodder that proved to be a significant factor in the great epidemic of the following summer. Over 8,100 dead were officially enumerated in the 1853 yellow fever epidemic, 7,000 of whom were natives of Europe, and half of those were said to have come in with the previous winter's immigration. Unofficial estimates of the death toll ranged from 9,000 to as high as 11,000. At the time this epidemic struck, the population of New Orleans was 145,449, according to U.S. Census figures.[8]

In terms of absolute mortality, the pestilence of 1853 was the worst mauling the Crescent City ever suffered at the hands of Yellow Jack. As if to emphasize its inscrutable etiology, the fever's first recognized victims in the city were among the crew and passengers of an immigrant ship that arrived in May directly from Bremen, Germany. Those reports were soon followed by cases among immigrant workers on the waterfront, but any direct connection with infected shipping remained unclear. Evidence that the disease might have been spreading through some mechanism of con-

6. John Harrison, "Speculations on the Cause of Yellow Fever," *New Orleans Medical and Surgical Journal,* III (1847), 563–92.

7. Carrigan, "Saffron Scourge," 68–82.

8. *Report of the Sanitary Commission of New Orleans on the Epidemic Yellow Fever of 1853* (New Orleans, 1854), 247–61.

tagion was weakened when other cases developed well away from the wharves in the vicinity of "Gormley's Basin," a large, polluted sump in the rear of the city, where drainage from many of the street ditches collected and stagnated. A doctor described the conditions favoring the evolution of fever in this part of the city in these terms: "The appearance of the hot sun after a rain speedily covers the cauldron with a deep green mantle, which a few hours of solar action converts into an elevated black foam. . . . To crown all, the whole district is occupied by a series of soap factories and tanneries, which no precaution can prevent from exhaling an offensive odor, as stale animal matter is here the material operated on." The pattern was further complicated when the sickness broke out at a boardinghouse on Tchoupitoulas Street. Here it was concluded that the occupants had not been exposed to infection or contagion "in any way whatsoever," and it was observed that the general neighborhood of the place was distinguished by numerous piles of "stinking rubbish." All these facts would later be cited as proof that the epidemic had not derived from an imported infection, but had blossomed spontaneously from local conditions in the city.[9]

The disease, still not generally called by its proper name, continued to spread and smoulder through the month of June, and public feeling grew increasingly nervous. "Worse and worse," one of the newspapers complained in an editorial on June 22. Under the heading "A Matter of Self-Preservation," it demanded immediate sanitary action. "The late rain has only stirred up the sinks. Filth, dirt, decayed vegetables, dead dogs, and worse, are the fascinating ornaments of our thoroughfares." At a meeting of the city's Physico-Medical Society on July 2, doctors reported that "bilious fever" was fairly widespread in the area of Mandeville and Esplanade streets, as well as along Bacchus and Religious streets, and was also present on some of the steamers lying opposite Jackson Square. In the weeks immediately following, the epidemic burst out ferociously. In the last week of July, 692 deaths from yellow fever were registered, though some consolation was taken from the fact that the sickness was still confined chiefly to "the unpaved and least improved parts of town." Thereafter it began to close in on the central part of the city, and in the second week of August,

---

9. *Ibid.*, 1–26, 477–503, 525–27; E. D. Fenner, *A History of the Epidemic Yellow Fever at New Orleans, La., in 1853* (New York, 1854), 10–31.

1,288 fever deaths were recorded. "At this period the epidemic raged most awfully," Erasmus Darwin Fenner later wrote. "The public consternation and distress were indescribable." On August 18 the mayor of New Orleans ordered cannon fired at sunset and tar fires burned in the streets all night, in a lilliputian effort to shake off the epidemic atmosphere.[10]

By the end of August the epidemic had taken more than 6,000 lives in the metropolis and had also begun diffusing to numerous places in the interior. An indication of what was transpiring in the hinterland was received when the mail bill from Thibodaux came back endorsed as follows: "Stores closed—town abandoned—151 cases of yellow fever—22 deaths—postmaster absent—clerks all down with the fever." Yellow fever of amazing virulence spread to an unprecedented extent in the region that fall. In Louisiana the small towns along Bayou Lafourche and Bayou Teche suffered most grievously, and outbreaks were reported along the Red River as far up as Shreveport. Communities along the Mississippi were stricken as far north as the village of Napoleon, Arkansas, at the mouth of the Arkansas River 200 miles below Memphis. In Alabama, the sickness spread up the Tombigbee River as far as Demopolis, and up the Alabama River as far as Montgomery. Pensacola, Florida, was badly scourged, as was Galveston, Texas. Mobile, Alabama, a city of about 25,000, reported a mortality of more than 1,000, while at Vicksburg, Mississippi, there were at least 500 deaths in a population of 5,000. Yellow fever reached many of the region's smaller, more distant towns for the first time ever in 1853, and in those highly susceptible communities the death toll was most frightful. "Certain it is," Dr. Josiah Nott reflected, "that in many villages around the Gulf States, this fearful epidemic committed ravages far beyond decimation." Perhaps the worse proportionate mortality was reported at Clouthierville on the Cane River in Louisiana, where 68 of the village's 91 inhabitants were said to have been lost to yellow fever.[11]

The experience of 1853 does not appear to have lessened or deflected much of the immigrant stream from New Orleans, however, for the cotton market was still booming and the city was still flush with tropical trade

10. Fenner, *Yellow Fever at New Orleans*, 35–49; John Duffy, *Sword of Pestilence: The New Orleans Yellow Fever Epidemic of 1853* (Baton Rouge, 1966), 31–97.

11. E. D. Fenner, "Report on the Epidemics of Louisiana, Mississippi, Arkansas, and Texas in the Year 1853," *Transactions, American Medical Association*, VII (1854), 500–34; Duffy, *Sword of Pestilence*, 115–28.

and western traffic in the aftermath of the Mexican War and the California gold rush. For the rest of the decade Yellow Jack continued sorting through the concourse of unacclimated newcomers in the city: over 2,400 died in 1854, over 2,600 in 1855, and over 4,800 in 1858, the latter epidemic vying with that of 1878 as the second-worst in the city's history. The extraordinary mortality of 1853 did rouse the city council from its usual fatalistic and temporizing attitude toward the disease, and in the fall it voted funds for a special Sanitary Commission, to research the cause and cure of yellow fever. The five-member group was chaired by Dr. Edward Hall Barton, professor of clinical medicine at the University of Louisiana and president of the Louisiana Academy of Sciences. Barton was a figure of more than local prominence, having recently served as chairman of the American Medical Association's Committee on Epidemics, and as chief health officer at Veracruz, Mexico, during the American military occupation. The Sanitary Commission immediately set to work combing the published literature on yellow fever, reviewing the history and statistics of the recent epidemic at New Orleans, and soliciting opinions and observations from doctors wherever the fever had been reported that summer, from Arkansas to Barbados. The final report of the Sanitary Commission, published in 1854, was largely written by Barton and was carried by him through two subsequent printings. By and large, the work got a favorable reception—philosophically, at least, for financial stringencies kept the city from ever giving its ambitious proposals for sanitary reform a real trial. It may be taken as the most comprehensive local testament on the etiology of yellow fever prior to the advent of the germ theory.

The Sanitary Commission opened and concluded its report by emphasizing the controlling influence of what it called "the epidemic constitution of the atmosphere." In fact, the report was an elaborate affirmation of the miasmatist and noncontagionist ideas that were already embraced by most of the profession at home and abroad. Since all conditions perceived as essential to the development and spread of yellow fever pertained to the atmosphere, it seemed clear that the essential cause must be developed in the atmosphere, and not in the human body. If no degree of contact or association with the sick could spread the disease in a locality that lacked the necessary combination of warm, damp air and "local impurities," it appeared to follow that the disease was propagated solely by alteration of the atmosphere and not personal contagion. Dr. Barton cast the guiding thesis in this florid but compelling language:

It has been as truly as beautifully said, that though we do not see the air we feel it, and what is more, we breathe it. We live by breathing it, insomuch that is has been well said, that as plants are the children of the earth, so men are plants of the air; our lungs being as it were roots ramified and expanded in our atmosphere; and this in fact is the chief means by which the filth and damp of towns that are not well drained and cleaned introduce their poison into the human constitution. The putrefying refuse, whether animal or vegetable, solid or liquid, becomes dissolved into various kinds of gas, all the more commingled with the common air as this is damp and warm. These principally constitute the special difference between the air of urban and rural districts.[12]

At New Orleans in 1853, "a disruption of the ordinary concatenation of the seasons was early apparent." A remarkably mild winter had been followed by an early spring, culminating in a summer atmosphere that was unquestionably "in a stagnant condition, hot, saturated, and filthy." When at length the fever erupted, it gained "a speedy prevalence over the city, breaking out in distant and disconnected points at the same time," a fact that seemed to discountenance any suggestion that the sickness could have been contagious in nature. In addition to the prevailing malady, there had been other tokens of a seriously distempered atmosphere that summer at New Orleans. The general appetite for food and drink diminished sharply, and doctors noted an increase in diseases of the skin. Market gardeners around the city complained that much of their produce was blighted in the field; meat in the butchers' stalls appeared more prone to spoil; wild birds seemed to withdraw back into the swamps and woods. Communications from elsewhere in the region revealed other omens and symptoms of a pervasive "epidemic atmosphere." Chickens were said to have had a very sickly summer at Natchez; the peaches and other orchard fruits were infested with worms at Baton Rouge; at Bayou Sara, the China trees mildewed. And at a great many places, it is interesting to note, the "musquetoes" were reported as remarkably numerous. The Sanitary Commission did not go so far as to insist there was any direct or necessary connection between any of those phenomena and yellow fever, but submitted the facts as indications of uncommonly damp and stagnant air, an unusually high degree of solar radiation, and a reduced level of "ozone" in the atmosphere.[13]

12. *Report of the Sanitary Commission*, 346–47.
13. *Ibid.*, 229–47, 261–80.

The Sanitary Commission considered it amply demonstrated that the exhalations and excretions of a yellow fever victim could not produce the disease in others, so long as the exposure occurred "out of the sphere of the epidemic atmosphere." They referred to some dramatic self-experiments performed by noncontagionist doctors in Philadelphia earlier in the century: "All the secretions and products of the disease have been over and over again inoculated into susceptible bodies. Even black vomit itself has been tried in every way, and all with impunity." And from the record of the past season, numerous examples could be cited where active cases of yellow fever had been removed to places presumably lacking the necessary "epidemic atmosphere" without the disease ever being communicated. By official count, sixty-two cases had occurred among the refugees who had fled to Memphis, Tennessee, four hundred miles to the north, but the disease had shown no tendency at all to catch or spread in that city: "The place was far from clean, but there is no proof either of high saturation or elevated temperature." Such behavior clearly removed yellow fever from the category of "contagious" disease, as the term was narrowly understood at the time. "The special characteristic attribute of contagion is that it is irrespective of external conditions; it pays no respect to climate, zones, or seasons; it requires no special atmosphere, and yields to none; it is self-propagating and progressive, and dependent upon its own creative and self-sustaining powers." Syphilis was obviously such a disease, and so too, by all appearances, were smallpox, measles, and scarlatina. "To none of them has yellow fever any similitude."[14]

Testimony in favor of noncontagion and local causation always seemed to outweigh any evidence to the contrary in the estimation of the Sanitary Commission and its correspondents. All showed considerable nimbleness and imagination in finding causes, remote or immediate, to fit their interpretation of consequences. In mid-September yellow fever had broken out at Hollywood, Alabama, a little beach resort on the east shore of Mobile Bay. It was acknowledged that some refugee cases from New Orleans and Mobile had been accommodated at the local hotel three weeks before, yet the doctor filing the report from Hollywood positively stated that there had been "no intercourse" between them and the first local cases, either direct or through fomites. He confidently declared that contagion was

14. *Ibid.*, 113–24.

therefore "an impossibility," and the outbreak of fever at Hollywood could only have been due to "local and atmospheric causes, and none other." Hollywood occupied a breezy, piny location and was free from stagnant waters, but it was pointed out that just prior to the appearance of the fever a well had been dug and the malodorous bore tailings had been spread over the ground.[15]

A similar set of evidence was collected at Lake Providence, Louisiana, where the fever had broken out toward the end of August and ended up killing 165 of the town's 1,000 people. Steamboats had landed at the town almost every day, and it was established that at least one traveler suffering from evident yellow fever had stayed at the town's hotel earlier in the month, but those facts were shrugged off as no sure evidence of contagion. Many people later fled from the infected town into the surrounding country, many with the sickness on them, but not a single farm or plantation around Lake Providence reported yellow fever subsequently. Two of the town's three doctors were of the belief that the disease had originated there spontaneously, the other saying he had formed no opinion on the matter. A dry-goods merchant acknowledged that he had received merchandise from New Orleans all summer, but did not think the fever could have been introduced that way. He had noticed that mildew had formed on his shelves to an unusual extent, however, and he also recalled "a very unusual and remarkable odor" which had seemed "to run in veins through the town." A judge recollected that his fig trees had produced little fruit, but his bermuda grass had grown "remarkably fast," the wild mockingbirds had been strangely absent, and his backyard chickens had looked "poor and lean" and had "a disagreeable flavor."[16]

The Sanitary Commission received similar statements from reliable authorities at many other afflicted places, all assuring that the first cases of yellow fever that summer had developed under unusual atmospheric conditions, and "without any possible intercourse or communication from abroad, or from any extraneous source whatever." A physician at the town of Centerville in St. Mary's Parish had perceived "no disposition to contagion" in the fever as it occurred there and noted that it broke out after an impromptu citizens' quarantine had been in force at the mouth of

15. *Ibid.*, 47–57.
16. *Ibid.*, 40–41, 60–63.

Bayou Teche for more than a month ("Think of that, ye advocates of quarantine laws!" he said). The first recognized case was a mulatto boy who had not been around any person suffering from yellow fever, and had not been away from the neighborhood to be exposed to any locality where the fever was prevailing. "I regard this case, beyond a doubt, as having originated spontaneously here, without any suspicion of intercourse with other cases of the disease," the doctor corresponding from Centerville declared. By way of offering an explanation for the Centerville outbreak, he observed that there had been considerable ditching around the town that spring, with consequent "stirring of mud," also a prevalence of northerly winds, and "more musquetoes this past summer than I have ever noticed in any previous year." He also noted that for a long time it had been customary to dump chips and shavings from the local sawmill over the streets and in low lots around the town, and this accumulated refuse was in "a very decayed condition."[17]

"The admission of a widespread atmospherical element in yellow fever," as Dr. Barton observed, indeed seemed to be "a conclusive answer to all averments of its contagious qualities." His concept of an "epidemic atmosphere" appeared to be flexible and amorphous enough to explain away almost any anomaly. The general cause of yellow fever was postulated in advance, and when the effect appeared, almost any local condition or circumstance could be indicated as a sufficient precipitating factor. In instances where the assumed cause existed in the greatest concentration without the development of any effect whatever, some assumed contingency could always be hunted up to counteract its power. At Trinity, Louisiana, the fatal sanitary factors seemed to be in as plentiful supply as at any of the other places, "for saw-dust was used to fill up low places in the streets, and even the earth dug from the foundation for a warehouse was spread upon the streets," but there were no indications of a deranged condition in the overlying meteorology: "There was no evidence of the existence of extreme heat, direct radiation or indirect, or proof of unusual moisture. On the contrary, no epidemic influence noted on the fruit, which were fine and healthy, musquetoes not so troublesome as usual, mould less than common (proof of dry air)." Consequently, the disease failed to propagate in Trinity, despite the town's exposure to a number of

17. *Ibid.*, 278.

imported cases. Discussing why yellow fever only recently had appeared at Rio de Janeiro, when the same filth conditions had existed there on the same scale for many years, Dr. Barton tendered the incredible statement that "the broad features of the climate of Brazil had altered strangely, old residents declaring that the seasons were no longer such as they remember them to have been. . . . Nor do we yet know of the presence there of a faithful notary of science, to record those important observations that instrumental readings alone can render valuable."[18]

Over two hundred pages of testimony like the above were printed up in the final report. The Sanitary Commission was satisfied that its copious documentation of noncontagion and local origin was enough to settle the question: "If a case of yellow fever proceeding from a locality where the epidemic atmosphere prevails is conveyed to another where it does not, it must terminate with that case, as has been eminently illustrated this last year on the various marginal limits of the epidemic. . . . If a case is carried from an infected locality to one that is pure it does not spread, but if conveyed to a place where there exists a kindred, foul, epidemic atmosphere the disease is propagated, and seems, to the superficial observer, 'contagious.'" In other words, instances of yellow fever's apparent transmission were really mere coincidences, which signified nothing when the disease was spontaneously springing up all around. Accordingly, the commission concluded: "The very idea of transporting an epidemic, which is mainly atmospherical, from one country or locality to another, is an absurdity upon its face."

Not all respondents had subscribed to the atmospheric doctrine so uncritically, however, and doctors at a number of places, notably Vicksburg, argued for the contagion theory. Some of them did a creditable job of retracing the disease's spread from place to place and from person to person. Dr. Josiah Nott maintained that yellow fever was propagated by "infusoria" (meaning germs), and a communication from him repeated some of the arguments he had developed in an article published several years before. Among other curious facts, he observed that the disease had appeared at Mobile in August and up-country at Montgomery in September, while many places in between were not stricken until October or escaped altogether—how, he wondered, could that erratic diffusion possibly

18. *Ibid.*, 287.

be explained terms of gaseous emanations or differences in climate? He also thought it very significant that places not visited by steamboats had been uniformly exempt from yellow fever. "A disease may not be contagious in the proper acceptation of the term, that is, communicable from one human body to another like smallpox, and still it does not follow that the germ or materies morbi may not be transported from one place to another in a vessel or baggage car, and there be propagated."[19]

Whenever it was confronted with such incongruities, the Sanitary Commission was ready to stretch its elastic doctrine to almost any length to provide an answer. It could not but acknowledge that the arrival of a boat from an infected place was often followed by an outbreak of yellow fever, but considered it more significant that equivalent exposure on many other occasions had failed to introduce the disease. Dr. Barton cleverly suggested the apparent transmission only occurred in cases where the boat's hold contained the exact addition of confined and corrupt air needed to tip the local atmospheric balance and create an "epidemic atmosphere" in the town. Nonconforming facts could always be adjusted or obfuscated by scratching up more agreeable testimony. Against Nott's assertion that the sanitary condition in Mobile prior to the appearance of the fever was as good as foresight could have made it, the Sanitary Commission could counter with a letter from another physician stating that there had been "extensive excavations" in the city that spring. In fact, a "much larger surface of fresh earth" had been exposed in 1853 than at any time since the epidemic year of 1825. "There are more false facts than false theories," Dr. Barton rather breezily decided. Such was the combined force of *post hoc* reasoning and a preconceived idea.[20]

Since ancient times, physicians had discussed the medical effects of "miasma" without ever specifying its composition. So too the Sanitary Commission of New Orleans could only indicate the general ingredients of the "epidemic constitution of the atmosphere" that produced yellow fever. High temperature was an obvious factor, not only because it produced the predisposing conditions of "languor and prostration" in unacclimated humans, but because it represented an elevated degree of solar radiation that decomposed "ozone," which, according to the Sanitary

19. *Ibid.*, 95–105.
20. *Ibid.*, 110–113.

Commission's theory, was a great neutralizer of corrupt gases. Heat evidently had to be qualified by high humidity, which was supposed to diminish the healthy, eliminative function of the lungs and skin and also increase the "solvency" of the air, making it a more receptive vehicle for the introduction of volatile toxins and impurities into the body.[21] Those atmospheric factors, however, made up only one of the environmental constituents required to develop yellow fever, or just one blade of the "Shears of Fate," as Dr. Barton expressed it. It was in elucidating the other constituent, the "terrene," that the Sanitary Commission attempted to enter yellow fever on the ledger of preventable diseases and link its conclusions to the sanitary gospel then ascendant in public health thinking in Europe and America.

In addition to defining the weather conditions that governed yellow fever, the Sanitary Commission declared that its investigations had uncovered "the more important and impressive truth, that it is concentrated filth which localizes it." It was clear that the special terrene agent concerned in yellow fever was uniquely concentrated in towns and cities, whose atmosphere was differentiated from that of the countryside by its peculiar concentration of "exhalations of all kinds," including not just the grosser stenches but also many more subtle impairments of air purity. It was maintained that the poison derived not from any one substance but rather from the complex mixture of "all foul, filthy organic matter passing through its decomposition," the sum of which apparently comprised, *pro tanto*, "the miasm, or rather the *mal-aria*, of yellow fever." What exactly the fatal compounds might be was a matter left for future chemists to discover, but the poisonous qualities of "ammonia," "sulphuretted hydrogen," and "carbonic acid gas" were suggested. The immediate sources of the effluvia in the city were more important to the practical sanitarian, and much easier to specify. There were the vast accumulations of manure, animal and human; vile open gutters, "reeking and bubbling" under the hot sun; thousands of moldering bodies packed in leaky crypts and shallow graves in a dozen municipal cemeteries; masses of rotten garbage dumped lawlessly in vacant lots and on the riverbank. The quantity of night soil generated by New Orleans every year was calculated at 5,000 tons, and most of that was imperfectly disposed of. When the total volume of manure, gutter

21. *Ibid.*, 281–308.

sludge, human and animal remains, slaughterhouse and kitchen offal, and tannery and cotton-press refuse was figured up, it amounted to the "frightful aggregate" of 300,000 tons of decomposing organic matter on and under the city's soil. The Sanitary Commission analyzed the mortality reports of the recent epidemic by district and ward and demonstrated how the worse "fever nests" had indeed coincided with the worst concentrations of palpable filth.[22]

The Sanitary Commission concluded with a long discussion of what had to be done to abolish yellow fever from New Orleans. They urged the restriction of tallow works and other noxious industries, a thorough scouring of the gutters, and an improved system of garbage collection and night scavenging. Cemeteries should be removed well outside city limits. The foul basins in the rear of the city should be filled in and planted, and converted into parks. Special measures were advised to keep town filth from getting into the subsoil, from which it would be given back in the form of dangerous gases. The common practice of spreading gutter sludge over the dusty roadbeds should immediately be stopped, and all the streets should then be paved with stone. It was observed that Norfolk, Virginia, had frequently been subject to yellow fever in the past, but since its streets were paved it had become "entirely salubrious." (In fact, Norfolk was terribly scourged by yellow fever the very next year, in 1855, suffering over 1,800 deaths in a population of 16,000. In the 1857 edition of this report Dr. Barton would charge that outbreak to the fact that the city had made the deadly error of using green brush and garbage for landfill along its waterfront.) The Sanitary Commission even recommended that the yards of all private residences in New Orleans be completely paved over, front and back, a measure that would have given the city a unique physiognomy if it had been carried out.

All digging and excavating in the city's "native soil" should be forbidden in the hot months from May to October—the Sanitary Commission was sure that dredging in the basins behind the city, trenching for gas and water pipes in the downtown area, and levee making across the river in Algiers had been potent influences in generating the 1853 epidemic. As a point of history, it observed that "extensive disturbances of the native soil"

---

22. *Ibid.*, 309–414. Compare René LaRoche, *Yellow Fever, Considered in Its Historical, Pathological, Etiological, and Therapeutic Relations* (2 vols.; Philadelphia, 1855), II, 369–403.

had accompanied every recorded epidemic of yellow fever at New Orleans as well as at Natchez, Mobile, and Charleston—gliding over the fact that in the young, prosperous, upbuilding towns and cities of the period, "extensive excavations" of one kind or another had undoubtedly gone on every year, whether accompanied by yellow fever or not. The Sanitary Commission noted the coincidence of yellow and other fevers with the receding of the Mississippi in late summer, and advised that the swamp and overflow lands surrounding the city be thoroughly cleared and drained—a recommendation that was sound as to malaria but perfectly irrelevant as to yellow fever. They urged that the wild brakes and forests around New Orleans be cut down to facilitate the free sweep of winds and breezes, while advising, paradoxically, that more trees be planted inside city limits to neutralize bad air. The use of wood in construction was be discouraged, because it was feared dry lumber would tend to absorb, accumulate, and finally remit atmospheric impurities. The Sanitary Commission made many other recommendations for the better sanitation and ventilation of the city—the building of a huge shed or awning the whole length of the riverfront to reduce air temperatures was one of the more quixotic.[23]

A favorable review of the Sanitary Commission's report in the *Boston Medical and Surgical Journal* affirmed the currency of its ruling concepts. Its "orderly classification of facts" and its "clear and cogent reasoning" were praised, and its conclusions commended. "Dr. Barton can do no more to enlighten the public or direct the magistrates. By following out in detail the inferences which he has drawn from the facts presented, and on which this report is based, New Orleans may yet establish a reputation for cleanliness and exemption from fatal epidemics." Dr. René LaRoche of Philadelphia hailed the report as "a capital work" that "will compare advantageously with anything of the kind I have seen."[24] There were a few critics at home who did not accept the "facts" and inferences of the report so easily, however. A number of mordant commentaries published in the *New Orleans Medical and Surgical Journal* by Dr. Morton Dowler over the next several years made perfect nonsense of the Sanitary Commission's proofs and ratiocinations. While personally a dogmatic believer in "the

23. *Report of the Sanitary Commission,* 414–58.
24. "Notices of the Report of the Sanitary Commission," in E. H. Barton, *The Cause and Preventions of Yellow Fever at New Orleans and other Cities in America* (New York, 1857), 5, 8.

unequivocal local origin of yellow fever," Dowler made it clear that he was not just skeptical but contemptuous of any study that pretended to reveal with scientific precision the unsearchably complex etiology of this disease. He insisted that hard evidence of a specific "sky-cause" or "ground-cause" was confirmed by neither general experience nor official records, in 1853 or any other epidemic year. "Each of these agencies, separately as well as conjointly, have been upon insufficient proofs assigned by medical philosophers for hundreds of years as the causes of epidemics. Without, therefore, the discovery of some new law determining the modus operandi of these agencies, there can be nothing satisfactory in such an aetiology." He produced weather records for the summer of 1849—by all accounts a remarkably healthy summer at New Orleans—and showed that the mean monthly temperatures recorded in 1853 were virtually the same, while total rainfall differed by a mere fraction of an inch. He noted that similar medical commissions organized at Gibraltar in 1850 and at Norfolk in 1855 had thoroughly examined meteorological variations but had turned up no satisfactory information regarding the ultimate cause of yellow fever. And he laughed that the Sanitary Commission of New Orleans "did not pass lightly over the signs, wonders, and prodigies that fitted through the distempered imagination of the excited public," but instead had eagerly seized on the ridiculous information to undershore its extravagant theories.[25]

In fact, countercurrents were already in motion that would gradually override the miasmatic theory of yellow fever. In 1848 a "long and rambling essay" was published in the *New Orleans Medical and Surgical Journal* by Dr. Josiah Nott, critical of what he called "the malarial hypothesis." He pointed out some of its manifest inconsistencies: how "offensive effluvia" abounded every summer, but yellow fever was only an occasional visitor; how the disease always erupted at an identifiable "focus of infection" and spread steadily outward regardless of air movements and prevailing winds, which could not happen if the poison were really "united to the atmosphere"; how despite the "wonderful perfection" of chemical science, "the laboratory has not succeeded in bringing to light any gas or product of putrefaction which can produce in the human frame a train of symptoms resembling those of yellow fever." After closely observing the course of

25. M. Morton Dowler, "Observations on Yellow Fever," *New Orleans Medical and Surgical Journal*, XVI (1859), 305–24.

five recent epidemics in Alabama, Dr. Nott could not accept that yellow fever arose from strictly local causes and was nontransportable; on the contrary, he asserted that it was "literally and truly a migrating disease, possessing an inherent power of reproduction and progression irreconcilable with any known laws of gases, emanations, vapors, or dews." Yellow fever's irregular occurrence from place to place and season to season, its periods of "activity and repose," and its evident property of self-multiplication, "propagating as it travels and scattering the seeds of reproduction behind it," could not be explained in terms of the physical laws of gases, but did seem to accord in many respects with the vagaries witnessed in outbreaks of the teeming insects. Nott drew a persuasive analogy between the occurrence of yellow fever in human populations and the occurrence of army worm in cotton: "Some years there may be an entire exemption from these insects or to use a medical phrase, there may be a few 'sporadic cases.' At another time worms may appear at a single point, and from this focus will spread slowly over a portion of a field, leaving the other portion almost untouched. In another year worms come like a great 'Epidemic,' appearing at many points in rapid succession or simultaneously, and ravaging not only a single plantation but laying waste the cotton region for several hundred miles." In developing his argument, Nott went on to draw parallels with various peculiarities of moths, aphids, and a variety of other insects, including mosquitoes. His article is often erroneously identified as the first statement of the insect vector theory. In fact the Alabama doctor had been influenced by recent publications of the German microscopist Christian Ehrenberg and the British medical philosopher Sir Henry Holland, and was simply following their example in applying the term "insect" to microbial life, as the closest thing that would be understandable to his readers. Good compound microscopes had only been available since the mid-1830s, and it was only in recent years that a specific microscopic parasite was first identified as the cause of a human disease (ringworm, the fungal disease of the skin). The science of microbiology was just being born, and its terminology as well as its techniques were still quite unfamiliar, even in professional circles. Later on in his essay, Nott began to use "insect" interchangeably with "animalculae" and "infusoria," and it becomes clear his reference was to what would later be generally denominated "germs." "The habits and movements of larger insects are obscured by numerous impediments," Nott speculated, "but how much more perplexing must be the natural history of those which can only be reached by powerful microscopes?"[26]

While it is incorrect to regard Nott as the author of the insect theory as we understand it, his article does have great significance as the first serious consideration of yellow fever being a germ-caused disease and not merely an aggravated phase of "malarial" or miasmatic poisoning. The idea slowly put down roots among doctors and scientists in the region, reinforced as the discoveries of Ehrenberg and other European microscopists gained wider circulation. In 1850 a chemistry professor at the University of Louisiana, J. L. Riddell, wrote of "motes of organic life . . . living corpuscles in the miasmatic air . . . the living cause of yellow fever" and published his design of an alembic device that would be used "to investigate the organized matter contained in the atmosphere during the prevalence of yellow fever in New Orleans." It is not known whether his invention was ever tested; if so, it would have anticipated by fifteen years a similar experiment by a committee of French scientists, one of them Louis Pasteur, to analyze samples of the air in Paris during the cholera epidemic of 1865.[27]

Dr. Riddell was appointed to the Sanitary Commission of New Orleans in 1853, evidently found himself at variance with the dominant views of Dr. Barton, and seems to have felt obliged to publish a two-page dissenting opinion in the *New Orleans Medical and Surgical Journal* in 1854. The propositions or "inferences" he submitted are important because they represent the first clear enunciation of the concept of infection, which would dominate medical views of yellow fever by 1878. Riddell agreed that the disease was not contagious, in that it "does not emanate in an active condition from the person of the patient laboring under the disease," yet he insisted that it was characterized by a certain "infectious communicability . . . the poisonous matter (doubtless some species of living organism) maturing its germ or spores on the surface of solids devoid of life, surrounded by confined or impure air, which germs become diffused in

26. J. C. Nott, "Yellow fever contrasted with Bilious Fever—Reasons for believing it a disease sui generis—Its mode of Propagation—Remote Cause—Probable insect or animalcular origin, &c.," *New Orleans Medical and Surgical Journal*, IV (1848), 563–601.

27. J. L. Riddell, "A Plan to be Pursued, to Investigate the Organized Matter, Contained in the Atmosphere During the Prevalence of Yellow Fever, at New Orleans," *New Orleans Medical and Surgical Journal*, VII (1850), 172–76.

the impure atmosphere." He thought this growth and diffusion was promoted chiefly by "abundant emanations from decomposing and disintegrating organized matters, complex products, gaseous, liquid, and solid, the pabulum or blastema of cryptogamous growths." Apparently, Riddell conceived of the infection as a kind of invisible smut or mildew, shedding its infectious spores into an atmosphere clabbered with the vapors of putrefaction. To that extent he was reconciled with the Sanitary Commission's general hygienic recommendations for the city. Dr. Riddell's concept of "infectious communicability," however distinct from the classical idea of contagion, still carried with it the recognition of yellow fever's transmissibility and transportability. He asserted that "the towns and plantations of the Southwest have this year derived their yellow fever from New Orleans," and that the infection in New Orleans had in turn "probably been derived from countries farther South."[28]

The southern medical establishment was generally unmoved by such suggestions. Dr. Erasmus Fenner, one of the founding editors of the *New Orleans Medical and Surgical Journal,* published his own book on the 1853 epidemic at New Orleans corroborating local causation and noncontagion. The journal published letters by two prominent physicians of Memphis, Tennessee, supporting the local-origin position and commended them to the "special attention" of its readers. These communications noted that Memphis had instituted no special quarantine regulations or sanitary measures: "Boats freighted with merchandise, saturated with the atmosphere of an infected city, landed at our wharf almost every day, and any number of persons affected with the disease were carried through our streets to the Hospital, and some of them dying in private families, and yet not a case was communicated to any of the nurses, friends, or physicians. . . . Does any person suppose for a moment that there could be brought into our city such a number of cases of any of those diseases ordinarily termed contagious, without the occurrence of a single instance of communication to the unprotected and exposed?" The conclusion was that Memphis enjoyed this exemption because it lacked the necessary "atmospheric constitution" to produce yellow fever, and that "without the prerequisite conditions of atmospheric and climatic derangement, yellow

28. "Professor J. L. Riddell's Opinion on the Causes of Yellow Fever," *New Orleans Medical and Surgical Journal,* X (1854), 813–14.

fever is no more liable to be communicated from one subject to another than gout or rheumatism."[29] In a long report to the American Medical Association in 1854, Dr. Fenner reaffirmed the formula of "local causes" plus "a peculiar state or constitution of the atmosphere." He decided that occasional stories of yellow fever introduction via personal contact or fomites signified little when set against the many instances where the disease had entirely failed to spread from similar exposures:

> It is sometimes extremely difficult to decide whether certain phenomena be mere coincidences, or hold the relation of cause and effect. Now that at least one case of yellow fever was actually introduced this year into a great many places previous to the outbreak of the epidemic is an undeniable fact. Such was the case in sixteen out of twenty places that have been noticed in this report, but does it thence follow necessarily that the epidemic broke out as a consequence of such introduction? If this were so, and the extension of the disease beyond New Orleans was attributable alone to infectious communication, it follows that wherever such communication existed the disease should have prevailed in at least a majority of instances, and it should have prevailed nowhere else. But such was not the fact. We have given instances, and might have given many more, in which the disease failed to extend itself under the most favorable auspices of this nature, and others in which it appeared to arise spontaneously, without any traceable connection with infected places. Now, if it is possible for yellow fever to originate from a local cause, under a certain condition of the atmosphere, at one place, it may have done so at all; and the fact that the epidemic broke out about the time that cases of the disease were introduced, might have been a mere coincidence, because a like result has failed to follow in hundreds and thousands of instances of equal exposure.[30]

Some medical practitioners—and, it seems, many nonmedical people as well—were nevertheless beginning to shift moorings on the subject of yellow fever. In 1854 the *New Orleans Medical News and Hospital Gazette* published a very interesting article by A. P. Jones, an observant country

29. Geo. A. Smith and W. J. Tuck, "Letters on Yellow Fever at Memphis, Tennessee, in 1853," *New Orleans Medical and Surgical Journal,* X (1854), 662–67.

30. Fenner, "Report on the Epidemics, 1853," 538.

doctor in Jefferson County, Mississippi, who related that "the practitioners of this section, with one exception, have heretofore been non-contagionists—local-origin men—now, with one exception, they are all the other way. . . . As to the laity, noted for a high degree of intelligence and general information, all the doctors in the valley of the Mississippi could not persuade them that this fever was not 'catching' and 'terribly killing' too, as they express it." Dr. Jones had difficulty connecting the diffusion of the late epidemic to the ordinary rural malaria, to emanations from filth and decay, or to atmospheric influences of any sort. He said seventeen plantations in Jefferson County had been visited by yellow fever in 1853, and at least thirty deaths were credited to the disease, despite the fact that for some years the area had been enjoying "a rather more than common immunity from the climatorial diseases of the season." He recalled that when he first came to practice, twenty years before, much new land was being opened, and slash and dead timber were everywhere. The maiden soil was washing from the hills into the valleys, "where covering and mixing with the debris of timber and rank vegetation it became a hotbed of malaria. . . . I think no part of the South would exceed it for fever." More recently, however, the planters had been abandoning their worn-out and gullied lands for more productive fields in the Louisiana bottoms and the prairies of north Mississippi and Texas, and the hills and valleys were being reclaimed by native trees and grasses. "Dead and decaying timber has disappeared, and the country has generally become healthier, insomuch that most of the country practitioners remaining have found it necessary to resort to other pursuits for a living."

Jones made an effort to retrace the diffusion of yellow fever in his home county in 1853, "showing the inlet of the disease and its progress thereafter." In using phrases like "focus of infection," he revealed the influence of Josiah Nott. The doctor observed that yellow fever broke out at one plantation after a visit by a drover from Port Gibson who had been "complaining" but was "not thought much ill." Jones showed that he was alert to the epidemiological problem posed by mild and unrecognized cases in a way most members of his profession would not be for another half-century. In recounting the story of the unfortunate "Jew pedlar" who was shunted from farm to farm in his illness, with the infection breaking out in his wake after an interval of two weeks, Jones submitted a perfect description of the phenomenon of extrinsic incubation, forty-five years before H. R. Carter's landmark study:

> A somewhat similar fact happened in the family of Adolph Heath, Senr.: a Jew pedlar, recently from Port Gibson, was seized with fever while on his rounds, and evidently infected three families; he was literally driven from one to the other till he got to Heath's, where being too ill to go back to town, he was put in a back shed room of the dwelling, and died of black vomit on the 10th of September. So much were the people of the house alarmed that the corpse was hurried into a coffin without un-dressing; his pocketbook full of papers, purse of money, and everything on his person were buried with him. The weather-boarding and gable-end of the room were knocked off to let in air and rains; the bedding and furniture were burned, only a few pieces of the best were allowed to lie out, one or two hundred feet from the building; meantime no one sick-ened. At the end of two weeks the bed clothes were brought in, boiled, wrung out and dried about the house, Mrs. Heath seeing to it. Within eight days from that time, and twenty from the death of the poor pedlar, Mrs. Heath, her husband and son, the woman who washed the clothes and several servants, sickened; the first two died—the others recovered.
>
> At a widow Perkins, where this pedlar staid the night before he went to Heath's, and was very ill all night with fever and vomiting, but well enough at daylight to mount his pony and ride a few miles, a little negro boy was seized with fever, sixteen days from the time the pedlar left. He died with black vomit and convulsions. Sixteen days from his death his mistress was taken and died similarly. I neglected to mention the pedlar's pack was left and remained all this time in the dwelling. There were other cases who recovered. The well were sent away, but returned after the frost of 25th October, and several of them had fever lightly.

Regarding this account, Dr. Fenner remarked: "If Dr. Jones's conclusions were correct, yellow fever must be a far more infectious disease than small-pox or any other that is known. The time between exposure and attack in his cases was much longer than is generally claimed by the advocate of infectious communicability." It will nevertheless be observed from the above quotation that common people were already beginning to react to yellow fever as though it were communicable through fomites as well as personal contact. "The experience of the last season has much weakened the confidence of many of our most intelligent planters and businessmen in the capacity of the medical faculty to teach them how to avoid the inroads of epidemics," Jones advised, "and the pertinacity with which some of the leading practitioners and ablest writers of New Orleans still cling to the local origin doctrine is still further impairing public confidence." He concluded his article by remarking: "Yellow fever is certainly spreading farther and farther from the great focus of infection of that city every visitation." He predicted that after the many new railroad lines then being built were completed, all inland towns having direct and rapid communication with New Orleans could be threatened by the disease, from the Alleghenies even to the Rockies: "We of the country will be compelled in self-defence to devise and adopt measures to keep it away."[31] It is interesting to note that Memphis, Tennessee, was connected by rail with New Orleans in 1855, and that same year happened to be visited for the first time by yellow fever in epidemic form: there may have been as many as two hundred deaths. Memphis' first epidemic was confined to the waterfront and was blamed on an infected steamboat, but it is certain that the railroads would be a most potent factor in expanding yellow fever's range in the region, both by spreading *A. aegypti* to more remote places, and by enabling human cases, carrying the virus in their blood, to reach those places while still in the incubative stage of the disease.[32]

In a follow-up report to the American Medical Association in 1856, Dr. Fenner pondered the recent appearance of yellow fever at Memphis and concluded that "some change must have recently taken place in the locality of Memphis, which either caused the disease to spring up spontaneously, or furnished a nidus favorable to its regeneration and extension when once introduced from abroad."[33] Some of the local accounts transmitted to the association by Fenner illustrated the shift in perception that was under way. In 1854 the fever had raged in a settlement of Negroes at a landing below Franklin, Louisiana, where an infected steamboat from

31. A. P. Jones, "Yellow Fever in a Rural District," *New Orleans Medical News and Hospital Gazette,* I (1854), 180–89, 205–209.

32. L. Shanks, "A Brief History of the Commencement and Progress of the Yellow Fever in Memphis, Tenn., in 1855," *Memphis Medical Recorder,* IV (1856), 204–45; John Huber Ellis, "Yellow Fever and the Origins of Modern Public Health in Memphis, Tennessee, 1870–1900" (Ph.D. dissertation, Tulane University, 1962), 25–33.

33. Erasmus D. Fenner, "Report on the Epidemics of Louisiana, Mississippi, Arkansas, and Texas," *Transactions, American Medical Association,* IX (1856), 624.

New Orleans had been tied up. The doctor who described this outbreak reflected: "I do not believe that yellow fever is contagious; that is, that one person having the disease can under ordinary circumstances communicate it to another. But here the cause of the fever, whatever it may have been, was evidently in the vessel, and was evidently communicated not only to those who cleaned the hold, but also to all persons in the vicinity. The cause remained after the vessel had left, and evidently increased in intensity."[34] Fenner was forced to acknowledge that "the experience of the last three years has greatly modified opinion on this subject":

> Some physicians still deny in toto the contagion of yellow fever, but I think the majority of those who have recently been brought into contact with it in this region now admit that under favorable circumstances and within a limited region the morbific cause may be conveyed from one place to another and take effect on persons thus exposed to it. The mass of the people who have been the sufferers are almost unanimous in this belief. But to the philosophical inquirer after truth is presented an array of facts apparently of the most contradictory character in relation to this question. Why should the disease be contagious at one place and not another? in one season and not another? Why should it now prevail epidemically for the first time at a town or plantation on the Mississippi River which has always been in direct communication with New Orleans, and into which cases of the disease and all sorts of goods have been introduced from an infected district, hitherto with impunity? Formerly, when it broke out at one of its old habitats, as New Orleans, Mobile, or Natchez, cases might be taken thence into the neighboring country without endangering the inhabitants; but not so now. It seldom fails to spread when taken to the neighborhood of those places.
>
> When the disease now breaks out for the first time at a town far up one of the navigable streams the inhabitants flee with consternation to the surrounding country, carrying in their systems the seeds of infection which then mature and develop the fatal fever, but incapable of spreading among the attendants on the sick; but perhaps a like immunity will not be observed a few years hence. Such are some of the curious and apparently antagonistic facts that require to be reconciled and explained before we can claim to understand the true nature and character of yellow fever.[35]

34. *Ibid.*, 662–64.
35. *Ibid.*, 626.

Public insistence prodded the Louisiana legislature into reinstituting a general maritime quarantine of the state in 1855, requiring all ships with evidence of infection to be detained ten days at Buras Station, eighty miles below New Orleans, before being allowed to proceed to the city. In 1858, New Orleans suffered another destructive epidemic, which the state's new board of health had no hesitation about tracing to an infected ship from St. Thomas that had slipped through the Buras defences. The board's president (a former member of the Sanitary Commission of New Orleans, it is interesting to note) proposed a more radical quarantine law that would have forbidden all vessels from infected ports from passing up to New Orleans anytime from May to November, compelling them to discharge their cargoes at special warehouses at Buras Station, from which consignees could only ship goods to points beyond the borders of the state. This potentially expensive and commerce-crippling measure was not enacted then, nor would it be when it was suggested again in the wake of the 1878 epidemic. In the pages of the *New Orleans Medical and Surgical Journal*, meanwhile, John Riddell and Josiah Nott reiterated their arguments for the germ theory and the "infectious communicability" of yellow fever.[36]

By now, in America as well as Europe, many of the more progressive medical thinkers had started drawing away from the physico-chemical doctrine of yellow fever and other epidemic diseases and had begun moving in half-circles toward what was to be known as the germ theory. In his two-volume, 1,419-page treatise on yellow fever, published in 1855, Dr. René LaRoche, an authoritative miasmatist and noncontagionist from Philadelphia, unbent so far as to allow nine pages for a consideration of the new "cryptogamic" and "animalcular" theories of yellow fever's etiology: "In this field of interesting inquiry and hypothesis the suggestion is offered, as at least a reasonable conjecture, that in the animal exhalations, infinitely abundant and varied, that are collected about the dense population of a crowded city, these organic germs may find occasionally all the elements essential to their germination and growth, and may propagate

36. "Synopsis of the Report of the Board of Health to the Legislature of the State of Louisiana for the Year 1858," *New Orleans Medical and Surgical Journal*, XVI (1859), 370–73; J. L. Riddell, "Memoir on the Nature of Miasm and Contagion," *New Orleans Medical and Surgical Journal*, XVI (1859), 348–69; J. C. Nott, "Yellow Fever in Mobile, A.D. 1858," *New Orleans Medical and Surgical Journal*, XV (1858), 819–24.

and multiply themselves in an atmosphere thus saturated with the pabulum adapted to their support and development."[37] During the 1860s, speculations about "germs" and "ferments" gained considerable acceptance as Pasteur and others demonstrated the role played by airborne yeasts and bacteria in the everyday phenomena of fermentation and putrefaction. Once it was shown how the rapid multiplication of a few foreign cells could curdle a jar of cream or corrupt a vat of wine, it was easy to conceive a larger role for them in the causation of epidemic disease. Sickness could readily enough be understood as a kind of fermentation or putrefaction of the living body, while the demonstration of an atmosphere swarming with animal and vegetable germs appeared to give a concrete basis to preexisting beliefs about the atmospheric origin of pestilence. *Zymosis,* from the Greek word for "ferment," appeared frequently in the medical literature as a term denoting infectious disease.

This point of view was soon being popularized by influential writers and lecturers. "Our air is full of the germs of ferments," the English physicist John Tyndall declared in one of his classic expository articles, and then proceeded to guide his readers' imagination from the stray thistle seed that lands on a patch of soil, reproduces itself, and soon overruns the garden, to the unregarded bacteria wafted as "invisible dust" onto the surface of a cup of beef broth, which before long is turbid and stinking with the proliferating particles. Tyndall then had his readers reflect on the probable action of those "special germs" that "sow pestilence and death over nations and continents."[38] The conjectured existence of "special germs" was raised to the status of a demonstrated fact as the new science of microbiology delivered its first crop of discoveries and pseudo-discoveries. During the 1860s and 1870s, pathologists in France and Germany successfully transmitted anthrax, tuberculosis, and diphtheria by inoculation and tentatively identified the specific germs of those diseases; meanwhile, other scientists were contentiously submitting their pet cryptograms and animalcules as

37. LaRoche, *Yellow Fever,* II, 587. LaRoche, however, decided the germ theory of yellow fever was either imadmissible, because the existence of the specific germ had never been demonstrated, or superfluous, because the deteriorated atmosphere on which the germ's operation was premised was already adequately accounted for by the miasm theory.

38. John Tyndall, "Fermentation and Its Bearings on the Phenomena of Disease," *Popular Science Monthly,* X (1877), 129–54.

the causative germs of glanders, whooping cough, malaria, cholera, and a host of other plagues.[39]

Compared with former assumptions about miasmatic emanations and impalpable gaseous influences, here was something at last that the imagination could readily grasp, something whose operation was clear and comprehensible to scientific and nonscientific minds alike. The spread of mold on a piece of cheese and the action of yeast in a lump of dough had obvious analogies to the march of infectious disease through a human population; the putrefaction and decay of meat had evident similarities to pathological changes in living tissue. Some physiologists were saying the phenomenon of fever could be understood in terms of the heat of fermentation. Others took the parallel further, and worried that the microbes that obviously propagated in dead and decaying substances could be imparted to the human system, and so actually be a source of infection—possibly the major source. One of those who expressed this idea most directly was William Schmoele, a Philadelphia sanitary writer, in an 1866 pamphlet: "The parasites inducing epidemic diseases in living organisms of a higher nature are identical with or homologous to the parasites known as the causes of putrefaction of dead animal and vegetable substances." According to Dr. Schmoele, the set of conditions essential to a yellow fever epidemic, like those essential to ordinary putrefaction and decay, required first of all the specific "living germs or seeds" of the disease, the presence of a "nutritive substance" suitable for their ripening and development, and the conditioning influences of moisture and "a certain degree of temperature." The germs of yellow fever obviously flourished best when deposited in "warm, damp, filthy localities, presenting all the conditions of development of minute vermin." Practical sanitarians were quite impressed by Schmoele's simple, cogent thesis, and he was still being cited in 1878.[40]

39. John C. Dalton, "The Origin and Propagation of Disease," in Smithsonian Institution, *Report for 1873* (Washington, D.C., 1874), 226–45; "The Influence of the Lower Organisms in the Production of Infectious and Contagious Diseases," *Philadelphia Medical Times*, V (1875), 761–64, 776–78, 793–95; W. B. Carpenter, "Disease Germs," *Popular Science Monthly*, XX (1881), 244–60; John Tyndall, "Progress of the Germ Theory of Disease," *Popular Science Monthly*, XXI (1882), 462–67.

40. See, for instance, "Weather and Disease," New Orleans *Picayune*, September 14, 1878; John M. Keating, *The Yellow Fever Epidemic of 1878 in Memphis, Tenn.* (Memphis, 1879), 17.

Undoubtedly, popular and professional acceptance of the primitive germ theory came about easily because it tallied in so many respects with the miasmatism it superseded. In fact, Schmoele's recipe for a yellow fever epidemic included the same atmospheric and telluric ingredients that had been specified by the Sanitary Commission of New Orleans twelve years before, only now they were placed on a different theoretical basis. Dampness and warm temperature were still important factors, because they favored the growth and proliferation of germs in the environment. The danger of rotting organic matter and its effluvia was if anything more keenly perceived, because it furnished the broth or culture medium in which the germs of infectious disease could develop. The success early laboratory scientists were having in culturing fungi and bacteria in crude nutrient solutions and pastes, and the demonstration about this time of the extrinsic transmission of an important animal disease (anthrax, whose hardy spores do persist for long periods in soil and on fomites), were considerations that encouraged the view that germs of all kinds readily flourished outside the living organism.[41] This was when the notion firmly took hold that disease germs could live in active or dormant form on inanimate objects, and so be transported and spread by means of fomites. This version of the germ theory also tended to substantiate the standing view of yellow fever as essentially an infection of places, not persons, as the president of the Louisiana Board of Health expressed in 1872: "The locality and not the individual is the seat of infection, the second case not being attacked by reason of proximity to the first but by exposure to the same causative infection."[42]

General belief in the extrinsic or extracorporeal origin of epidemics,

41. On the perceived relationship of germs to filth, see William Roberts, "The Doctrine of Contagium Vivum and Its Applications to Medicine," *Medical Times and Gazette*, August 11, 1877, pp. 138–45; J. L. Cabell, "Address on State Medicine and Public Hygiene," *Transactions, American Medical Association*, XXIX (1878), 551–83; Henry O. Marcy, "The Recent Advances of Sanitary Science—The Relations of Micro-Organisms to Disease," *Journal of the American Medical Association*, I (1883), 493–501; Theobald Smith, "Some Observations on the Origin and Sources of Pathogenic Bacteria," *Reports and Papers, American Public Health Association*, XIV (1888), 171–78. "At all events," concluded John Shaw Billings, "we have learned enough to know that the life which is born of, and nourished in, death and corruption may become the cause of disease and death in higher organisms" ("Germs and Epidemics," *Sanitary Engineer*, VII [1883], 390).

42. Louisiana Board of Health, *Report for 1872* (New Orleans, 1873), 22.

and in the contributing role of filth in their development, was in fact greatly strengthened and stimulated by the rise of the new germ theory. By 1880, Dr. Ezra Hunt was merely stating the conventional view when he wrote: "In respect to most if not all the particles which give rise to epidemics, it may be said that they are chiefly if not entirely dependent for their fertility and extended spread on the presence of filth. They are either bred or incubated chiefly if not entirely amid the putrefactive decompositions of vegetable and animal matter."[43] Just as the germ theory of disease was borne out by the actual discovery of virulent microorganisms in the tissues of the sick, so its corollary, the filth theory of epidemics, appeared to be substantiated when similar microbes were found in long-suspected sources of putrefaction and miasma. In 1879 a pair of investigators in Italy announced their discovery of "*bacillus malariae*," cultured in gelatin from samples of mud taken from a notoriously malarious marsh outside Rome, which they offered to the medical world as the specific cause of malaria. Dr. George Sternberg of the United States Army immediately duplicated their experiments with cultures of bacteria and fungi derived from mud and slime skimmed from foul gutters and basins in and around New Orleans. Injected into rabbits, this culture fluids produced a rather violent septicemia, fatal in twelve of thirty-seven cases, some symptoms of which indeed resembled those of malaria and yellow fever in human beings. Sternberg's findings were admittedly inconclusive, but he felt justified in declaring:

> The fact observed by myself that during the summer months the mud in the gutters of New Orleans possesses an extraordinary degree of virulence shows that pathogenic varieties of bacteria are not alone bred in the bodies of living animals. The more I study this subject the more probable it seems to me that in this direction lies the explanation of many problems which have puzzled epidemiologists and that the sanitarians are right in fighting against filth as a prime factor in the production of epidemics—a factor of which the role is easily understood, if this view is correct. The presence of septic organisms possessing different degrees of virulence depending upon the abundance and kind of pabulum furnished them and upon meteorological conditions more or less favorable constitutes, in my

43. Ezra M. Hunt, "Our Present and Our Needed Knowledge of Epidemics," *Reports and Papers, American Public Health Association,* VI (1880), 100.

opinion, the *epidemic constitution of the atmosphere*, which wise men were wont to speak of not many years ago as a cloak for ignorance. It must be remembered that the gutter mud of today with its deadly septic organisms is the dust of tomorrow, which in respiration is deposited upon the mucus membrane of the respiratory passages of those who breathe the air loaded with it.[44]

In its practical implications the germ theory brought a reinterpretation, but certainly not a devaluation, of the sanitary principles that had been founded on the now-obsolete concept of an epidemic atmosphere. "Whatever may be the theory as to the nature of the poison," one of the nation's leading medical journals would editorialize during the 1878 epidemic, "we do certainly know the peculiar way in which it is transmitted, and the special soil which it requires for multiplication. . . . In New Orleans we are told that parts of the city which furnished aliment for the disease in 1853 are in 1878 in just as filthy a condition, if not more so. Houses seem to have been adapted to keep out the fresh air and to receive the foul emanations from the sinks and garbage and offal in the backyards and alley-ways." At Grenada, Mississippi, the fever's appearance was tentatively blamed on a choked-up sewer running through the middle of town. "It collects the drainage of stables, cesspools, and probably of privies. Not uncommonly the hogs, which appear to be the natural scavengers of the place, found their way into its convenient openings, and failing in their efforts to get out again, died, leaving their carcasses to rot and pollute the air. . . . This sketch of a Mississippi town is said not to be exceptional. All sorts of refuse is thrown into the streets or into the backyards and alleys, making the very conditions that are known to favor the outbreak of an epidemic."[45]

At those and other places menaced by Yellow Jack, the most urgent efforts were concentrated on cleaning up and disinfecting the sewage, garbage, offal, and other varieties of "animal filth" through which the disease was supposed to propagate and spread. "Filth the Cause and Cleanliness the Cure of the Southern Pest," was the confident and alliterative headline of one sanitarian's homily in the Washington *Post* that fall. "Fetid organic

44. G. M. Sternberg, "Experimental Investigations Relating to the Etiology of the Malarial Fevers," in National Board of Health, *Report for 1881*, 91–92.
45. "The Yellow Fever Scourge," *Medical Record*, XIV (1878), 173–74.

matter is the most dangerous medium yet discovered to be a cause of disease, as it is in this noxious vapor that disease germs float, the same as the fine pollen of flowers or other germ elements that float in the air." "There is nothing whatever mysterious about this pestilence, its starting place is invariably some unclean locality for which man alone and not Providence is responsible," the New York *Bulletin* editorialized, while formal discussions at the New York Academy of Medicine agreed that the root cause of the plague then ravaging the South existed in "accumulations of filth and deviations from good sanitary conditions."[46]

The vision of disease-causing spores and animalcules with a vigorous saprophytic existence outside the human body ("germs" whose abiding place was "filth") cannot be given too much emphasis in explaining the methods and approaches of public health officials during the last half of the nineteenth century. The notion was especially forceful and relevant in the minds of those sanitarians who were grappling with the problem of yellow fever, which was at once the most obvious and the most perplexing example of an extrinsic infection. Two exemplary articles published during the 1870s can be taken to illustrate the general state of perception. In an 1878 lecture to the Philadelphia Social Science Association, Dr. Joseph Richardson of the University of Pennsylvania premised that epidemics were spread and propagated "by the transplanting of microscopically visible spores or seeds, which have a separate vitality of their own, and which are to be escaped just as we would escape swarms of insect pests, by shutting them out or killing them off before they can succeed in fastening themselves upon our bodies." Once such spores had fastened on the body the processes of disease were easily explained: "The gradual increment of the symptoms is attributed to the growth of the millions of minute fungoid plants, whose period of greatest luxuriance marks the acme of the attack. . . . Now these spores," Richardson advised, "just like the seeds of larger noxious weeds which when allowed to gain a foothold in our fields and gardens propagate themselves with such rapidity, can only develop if they meet with air, moisture, and congenial soil suited to their peculiar

46. "Pestilence Preventable," New Orleans *Picayune,* August 28, 1878, also "The Origin of Fever," September 6, 1878; "New York Academy of Medicine—Stated Meeting October 17, 1878—The Problem of Yellow Fever," *Medical Record,* XIV (1878), 335–37. See also Keating, *Epidemic of 1878 in Memphis,* 287–326; R. C. Kedzie, "The City of Destruction," *Detroit Lancet,* III (1880), 345–53.

requirements."[47] Franklin Barnard, the president of Columbia College, had interpreted the significance of the germ theory in similar terms in an address before the first general meeting of the American Public Health Association in New York City in 1873. He saw the essential mission of modern public health as consisting in the "severe exclusion" from towns and cities of "noxious gases and offensive effluvia, especially such as arise from decaying organic matter." This was to be secured by a rigid sanitary policing of communities, aimed at achieving pure soil, air, and water, thorough drainage, and strictly enforced cleanliness in all respects. Also vital to a well-founded sanitary program, according to Dr. Barnard, was "the prompt and complete disinfection of every spot where pestilence may lift its head, and of every article and substance which may serve as a vehicle for the disease."[48]

Having persuaded themselves that infective and fermentative germs suspended in the environment were the true cause of yellow fever and other epidemic diseases, scientists next began to examine the idea that an unwholesome environment could be "disinfected" by applying chemicals destructive to those "low forms of life." Many different substances were tested in this connection; gradually carbolic acid (phenol derived from coal tar) emerged as the most promising. The first extensive experiments with this compound were undertaken by the eminent chemist, William Crookes, during the rinderpest outbreak in Britain in 1865–1866. Crookes, not a medical man by training, contemplated the new germ theory and decided that it "certainly includes and explains a far greater number of the phenomena of disease than any other hitherto propounded." In his laboratory he began studying the effects on minute life of various antiseptic and deodorant chemicals, paying particular regard to carbolic acid in view of the apparently favorable results of recent French experiments with it. Crookes exposed crickets, fleas, moths, and other insects to the fumes of carbolic acid and found that it "proved quickly fatal." He added a few drops to water in which minnows were swimming, with the same results. Applying a dilute solution to "animalcules" swarming in smears of putrid blood, sour paste, and decayed cheese, he reported that "in every instance

47. Jos. G. Richardson, "The Germ Theory of Disease, and Its Present Bearing on Public and Private Hygiene," *Medical Record*, XIV (1878), 362–66.

48. F. A. P. Barnard, "The Germ Theory of Disease and Its Relation to Hygiene," *Reports and Papers, American Public Health Association*, I (1873), 70–87.

the destruction of vitality and the arrest of putrefaction have been simultaneous." Carbolic acid also destroyed the vitality of both dry and active yeast, Crookes determined. "In most cases its action is characterized by the certainty and definiteness of a chemical reagent. In the presence of carbolic acid the development of embryotic life is impossible, and before its powerful influence all minute forms of animal life must inevitably perish."

Crookes went on to undertake practical experiments at cattle farms in Yorkshire threatened by the rinderpest. At one establishment a barn was cleaned out and prepared by the burning of sulfur and sprinkling of carbolic acid; all exposed wood surfaces were whitewashed (it was thought the lime in the whitewash would have a supplemental disinfecting action), and fabrics soaked in carbolic acid were hung from the rafters. Two dozen healthy cows were led into the barn and kept there after being brushed down and sprayed with dilute carbolic acid. Although the epizootic was soon making "terrible ravages" all over the neighborhood, these animals escaped the disease—undoubtedly because of strict isolation and sheer good luck and not because of the "disinfecting," but the results were deemed persuasive just the same. Crookes proceeded to perform more tests at farms where the disease had already taken hold. Sick and healthy cows were brought in from the fields and tethered near each other in sheds that had been similarly disinfected. Nearly all the well animals sooner or later developed symptoms of the sickness and most of them died, but Crookes was sure the influence of carbolic acid had retarded the incubation of the disease and reduced its malignancy. It was observed that wool daubed in the slobber and discharges of infected animals would communicate the plague to other beasts, but if it was subsequently steeped in carbolic acid, it lost its infectiousness. The members of the Royal Commission on the Cattle Plague pronounced these results "very encouraging" and said, "it is very desirable that the use of carbolic acid should become general throughout the country."[49]

In the course of the decade many up-to-date doctors began using carbolic acid to dress wounds and as a dip to sterilize their instruments; progressive hospitals were also using it in dilute solution to wash bedding and other contaminated articles. Hopes that the compound could be used on

49. William Crookes, "On the Application of Disinfectants in Arresting the Spread of the Cattle Plague," *Chemical News,* XIII (1866), 242–44, 254–58, 268–72.

an expanded scale in the control of major epidemics were further stimulated by the studies of Dr. Arthur Sansom, who with the famous Lord
Lister had been one of the pioneer advocates of antiseptic surgery. In
mashes of egg and flour, Sansom prepared cultures of assorted fungi and
bacteria, then exposed the growths to the vapors of pure carbolic acid,
which effectively killed them. He believed his evidence "fully shows that
the presence of certain volatile or gaseous antiseptic agents in the air is
sufficient to poison the lowest forms of organisms, to prevent the appearance and development of fungi, and to arrest the putrefaction of organic
material." Sansom repeated that the "subtle poisons of disease" consisted
of "minute particles of living matter" that were "contained in and wafted
by the air. . . . We do not pretend that they are equally numerous with the
harmless germs of living things which the air normally contains, but they
are with them and among them. We show that the presence of antiseptic
agents in the air destroys the harmless germs, and we contend that it is
probable that it destroys the disease germs, which have strong analogical
relations with the former, which certainly do not exceed them in bulk, and
are probably far more minute than those which are obviously destroyed."
Among the various volatile antiseptic agents he had worked with, Sansom
had found carbolic acid to be "the most efficient and the most manageable
of all."[50]

New Orleans had enjoyed a remarkable respite from yellow fever during the Civil War period, with a total of only 11 deaths recorded between
1861 and 1865. The scourge quickly reasserted itself, however, with the revival of commerce and immigration after 1865. The epidemic of 1867 swept
away more than 3,100 lives in the city. It made its second appearance at
Memphis that year, claiming at least 200 lives. New Orleans began to
manifest a particular interest in the theory and practice of air disinfection,
and by 1870 the city's board of health was ready to commit itself to the
systematic use of deodorant and disinfectant chemicals in its renewed
struggle with yellow fever. The board frankly admitted that the work was
experimental and said it would be kept open to the logic of facts, but
expressed its earnest hope that "though the ferment of yellow fever be not

50. A. Ernest Sansom, "On the Disinfection of Air," *British Medical Journal*, October 5,
1872, pp. 375–77.

discovered and isolated, empiricism may find the method of ensuring its destruction." The city was severely visited by yellow fever in 1870, with 587 deaths officially recorded. Municipal sanitary crews, working under the direction of medical doctors, treated 1,470 infected premises over the course of the season, mostly in the Second District, where incidence of the disease was worst. After removal of the sick, the infected apartments were fumigated with "sulphurous acid gas," generated by burning raw sulfur, and "free chlorine gas," evolved by mixing manganese peroxide, sulfuric acid, and common salt in water. Carbolic acid was sprinkled around the yards and distributed along the gutters; copperas (vitriol of ferrous sulfate) and zinc-iron salts were poured into sinks and privies; lime was scattered over adjoining streets.

More than 2,000 gallons of carbolic acid were used during the month of September, but in spite of that liberal and energetic disinfection, yellow fever mortality actually increased in the following month, with 242 deaths, 165 of them in the Second District, where disinfection efforts had been most intensive. It was easy for the proponents of disinfection to defend their stance by claiming that mortality would have been much worse without carbolic acid. And there were bound to the instances—purely coincidental, of course—where the chemical treatment had seemed to be very effective in stamping out the disease, and those could be picked out as striking examples of carbolic acid's potency. On Chartres Street in the Second District, for example, 44 cases of yellow fever had suddenly appeared in a tenement house occupied by 183 Italians and Maltese, mostly recent immigrants and therefore mostly unacclimated. The place was thoroughly disinfected by a city crew and reoccupied, and only two cases subsequently occurred. Taking such reports into consideration—and, perhaps, hoping against hope—the board of health declared that it felt "encouraged to persevere" in the disinfection program.[51]

Yellow fever seems to have gone into another of its brief periods of abeyance the two following years. Only 114 cases and 54 deaths were reported in New Orleans in 1871, and only 83 cases and 39 deaths in 1872. In both years the outbreaks of the disease were concentrated in the Fourth

51. Louisiana Board of Health, *Report for 1870* (New Orleans, 1871), 9–12, 24, 26, 32, 40–43.

District of the city, and were promptly attacked with carbolic acid: "It was freely applied to the filthy streets, unpaved yards, alleys, stagnant gutters and ditches, by which all the streets and many of the houses are surrounded, as well as to manure heaps, collections of refuse, and other nuisances which abound in those neighborhoods. Carbolic acid was chosen for this purpose as the best disinfectant known, as it coagulates all albumen and is certain to destroy all the lower forms of life. It volatizes easily and freely and thus attacks the hidden germs of disease that float in the atmosphere." The "crude carbolic" used on the streets was actually a form of creosote, and it drew complaints of nausea and headache from sensitive residents, but the city persisted in the work. Sprinkling was usually performed in the evening hours to minimize wasteful evaporation. These treatments were "almost completely successful," the sanitary inspector of the Fourth District averred, maintaining that the malady had been "checked in its outward course, and a malignant and widespread epidemic averted." The doctors on the board of health were satisfied at the apparently successful containment, confinement, and destruction of the yellow fever germs. Here again, in those instances where the disease broke out anew after the application of carbolic acid, it could easily be explained that the treatment had not been continued long enough or that some infectious particles had inadvertently been "left beyond the circle of its operation" for lack of understanding of the germ's invisible movements. It was expected that practice and experience would gradually make disinfection more effective.[52] The president of the board offered this tentative explanation of how yellow fever spread and how it could be stopped:

> It is not supposed that the patient himself breeds the poison, but that he suffers from its presence in that locality, or that he may have brought, by baggage or otherwise, those seeds of the disease which, finding a congenial soil and climate, multiply and enlarge the circle of poisonous infection in perhaps every direction. . . .
>
> The peculiar localization of yellow fever as observed in previous years, and its slow and regular march forward in those localities, suggests that if it be the multiplication and spread of either animal or vegetable life, that agents powerfully inimical thereto, although not able to reach

52. Louisiana Board of Health, *Report for 1871* (New Orleans, 1872), 17–20, 25–26, 64–71.

all hidden and enclosed places and thus utterly destroy all germs, might at least destroy those likely to be carried about or wafted on to infect neighboring localities. If the poisonous or poison-causing agent spread along the ground, it seemed not unreasonable to hope that a powerful agent like carbolic acid, freely applied to the streets, would prevent its crossing them, and by its vapor rising into the air as it were wall in the infected places.

The effect of the thinnest possible film of corrosive sublimate in preventing insects from crossing into safes and cupboards is a fact of domestic economy well known. There may be remedies of analogous action towards the cause of yellow fever.[53]

The board of health increasingly pinned its hopes on carbolic acid. In 1872 the compound was used indoors for the first time to disinfect sickrooms. A 2 percent solution of the pure acid in water would be heated in a small copper vaporizer, and with a quarter-inch hose the steam was directed "into every part of the room, upon the walls, ceiling, furniture . . . into every crevice and fold." The sanitary inspector of the Fourth District confidently stated that this procedure "certainly destroyed a large number of disease germs." As a follow-up measure, a pound or two of sulfur would be set alight in a brazier and the room closed up for a few days.[54] Sulfur had a more ancient pedigree than carbolic acid; it had been burned for centuries in the hospitals and lazarettos of Europe and the Levant, with vague ideas of dispersing the "miasma" or "contagium vivum" that was believed to collect where sick people were concentrated. It might have done some real good against yellow fever if it had been more generally applied, for sulfur smoke happens to be a fairly effective insecticide—it became, in fact, the favorite fumigant of twentieth-century yellow fever sanitarians up until the introduction of DDT.

In its annual reports, the board of health also began emphasizing the role of sewage, kitchen garbage, and other varieties of decomposing filth as the essential habitat and pabulum of yellow fever germs. The accumulations in streets and drainageways of "offensive black mud" (actually comprised in large part of human ordure) were indicated as particularly dangerous, but the "most injurious effluvia" were believed to arise from

53. *Ibid.,* 17–18.
54. Louisiana Board of Health, *Report for 1872* (New Orleans, 1873), 95–98.

the gutters, which were said to have "never before been in so bad a condition" and were described as choked along their whole extent by "a slimy mass, green, and offensive to both sight and smell." In 1871, special reports submitted to the city council by certain of the sanitary inspectors recommended a regular program of sprinkling the street ditches with carbolic acid and also advised that large, gated siphons be installed along the levee to copiously flush the gutters with fresh river water as the need arose. That summer the board of health published a circular for the general public, urging householders to pay better attention to the state of their privy vaults and to get in the habit of using disinfectants around their yards.[55]

On August 20, 1873, three tramps died at Shreveport, Louisiana, with symptoms of yellow fever. While local doctors debated over the correct classification of the early cases, the sickness rapidly extended itself over the town. Within a few weeks more than 100 Shreveport people were dead, and the city was firmly in the grip of the worst yellow fever epidemic any inland community had experienced up to that time. A letter to New Orleans explained the distress that welled up when the true character of the plague became evident: "The yellow fever has come and like some awful black pall spread its pestilential folds about us spreading fright, terror, and death amongst us. The town is nearly depopulated by stampede and sickness." The New Orleans *Picayune* observed that perhaps 4,000 people were at risk in Shreveport and 22,000 in Caddo Parish generally, but submitted the "hopeful reminder" that Shreveport's "latitude" (over 300 miles northwest of New Orleans) and the "general purity of its country air" were regarded by medical authorities as "unfavorable to a violent spread of the complaint." The fever nevertheless did spread violently, prostrating most of the white people who remained in the city and taking no fewer than 759 lives before the season was over. "The situation is simply fearful," marveled one correspondent, "Nothing like it has ever been here." By the end of September, outbreaks were being reported in most of the smaller towns of Caddo Parish, and sporadic cases were sparking panics all over this quarter of the state.[56] A correspondent of the *Picayune* found the town of Coushatta, 40 miles below Shreveport, "entirely deserted," its inhabi-

55. Louisiana Board of Health, *Report for 1871*, 32, 118–20, 122–29.

56. U.S. Marine Hospital Service, *Report for 1873*, 110–11; Joseph Jones, "Yellow Fever at Shreveport, La., 1873," *Boston Medical and Surgical Journal*, XC (1874), 73–74; New Orleans *Picayune*, September 12, 16, 27, 1873.

tants having precipitately fled to "out of the way pine-hill places. . . . The greatest excitement prevails throughout the whole Red River Valley—a perfect panic. The country looks desolate, worse than ever it looked during and after Banks's raid through Red River. From Campti to within eight miles of here you cannot find a white family, with very rare exceptions. This is a distance of fifty miles through a very thickly-settled country, where you can see farm houses in sight of each other continually." [57]

There was an unprecedented outbreak in the heart of Texas, on the Brazos River below Waco, evidently carried there by Shreveport refugees. The town of Calvert was evacuated in "a perfect stampede. . . . Hearne has emptied itself. Bryan is following in its wake. Wagons command high rates. Most families are going to the country." Public clamor at Dallas and Corsicana forced the Texas Pacific Railroad to stop running its trains into northwest Louisiana, and a wide section of the region was reduced to wagons alone for overland transport. Spontaneous flight from towns in the face of epidemic disease was certainly nothing new. There had been impromptu stampedes from Louisiana communities during the yellow fever of 1853; Boccaccio described the same thing in plague-stricken Tuscany five hundred years before that. Running away might be regarded as an almost instinctive human reaction to "pestilence that walketh in darkness and wasteth at noonday," and a true instinct needs no special urging. On several occasions early in the century, New York City officials had ordered the depopulation of neighborhoods infected with yellow fever with good results, and LaRoche in 1855 had endorsed the policy as a means of limiting the depredations of the disease. Yet it seems to have been in 1873 that medical and public health authorities first began advocating peremptory evacuation of whole communities as an effective measure against this infection in particular. On September 17, the secretary of the American Public Health Association cabled Louisiana authorities to advise the following: "Removed beyond the first line of plains and hills that skirts Red River in that region, entire security can be had a few miles beyond the river. Flight to a great distance will not give the kind of security that can be obtained at small cost and less than three hours travel. If $5,000 and an effective organization of nurses together with a well-devised plan for moving the unprotected were to be brought into effective service, the panic

57. New Orleans *Picayune*, October 2, 1873.

and pestilence would soon cease."[58] It was too late to extend that kind of relief in this outbreak, but we shall see how the strategy of systematic depopulation was put into operation at Memphis in the epidemic of 1878.

So severe an epidemic occurring so deep in the interior stimulated a certain amount of speculation about its origin, reflecting the transitions still under way in yellow fever theory. The old notions about local causes, miasms, and the spontaneous origin of yellow fever had not been in the tomb so long that they could not be plausibly resurrected. A correspondent of the Cincinnati *Commercial* who had visited Shreveport in June reflected back on "the prevailing filth which impregnated every cubic foot of the atmosphere"—fetid cisterns and reeking mud puddles in backyards; sewage rotting in the street ditches; stinking alleys where putrid garbage and the bodies of dead chickens, cats, and dogs were cast for the town's free-ranging hogs to feed on. (Of course, these were really just the ordinary sanitary delinquencies of the typical southern town of that period.) "Death and disease seemed to rise out of the very ground, or rather from the filth that was on the ground." To aggravate matters, in August a steamer towing a big shipment of Texas cattle had foundered in the river just below town, and the local blacks had fished the drowned beasts out to appropriate the hides, leaving hundreds of skinned carcasses to rot in the hot sun. Taking this array of "fearful stenches" into account, a prominent New Orleans doctor was forced to concede that "if it be possible to generate in this latitude yellow fever by a combination of filth, heat, and moisture, the conditions were certainly present for the origin of the pestilence de novo." Another popular explanation was that the fever was actually an "altered malignant malaria" generated by removal of the so-called Red River Raft, the vast floating braid of snags and driftwood that extended from above Shreveport almost to the Arkansas border. It was theorized

58. *Ibid.*, September 15, 30, 1873. See LaRoche, *Yellow Fever*, II, 747–51; John Duffy, *A History of Public Health in New York City, 1625–1866* (New York, 1968), 109–14. At the height of the great yellow fever epidemic at Buenos Aires in 1871, the local authorities belatedly resolved on a complete evacuation of the city but were unable to make good on the plan in any significant way. Following the universal pattern, most of the city's well-to-do, the *gente acomodada*, had already beat it to safety, leaving the *gente pobre y trabajadora* to contend with the fever's fires as best they could. More than 13,000 lives were lost in that horrific visitation; see Miguel Angel Scenna, *Cuando Murió Buenos Aires: 1871* (Buenos Aires, 1974), 339–42, 350–52, 420–30.

that when the government snag-boats set to work on the raft that spring, sudden exposure to the sun of accumulated muck and rotting vegetation had released a concentrated miasm. This suggestion tended to lose credit when it was pointed out that none of the men actually engaged in the operation had fallen sick unless they had been into infected Shreveport. Ultimately the germ theory and the principle of infectious communicability prevailed: a committee of local doctors decided the disease had probably come to Shreveport from New Orleans via one or another of the river packets.[59]

When yellow fever erupted in Memphis, Tennessee, doctors there were also able to discover an abundance of those "terrene influences" still widely supposed to generate the disease *de novo*. Along in August the inhabitants of Happy Hollow, a particularly nasty little slum underneath the bluff below Front Street, began to complain of "bilious fever" and "dengue" going the rounds among them, and even the city's doctors were slow to recognize the true character of the disease. Yellow fever had been recorded only twice before in Memphis' seventy-five-year history, and had never been too severe or become very prevalent. The Happy Hollow neighborhood consisted of a few acres of batture land that had formerly been used as a dump for the city's rubbish and offal carts. The rains had gradually spread and settled the refuse and mixed it with mud until a little stratum was formed, and this adventitious bit of ground, not covered by titles and not subject to rent or taxes, had been taken over by a collection of Irish and other poor whites, who lived there at the sufferance of city politicians. Dwellings of the cheapest order, patched together with all combinations of cast-off lumber and sheet metal, clung to the sides of the cove or perched on stilts over the landfill. Outfall from the gutters of Commerce and Exchange streets trickled down the bluff and kept the hollow perpetually sodden, with a "soft muddy appearance, the general effect of which is heightened by small sewers and pools of stagnant water covered with a green scum that looks very suggestive of death in every form," as one reporter expressed it. The Memphis *Avalanche* speculated that "the sun heating up the matter during the day and then cooling off at night causes a vapor to arise which necessarily is impregnated with all the poi-

59. New Orleans *Picayune*, October 1, 15, 1873; Jones, "Yellow Fever at Shreveport," 151–54. On the Red River Raft, see A. K. Lobeck, *Geomorphology: An Introduction to the Study of Landscapes* (New York, 1939), 428.

sonous qualities of the ground, and this being inhaled constantly must breed disease of a malarious nature." Lending further distinction to the local atmosphere were the stagnant waste ponds of nearby oil presses, "which are in themselves sufficient to kill any person who unfortunately comes in contact with them." "During the hot summer months this accumulated mass of filth had been festering and rotting in the sun," the president of the Memphis Board of Health would tell the American Public Health Association in New York City that fall, "exhaling mephitic gases which in themselves are potent enough to induce infection, only needing the germ of yellow fever to be sworn to yield all the fearful fruits of an epidemic. Such was its origin and such the locus from which it started."[60]

The Memphis Board of Health finally took cognizance of the bad situation that had developed in this neglected nook of the city and announced the presence of yellow fever on September 13, by which time at least thirty people had died. City workers immediately dug pits at the intersections of Happy Hollow lanes and set coal-oil fires burning in them around-the-clock in a crash effort to disengage the miasm and purify the air. Contemplating the clouds of tarry smoke one evening from the bluff at the foot of Main Street, one reporter was involuntarily reminded of "that other valley, the one of Death." Yellow fever nevertheless ascended the bluff, and by the first week of October was prevailing in a thirty-block area from Poplar Avenue to Bayou Gayoso. This was a lower-class tenement section, "inhabited mostly by our Irish and German population, many of the latter Hebrews," and from a sanitary standpoint was considered not too much better than Happy Hollow. At New Orleans and other cities prone to yellow fever, it had long been observed that the worst fever nests tended to be the neighborhoods of the "poor, filthy, and intemperate." This reflected a common medico-moral prejudice of the time, but in the case of yellow fever it also described a real convergence of epidemiological factors. The poor and dirty tended to be immigrants or country people, and therefore nonimmunes, and being without money they tended to crowd into the low-rent, waterfront districts, which were frequently exposed to infection from boats. The initial conjectures about the spontaneous generation of

60. Memphis *Avalanche,* September 15, 1873; John H. Erskine, "A Report on the Yellow Fever as It Appeared at Memphis, Tenn., in 1873," *Reports and Papers, American Public Health Association,* I (1873), 386; Y. R. Lemonnier, "Epidemic of Memphis, Tennessee, in 1873," *New Orleans Medical and Surgical Journal,* n.s. I (1873), 449–56, 673–78.

yellow fever in Memphis were revised later that year when official inquests revealed that back in early August, a New Orleans towboat had dropped off, at a Happy Hollow shack, a crewman dying with a "malignant malarial fever" whose symptoms, considered in retrospect, sounded suspiciously like those of yellow fever.[61] Steadily the germ theory and the concept of infection were penetrating the professional perception of yellow fever. In an 1874 article discussing this epidemic, one physician clearly expressed the transition in thinking:

> Yellow fever is peculiarly a disease of cities, where large numbers of people are crowded together and effete animal matters are allowed to pollute the atmosphere; but it is not proved that filth, garbage, or noxious gases from rotting animal or vegetable matter can any more produce yellow fever than they can smallpox; though it is almost certain that they do so vitiate the atmosphere as to render it a proper nidus for the reception and proliferation of the essential epidemic germ, be it what it may; whether of fungoid growths, or germinal masses derived from normal cells, or analogous to yeast or other ferment, which by virtue of catalytic action is capable of producing deleterious changes in the constituents of the body.
>
> Assuming that all the destructive changes which the blood undergoes in yellow fever are due to the contact of certain infinitesimal particles, it may be readily conceived that after entering the organism and affecting the vital constituents, they may reproduce themselves and from their extreme minuteness permeate the tissues, and escape from it by the skin, the breath, and the excretions. When without the body they may continue to multiply themselves indefinitely if the atmosphere be in a favorable condition; and floating about in the air impregnate water and food and attach themselves to clothing, bedding, or other material, and so admit of transportation, gaining access to the bodies of persons suitable for their reception.[62]

By the time frost came, in November, yellow fever had taken no fewer than 1,255 lives in Memphis. This was an unprecedented toll for an inland

61. Memphis *Avalanche,* September 14, 17, 1873; Erskine, "Yellow Fever at Memphis," 385–92; U.S. Marine Hospital Service, *Report for 1873,* 104–105; R. W. Mitchell, "Yellow Fever in Memphis in 1873," *Richmond and Louisville Medical Journal,* XVII (1874), 533–37.

62. C. Happoldt, "Remarks on the Yellow Fever Epidemic of Memphis, Tenn., in 1873," *Richmond and Louisville Medical Journal,* XVIII (1874), 134.

city, but the disease had pretty much confined itself to the district south of the bayou and north of Poplar, and never raged generally over the city. An unknown number of citizens—thousands, certainly, but no exact count was ever made—had fled the city when the appearance of Yellow Jack was announced in September, but these tended to be the relative few who could afford to leave their jobs or businesses for a season, and the evacuation was not nearly so clamorous and complete as the stampede that would take place in 1878. In October the *Avalanche* could cheerfully claim that the billiard and lager parlors still had their Saturday-night patronage substantially intact, and the churches their Sunday-morning congregations. The intensity of public reaction to yellow fever tended to be in direct proportion to the recency and severity of the last epidemic, and in 1873 the disease was still an unfamiliar visitor in Memphis. On October 5, however, the paper commented that "the question of tenting out on the public commons three or four miles from the city, where the air is fresh and unvitiated by noxious vapors or malarial poisons, is one that might well engage the attention of those whose circumstances are such that they cannot go any distance from this fever-scourged city." It recalled that in 1855 the inhabitants of several fever-stricken towns in Mississippi went out to the hills for a month or two and escaped the disease, while those who stayed in the infected towns "suffered immensely." It also noted the recent history of a battalion in the West Indies that was troubled by yellow fever: "The force was removed from their regular barracks to a tented field two or three miles off and the fever disappeared. Their barracks were then carefully fumigated and whitewashed, and upon the troops reoccupying them, the disease broke out violently. The soldiers took to their tents a second time, and the fever no longer annoyed them." The paper noted that several Memphis families were already camped out at the far end of the Poplar Avenue extension, "experiencing all the romantic delights of the nomadic habits of the Modocs, and the fashionable ways of the tenting Arabs," and suggested that others might go and do likewise, "in the woods a few miles off, where weather-proof tents could be improvised from blankets, canvas, brush, and a few posts, and so render themselves comfortable for a short time." Here, in a miniature, was a preview of the dramatic experiment in mass depopulation that would be undertaken in 1878. This idea was also catching on generally, and in 1874 a prominent New Orleans doctor was led to advise: "So far, we know of but one positive prophylactic means, which is to flee from the disease if you can. This is the only means of protecting one's self from yellow fever. No known agent will do this."[63]

The season at New Orleans, meanwhile, appeared to clinch the case in favor of disinfection. In terms of mortality it had been a relatively mild season, with only 226 deaths registered from yellow fever, even though the disease had appeared early and broken out virulently in all districts of the city, and daily temperature and barometric readings had matched those recorded at Shreveport and Memphis. The authorities could only conclude that the favorable difference in mortality was due to the other places' "neglect of sanitary measures" and to New Orleans' "full use of disinfectants," especially its "timely and free use of carbolic acid." One hundred entire city squares had been thoroughly disinfected during August, September, and October, requiring more than 7,000 gallons of carbolic acid besides large quantities of other chemicals. It so happened that new cases of yellow fever were reported on only 21 of those squares after treatment, and the members of the board of health waxed enthusiastic. Success had been most convincing in the Sixth District, where 27 separate outbreaks had been reported over the course of the season, and all had been immediately and energetically attacked with carbolic acid. In only two instances had yellow fever reappeared after disinfection of premises, and the disease was ostensibly stamped out by the end of September. "We can hardly suppose the sudden decadence of the disease was spontaneous," said the sanitary inspector of the Sixth District, "for the squares surrounding the above designated ones were as populous as those infected, and the residents as amenable to the disease as those on the opposite sides of the street. . . . An isolated instance does not substantiate a position, but a series of results, all analogous, must be admitted as good evidence."

The infection had been more stubborn in the Third District. Finally, in October, the sanitary inspector decided that "concealed, latent, retained, and infectious germs" must have found a "hiding place" in the trash and offal that had accumulated immemorially under the wharves along the river. He had a crew scrape out the filth and sprinkle the batture thoroughly with carbolic acid, and was "happily rewarded by finding a total cessation of the malady." Although confessedly "yet in the dark as to its etiology or causa causans," the sanitary inspector of the Second District

---

63. Memphis *Avalanche,* October 5, 1873; Lemmonier, "Epidemic of Memphis," 670.

reflected: "The results are or seem to be that this disease has been limited, restrained, lessened, or modified, if not eradicated." Perhaps, he thought, the "indefinite secret agency," or "peculiar something" that caused yellow fever, whether germ or poison, was "more or less controllable" after all. The sanitary inspector of the First District effused: "I cannot too strongly express the gratification I feel that chemical science has finally furnished us with an infallible process of neutralizing all noxious and malarial infections." In a communication to the surgeon general of the U.S. Marine Hospital Service in November, the supervisor of the Marine Hospital at New Orleans gave it as his opinion that, thanks to sanitary vigilance and the use of carbolic acid: "Yellow fever in this city has been greatly modified, if not completely disarmed of its subtile and terrifying power." Carbolic acid was employed for the first time at Mobile, Alabama, this year, and there too had won converts in high places. The president of the Mobile Board of Health affirmed that disinfection had effectively "hedged in the disease, and no epidemic resulted," and thought the success "too apparent to permit a doubt to remain in the mind of any honest individual."[64]

New Orleans was not much afflicted by yellow fever in the years immediately following 1873, and prima facie evidence in favor of carbolic acid continued to accumulate. Only eleven deaths from yellow fever were reported in 1874; sixty-one in 1875; forty-two in 1876. It surely seemed as though the fever's major inroads were being hampered by the chemical, and further instances could be cited where carbolic acid had appeared to completely arrest local outbreaks of the disease. "This may be called coincidence," the sanitary inspector of the Second District observed, "but if so it is singularly continuous." The sanitary inspector of the Third District thought the experience of these later years, added to that already cited in former reports, "must tend to remove all doubt" of disinfection's basic utility, "leaving only for study the improvements to be made." The sanitary inspectors were aware of the practical problem they faced in trying to intercept the movements of a germ that could not be seen, and whose behavior could only be traced through its effects. Since 1870 the board of health had been keeping careful records of the location and sequence of all yellow fever reports in the city. By 1874 the board believed it had enough

---

64. Louisiana Board of Health, *Report for 1873* (New Orleans, 1874), 46–57, 66–75, 158, 161–62, 172–76, 181–82, 189–91, 200–201; U.S. Marine Hospital Service, *Report for 1873*, 103, 108.

data to offer a working guideline for disinfecting crews: "The infection extends along the ground at the rate of forty or fifty feet daily." Doctors had begun to think that yellow fever was only secondarily an atmospheric infection, observing that the germ seemed to have a peculiar affinity for surfaces of all kinds—walls, for instance, which explained why the disease was so difficult to dislodge from houses—and preferred to propagate along the ground, which explained why the outward spread of yellow fever was so little affected by prevailing winds. The importance of thoroughly disinfecting streets and lanes came to be emphasized. In 1875 tank wagons fitted with booms and extension hoses were introduced for sprinkling streets and sidewalks; previously this work had been done with watering cans.[65]

There was still, however, more than a little practical and theoretical opposition to carbolic acid disinfection. In September, 1875, ten concerned physicians of the city held a symposium at the Medical Building of the University of Louisiana, the tenor of all their reports being unfavorable to the continued use of carbolic acid. One doctor stressed that air disinfection was essentially misconceived because any vapor was subject to immediate dilution and dissipation in the atmosphere. He asked, "Can carbolic acid be made to permeate our atmosphere in such a degree as to seize on disease germs and destroy them? Surely not outside the room, or at farthest the house, in which a man has been sick with the disease. . . . I can saturate a bowl of water with salt, but you cannot furnish me salt enough to saturate Lake Pontchartrain." Another maintained that the antiseptic action of carbolic acid was transitory, if not completely illusory, that it did not really destroy the infectious element but only suspended it, and he cited findings recently published in the *Lancet* that showed that the "vital principle" of smallpox vaccine was not at all impaired or diminished by exposure to carbolic acid vapor. He went on to speculate that a caustic chemical might indeed have the effect of hardening the germs—of "tanning" or "mummifying" them—and so actually serve to preserve infection in the city from year to year.

Some of the other doctors pointed to research showing that prolonged exposure of laboratory animals to the fumes of carbolic acid caused

---

65. Louisiana Board of Health, *Report for 1874* (New Orleans, 1875), 23–24, 108–11; Louisiana Board of Health, *Report for 1875* (New Orleans, 1876), 33–35, 108–13, 127–33.

intoxication and poisoning, and sometimes permanent injury to skin, lungs, and kidneys. They worried about the possibly pernicious side effects of the chemical on the city's people. The residents of streets where disinfection was applied had been complaining for some time that the naphtha vapors of the "crude carbolic" made them ill, and reports from the board of health during these years admitted that disinfecting crews had been meeting with considerable protest in some neighborhoods, and in a few instances had even been driven off by the "violent opposition" of the people. Other participants in the discussion pointed out that many sporadic cases of yellow fever had undoubtedly gone unreported or were misdiagnosed, and the localities were therefore never disinfected: why had no larger outbreaks developed from those focuses? Critics insisted that the disease's behavior had not been essentially modified by disinfection, and noted that there had been other times when yellow fever had mysteriously ebbed away from New Orleans for a number of years. They suggested the city was enjoying its present intermission because the sweeping epidemic of 1867 had probably acclimated most of the established residents, while fresh immigration to the city had diminished because of the general business recession. (This was forty-two years before H. R. Carter explained the phenomenon of "spontaneous disappearance of yellow fever by failure of the human host." An obligate virus circulating in a stable population would simply die out as the percentage of immunes rose to a level where effective transmission was improbable.)[66]

In the fall of 1875, one of the sanitary inspectors educated the New Orleans Chamber of Commerce on the question of carbolic acid disinfection. In confident language he reviewed its apparent successes, and asked rhetorically: "Is not the evidence of beneficial results sufficient to warrant continuation of the system? And may we not claim that the spread of yellow fever may be controlled? May we not hope to be able, ere long, to announce to the world that a general epidemic of yellow fever will never occur here again?" The mercantile interests of the city were naturally predisposed to the idea of disinfection, for the practical advantages of a quick sprinkling and fumigation of inbound ships and cargoes were obvious,

66. "Minutes, Meeting of Physicians to Discuss Carbolic Acid," *New Orleans Medical and Surgical Journal,* n.s., III (1875), 414–40. See also H. R. Carter, "The Mechanism of the Spontaneous Elimination of Yellow Fever from Endemic Centres," *Annals of Tropical Medicine and Parasitology,* XIII (1920), 299–311.

compared to the vexatious ten-day layover at the quarantine station then required by law. Also, any new development that could improve on New Orleans' image as a hapless pesthole would be good for business in general, and for real estate values in particular. The chamber resolved that the scheme of carbolic acid disinfection, "practiced with so much apparent success since 1870, should be continued and encouraged by the state and city authorities."[67]

It so happened that only one case of yellow fever was identified in New Orleans in 1877—a passenger off a steamer from Havana, who died just a day after landing in the city. The square where he died was immediately surrounded by a sanitary crew and treated with carbolic acid in the established way. The month was October, the weather was cool, and no other cases appeared. Officials were cheered by the headway they seemed to be making against the old incubus, Yellow Jack. In his report for 1877, the president of the board of health declared that, with the aid of carbolic acid, "we may reasonably hope to keep mastery over the pestilence which has made our city a dread to its inhabitants and an abhorrence to strangers, at incalculable cost to our commercial prosperity."[68] Such, then, was the confidence of the medical authorities, and such was their armamentarium, as they approached the year 1878 and their climactic showdown with the King of Terrors.

67. Louisiana Board of Health, *Report for 1875*, 15–23.
68. Louisiana Board of Health, *Report for 1877* (New Orleans, 1878), 13–15.

THREE

The Epidemic at New Orleans

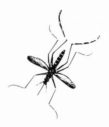

The great yellow fever epidemic of 1878 first manifested itself in the shipping at New Orleans, but the exact circumstances of the introduction are impossible to pin down. The three-way connection between a transient population, an invisible virus, and a particular species of mosquito is tenuous and complex under any circumstances, and it is all the more difficult to identify and trace through records from a period in which the true nature of the disease and its transmission was not yet suspected. At the time, opinion at large squarely blamed the *Emily Souder*, an oceangoing steamer that shuttled regularly between Cuba and New Orleans. This charge was advanced in the city newspapers as early as July, and the board of health, reviewing what evidence it had marshalled by year's end, concurred. Three days out of Havana, by way of Key West, on May 21 the *Souder* had cleared quarantine below New Orleans, having declared no sickness on board and having had the hold fumigated and the crew examined. The ship was passed on to the city with a clean bill of health. The quarantine physician later admitted that the *Souder*'s purser had complained to him of "neuralgia headache," and he had detected a slight fever in the man, but those vague symptoms were explained away at the time as mere hangover resulting from a spree two nights before at Key West.

On the morning of the twenty-third, the purser got off the boat feeling unaccountably feverish and restless and took a room at a boardinghouse on Claiborne Street in the First District. After suffering for two days with intolerable head and back pains and high fever, he died, in violent convulsions and delirium, very early on the twenty-fifth. The case was registered as one of "bilious fever" and the body was removed and buried later the same morning. That afternoon, the *Souder*'s engineer took to bed with the same complaint at his room at Front and Girod Streets. He died on the evening of the twenty-ninth. The symptoms worried the attending physician, and he forwarded the body to the city morgue and alerted health authorities. An autopsy was performed. Officials were alarmed to see that the skin had turned a "bright canary color," and upon opening the cadaver, they found the liver and kidneys discolored and congested, with the pathognomonic appearance of "fatty degeneration." When the two deaths from the *Souder* were considered together, a quiet order was issued that the yards, sidewalks, gutters, and privies around the victims' lodgings be sprinkled with carbolic acid. In retrospect, it was concluded that at this point, yellow fever had gained its foothold in the city.[1]

The official report of the Mississippi River Quarantine Station for 1878, however, clearly shows that Yellow Jack had been persistently knocking at Louisiana's door all season long. During February, March, and April, four steamships, all bringing cargoes of coffee from Rio de Janeiro, touched quarantine and reported single deaths from yellow fever en route to New Orleans. Another bark arriving in April from the same port reported three deaths on the voyage north. Those ships were duly fumigated and disinfected; their crews and passengers were given a cursory examination and pronounced healthy, and were admitted to the port of New Orleans without any period of detention. On May 21—the same day the *Souder* came in—another ship from Havana arrived and disclosed five cases of yellow fever on board. The vessel was detained eleven days, the sick were placed in the station hospital, sulfur was burned in the ship's hold, and pure carbolic acid was poured into the bilge. The ship was allowed to go on to the city on June 1. During the month of July, a bark from Havana and a schooner from Matanzas came in, and each reported two yellow fever cases on board; another coffee ship from Rio arrived and reported one death en route. All told, from the last week of May to the middle of July, customs officials at New Orleans recorded the arrival of eighteen vessels from Havana and another fifteen from Matanzas, Vera-

1. Louisiana Board of Health, *Report for 1878* (New Orleans, 1879), 1–4, 8–10; E. S. Drew, "The First Case of Yellow Fever in New Orleans, 1878, by the Physician Who Attended It," *Sanitarian*, VIII (1880), 35–36.

cruz, Tuxpan, Progreso, Kingston, Rio, and other infected or potentially infected ports. There is a strong probability that among these ships there were several, perhaps many, unrecognized sources of infection.[2]

In the first week of July, illness of a pronounced or suspicious nature began coming to light in the First District of the city, on certain blocks off Claiborne Street south of Canal and also around the foot of Girod Street. These reports were all within one-quarter mile of the houses where the sick men landed by the *Emily Souder* had lodged in May, and the board of health considered the "line of infection" from the presumed infecting cases to these subsequent outbreaks to be "tolerably clear" though admittedly "long latent." More puzzling was a simultaneous eruption of cases on the other side of the district, on Constance near its intersection with Terpsichore, which was almost a mile from the nearest recognized focus of infection on Girod. This gave the fomites theory an opportunity to demonstrate its ruggedness. Officials eventually decided that the infection had been carried into that locality in the clothing of a tugboat engineer whose vessel had taken the *Emily Souder*'s slip at the Calliope Street wharf on June 1, a few hours after the *Souder* departed for Cuba. The boatman himself did not develop the disease until later in July, but his mother-in-law was stricken with it at the end of June, along with some neighbor children who had played under the clothesline where the laundry was hung to dry. About the middle of July, a number of cases turned up in the Fourth District along St. Patrick and St. Phillip streets, all seemingly traceable to direct personal exposure to the Constance Street focus. One of the first victims in this neighborhood was a laborer who had walked along Constance to and from his job each day; two others were bakery employees who had been delivering bread in the area. Those reports were soon followed by cases at various spots below Washington Street, where the source of infection could not be clearly determined. The official report reconciled the facts this way:

2. Louisiana Board of Health, *Report for 1878*, 19–24; S. M. Bemiss, "Report upon Yellow Fever in Louisiana in 1878, and Subsequently," *New Orleans Medical and Surgical Journal*, n.s., XI (1883), 82–86. By June yellow fever was prevalent in both Havana and Key West; see "Abstract of Sanitary Reports, July 13, 1878," in *Bulletins of the Public Health Issued by the Supervising Surgeon-General, Marine Hospital Service* (Washington, D.C., 1881), 7; R. J. Perry, "Yellow Fever at Key West, Florida, 1878," in U.S. Navy, Bureau of Medicine and Surgery, *Hygienic and Medical Reports, 1879*, 729–36.

It must be granted that we should naturally expect to find intervening cases in both space and time, but we are here confronted with no greater mysteries than we find in other infectious diseases. . . . Grant that a certain number of the germs were reproduced, either inside or outside the human body; that they multiply in rapid geometrical ratio by repeated generations at short intervals; that a new generation brought to life in hot weather is not only vastly more numerous, but more energetic individually than its predecessors; that these germs are capable both of spontaneous locomotion along the ground and other surfaces, and of transportation in the clothing of persons. Grant these conditions, which are quite in harmony with the known behavior of animalcular beings, and the difficulty of missing links in the chain of evidence is reduced to mere cavilling.[3]

By the last week of July, yellow fever cases in New Orleans had swiftly and undeniably begun to multiply. On the twenty-fourth, the *Picayune* was obliged to follow up on the prevailing rumors and announced the presence of Yellow Jack in the city, tallying fourteen cases and seven deaths up to that date. It was careful to blend in the comforting intelligence that all cases so far had involved only "strangers" and were thought to be "sporadic in nature and in no wise threatening the general health." The paper pledged itself to a whole-truth policy concerning the situation and urged the city government to do the same as the only way to quelch "exaggerated and injurious reports" about the bad state of the city's health. The matter was finally broached in the newspapers, and the board of health began discussing the menace publicly and advising on preventive measures. The board believed all cases so far were traceable to the infection brought in by the *Emily Souder* in May, but also took the occasion to reprimand the city's produce dealers, who were widely suspected of flouting the quarantine law by falsely declaring the origin of fruit from infected ports. It counseled the people to avoid night air as a general rule and to stay away from infected areas at all times, and resolved to distribute a flier describing the fever's premonitory symptoms and outlining the approved therapy. It directed the police to keep street vendors, organ-grinders, and others like them out of infected neighborhoods. The board also announced its inten-

3. Louisiana Board of Health, *Report for 1878*, 4–8, 81–82; see also Bemiss, "Yellow Fever in Louisiana," 86–88.

tion to order the administrator of improvements to begin flushing the gutters with fresh river water.[4]

For some weeks the fumes from carbolic acid spot treatments could be whiffed in the infected localities, and one of the board's first recommendations was an enlarged scheme of outdoor disinfection, such as had served the city so well in outbreaks earlier in the decade. Householders were urged to obtain carbolic acid from retail sources and to begin treating their yards and privies with the compound, and city authorities were directed to embark on an expanded program of "carbolizing" the streets. In his official report for 1878, the president of the board of health reiterated the theory on which the scheme of carbolic acid disinfection was founded—a theory, it bears emphasizing, that tended to regard the locality rather than the sick person as the infectious element:

> It is based upon the hypothesis that the materies morbi of yellow fever consists of living germs, probably animalcular. The object is to attack these germs, wherever existing, by some agents destructive to low forms of life, without being injurious to their habitat. . . . With regard to outdoor localities, it is supposed that the yellow fever infection progresses from an established focus by a spontaneous movement. From repeated observations of the sick with yellow fever conveyed from an infected locality to a healthy one, without communicating the disease to those around them, it is reasonable to conclude that these germs do not multiply by reproduction within the human body. The supposition is therefore ventured that the germs of yellow fever are wingless animalcula.

Accordingly, once a "focus of infection" had been identified by the sanitary inspectors, the plan of attack was first to calculate "the probable extent of progress of the infection since its inception" (the rule of thumb was about forty feet a day) then, for blocks around if need be, to begin wetting down streets, sidewalks, and gutters with a 5- to 10-percent solution of carbolic acid in water. After this cordon sanitaire had been blocked out, the work was carried inward to the infected residence, treating streets and alleys as before and also entering private yards to sprinkle by hand. The solution was doubled in strength closer to focus of infection, and fortified with copperas when poured into privies. By July 27, the city had

4. New Orleans *Picayune,* July 24, 26, 1878.

a dozen tank wagons and crews engaged in this operation, and the sanitary inspector of the First District was said to have had his hands full supervising the work. It was believed the disease had been checked at all points on Constance Street, and although a new focus of infection had cropped up on Camp Street a few blocks back from the river, the president of the board of health was said to be "not at all alarmed" about any prospect of an epidemic developing. By the close of that day, a total of thirty-six cases with eighteen deaths had been reported in the city.[5]

Underlying the city authorities' reluctance to proclaim the appearance of yellow fever was the dread of quarantine by neighboring towns and cities, a blockade that indeed fell hard and heavy as soon as the truth of the situation leaked out. Shreveport and Pensacola declared rigid nonintercourse quarantines against New Orleans on July 26, commanding a peremptory and complete embargo of all persons, freights, and mails. They were followed by Galveston on July 29 and Mobile on July 30, those important centers strictly blocking out all contact with the Crescent City by land and sea. The two latter proclamations were especially galling to the interests of New Orleans—Galveston because it was the gateway to a large and lucrative trade with the Texas interior and Mobile because it sat athwart the New Orleans, Mobile & Ohio Railroad, one of only two overland trade routes (and, in this crisis, escape routes) to the north and east. Traffic on the line was shut down at Biloxi, Mississippi, just 80 miles east of New Orleans. The New Orleans Board of Health tried strenuously to persuade Mobile authorities to at least reopen through traffic on the railroad, pointing out that the part of Mobile the tracks ran through was an unpopulated section occupied mostly by warehouses and cotton presses, that the coaches were certain to be ventilated of any contagion after the 140-mile ride from New Orleans, and that kerchiefs dipped in dilute carbolic acid and inserted in the baggage would be more than adequate to destroy any concealed germs. The assurances of the New Orleans doctors were in vain, however, as were the railroad company's threats to sue for damages, and the city of Mobile maintained rigid quarantine until November and the first confirmed frosts. "There is nothing that deprives men of the natural use of their reasoning powers so quickly and entirely as fear," the *Picayune* expostulated. The estimated 20,000 to 30,000 refugees who

---

5. *Ibid.*, July 27, 28, 1878; Louisiana Board of Health, *Report for 1878*, 10–11.

had begun hustling out of New Orleans still had the Chicago, St. Louis & New Orleans Railroad open to them, as Jackson, Mississippi, in spite of its highly exposed position, continued to demur on the question of rigid quarantine.[6]

On July 31, the editor of the *Picayune*'s financial page expressed the metropolitan hope that "the cloud which has appeared above our city will pass away before the dreadful consequences to business apprehended." Many leaders feared that smaller towns of the hinterland would follow suit and join in a general "fever embargo" against New Orleans, an apprehension that largely came to pass during the first week of August. "Nominal" quarantines, which theoretically barred deliveries of goods and passengers but admitted through traffic, were soon in effect in all the parishes along the Lafourche and Teche bayous to the west of the city, including the important shipping points of Thibodaux, Houma, and Morgan City. The policy was also in force in the parishes along the lower Red River, up as far as Natchitoches where "rigid" quarantine, which shut out downriver contact totally, had been declared. The *Picayune*'s maritime column began carrying advisories on the closure of inland channels to steamboat traffic. On August 15, for example, pilots were warned that farmers and villagers along the bends of the Yazoo were armed, on full alert, and "perfectly wild" with dread of the fever, and that New Orleans packets attempting to put in even at remote woodyards had been precipitately driven off. As to navigation on the Red, it was simply reported: "No use to try to send boats above the mouth of Cane River."

Even people in the valley of the Ohio were restless, having been sen-

---

6. New Orleans *Picayune*, July 30, 31, 1878. Mobile became afflicted with the infection anyway; some yellow fever cases were rumored to be there as early as the last week of July, and the first confirmed case appeared on August 11; see T. S. Scales, "Municipal Sanitation as Practiced in Mobile for Preventing the Spread of Yellow Fever," *Reports and Papers, American Public Health Association*, VI (1880), 180–84. Galveston and Natchez appear to have been luckier; see "Quarantine at Galveston" and "The Quarantine at Natchez," unnumbered addenda to "Report of the Yellow Fever Commission on the Epidemic of 1878," in Record Group 90, National Archives. The "Report of the Yellow Fever Commission" consists of a collection of manuscript reports and letters, some numbered some not, forwarded to the National Board of Health by Dr. Jerome Cochran around 1880. The report was never completed and never published. See Charles Zaid, comp., "Preliminary Inventory of the Records of the National Board of Health (Record Group 90)," Preliminary Inventory 141, National Archives and Records Service, General Services Administration (1962), 11–12.

sitized to the danger of Yellow Jack by the first-ever occurrence of some cases at Cairo in 1873. One New Orleans packet, caught in the uproar while making its way up the Ohio River, relayed back its experiences along the Illinois shore: "At Mound City the citizens of that burg had the fire alarm bells rung and would not permit us to land. We next passed Shawneetown, where a skiff came out from the shore and informed us that the entire population of the place was on the river front and to land was out of the question. In fact an organized militia was on hand to dispute our landing at all hazards. This will give you an idea of how the yellow fever scare has traveled up the river." The pilot was dismayed at the reception and in all good faith could declare that he had "not a case of yellow fever on board," though he admitted a woman passenger from New Orleans had died of "bilious fever" on the way up and had to be buried in the riverbank below Paducah. By the middle of August, activity at the docks in New Orleans had fallen from "not very animated" to "scarcely worth noting," and local businessmen knew that the situation held but scant prospect for revival.[7]

On July 25, under the caption "Let the Authorities Look to It," the *Picayune* editorialized on "the effluvia arising from the gutters and the foecal deposits in streets and alleys. . . . Scarcely a square in any part of the city can be walked that the nostrils are relieved of the noxious odors." This was a standard summertime complaint in the city, no doubt gaining a measure of urgency after the most dreaded of "filth" diseases had asserted itself. The four hundred miles of open gutters and street ditches that gridded the city of New Orleans had been excavated casually over the years without reference to an established grade (indeed, a complete topographic survey of the city would not be available until 1893). Extensive pooling and stagnation of runoff was the consequence. Compounding the basic drainage problem was the fact that the public streets and way places were everywhere being used as a meet receptacle for the grossest kind of private filth and waste. It was not until 1876 that the New Orleans Board of Health managed to secure an ordinance forcing hotels and other downtown institutions to pipe away the discharge from their sinks and toilets, curtailing at last their oldtime privilege of running their slop and sewage directly into the street ditches in front of their establishments. The mandated pipes were just being laid in the spring of 1878.

7. New Orleans *Picayune*, August 1, 6, 8–10, 15, 16, 1878.

The law had always compelled private householders to dig backyard vaults and hire the services of night scavengers, *vidangeurs,* but the promptness and efficiency of rotational cleaning left much to be desired, and in an 1872 report the city chemist estimated that fully one-quarter of the town's kitchen, laundry, and chamber slop was eluding the attention of the excavators and finding its way into the gutters. It was only in 1870 that the city began requiring that newly constructed privy vaults be lined with brick or cement. The thousands of old-style vaults that still stored the vast proportion of the city's excrement had originally been installed as wooden boxes, but those had quickly rotted out, leaving only holes in the ground. In periods of wet weather and rising water tables, the contents of these sinks would well up uncontrollably and spill out, and there was nothing to do with the semiliquid ordure but sweep it into the convenient street ditches, ordinances to the contrary notwithstanding. Yard sweepings, stable manure, and other sediments added to the burden that accumulated year to year, until drains that could barely carry away normal surface runoff when clear became clogged and blocked in many places with drifts of malodorous sludge. When local outcry demanded it, the custom of the municipal street contractors was to rake and shovel up the worst accumulations of this mud and cast it out into the middle of the streets in piles, to be carted away eventually or simply left to be washed back into the gutters by the next rains.[8]

On July 26, the board of health ordered an immediate stop to such slovenly practices and initiated, as the other main thrust of its antifever campaign, a program to flush and purge the city's cloacal streets with fresh water from the Mississippi. The river had already receded so low that it could not reach the gravity sluices that had been installed along the levee for this purpose some years before, and the necessary water could only be had via the feeble pumps of an underdeveloped municipal waterworks. Street hydrants were turned on, starting along the levee front and around the public markets, and street contractors were ordered by the administrator of improvements to detail extra crews to work the gutters with brooms as the water ran down them. As it developed, the city mains were capable of delivering only some nine million gallons a day—not nearly enough to

8. *Ibid.,* July 25, 1878; Louisiana Board of Health, *Report for 1872* (New Orleans, 1873), 108; George E. Waring, *Report on the Social Statistics of Cities* (2 vols.; Washington, D.C., 1887), II, 276; "New Orleans Drainage and Sewerage," *Sanitarian,* XLIII (1899), 299–314.

do the work expeditiously on the scale contemplated. To attain even that volume the pumps were running at full capacity night and day, and the director of the Water Works Company expressed concern that the machinery would break down under the strain. On August 2, the city's fire engines were ordered to the upper ends of some of the streets in the Second District and pumped water straight from the river, directing it down the gutters. By August 8, it was obvious that all appliances so far deployed in the flushing project were totally inadequate. Local jobbers were engaged to move in a few of the big stationary drain pumps from the nearby rice fields to assist in the Augean task of "cleansing and irrigating the city." The administrator of improvements was given special permission by the mayor to divert money for this purpose from any city fund that showed a current surplus. A contractor had one of the monster machines in service at the head of Josephine Street two weeks later, throwing a fine volume of water, but it appeared that the apparatus was too heavy to be moved from one position to another efficiently.[9]

By the end of July, a total of 135 cases of yellow fever had been reported in the city, with 39 deaths. Day-to-day fluctuations in the fever's early progress were still being followed optimistically by the board of health and so reported by the *Picayune*. Eleven new cases and 5 deaths on July 30 were followed by 21 new cases but only one death a day later, and this was "encouraging" because "while the number of new cases may increase from day to day, the percentage of mortality will decrease." On the first of August, 31 new cases developed and there were 4 deaths; the next day 24 new cases were reported and the death toll reached 7, the highest daily total yet—but it foretold "brighter prospects" because the increase in new cases was "much less than anticipated." At a meeting on the evening of the first, the president of the board of health admitted that the germ appeared to be "exceedingly virulent" this year, but its confinement so far to a few parts of the First District and a section of the Fourth vindicated his faith in the efficacy of carbolic acid disinfection. The sanitary inspector of the Second District seemed less confident, noting that scattered cases were now beginning to appear on his side of Canal Street across from the infected areas of the First District, and he feared that within a fortnight there would be cases all over the Second District. In the Fourth District it was ranging

9. New Orleans *Picayune*, August 3, 8–10, 28, 1878.

along Erato, Felicity, Chippewa, Poydras, and Julia streets in a broad angle between Magazine Street and the river. The sanitary inspector of the Fourth District was engaged in supervising disinfecting operations and could not attend this meeting, but the officers of all other districts were present and reported that their jurisdictions were in good general health and free from yellow fever so far. All of them confessed, however, that their streets were everywhere in a bad condition, the gutters clogged with sludge and covered with green scum. Foul fishponds and vile hog yards here and there were indicated as other hazards that had to be abated in the face of the fever menace, and attention was also directed to the "disagreeable and sickening odors" arising from the stagnant Claiborne Canal.[10]

Before the week was out, new cases were being reported in the city at a rate of thirty to forty a day. From the sixth to the seventh, the reported deaths happened to drop from twelve to five. Still optimistic, the board of health trumped this as a "most hopeful" indication, showing that disinfection procedures were "decidedly justified" after all. The city council accordingly moved to replenish stocks by ordering fifteen thousand gallons of carbolic acid from the north, along with two thousand barrels of lime and a half a ton of copperas. Meanwhile, the city government was having to parry solicitations from all over for contracts to supply New Orleans with superior disinfecting compounds. An eager proposition came from a Charleston manufacturer offering his special blend of sulfur, iodine, and carbolic acid, which he touted as "a powerful fumigator that completely destroys all germs of infection in a house or in clothing." He promised: "I will furnish each house with five pounds for the purpose of fumigating, and will burn fifty barrels or more in different parts of the city. It may, perhaps, require 100 barrels to stop the further progress of the disease. It requires greater quantities when burned in the open air. I will only ask fifteen cents per pound." Sanitary advice of a gratuitous character was also in good supply. "If the Board were to take the matter in charge and have buried in the ground outside of the city the excrementatious matter of the sick, the producing cause of epidemics would be removed, and the disease would soon disappear," was the "belief amounting to positive conviction" of one helpful New Yorker. The city's residents seem to have been heartened by the board of health's repeated assurances of yellow fever's "early de-

10. *Ibid.*, July 31, August 2, 1878.

parture" and were participating in sanitary efforts with alacrity and imagination. One letter writer argued for a thorough fumigation of all buildings with burning sulfur. Another thought the best course of action would be to clean out and permanently do away with the city's noisome privy vaults, "those awful holes containing the accumulated filth of months," and replace them with dry earth closets. The interesting discovery by *vidangeurs* of human remains in the common privy of an Annunciation Street tenement was referred to the Police Department for investigation.[11]

The sanitary inspector of the Fourth District offered his belated report on August 8. He too submitted a favorable appraisal of the disinfection effort, relating that on the four squares initially treated with carbolic acid, only one new case of yellow fever had appeared so far. The board heard with satisfaction his conclusion that carbolic acid had rendered the germ "greatly modified in point of malignancy." The whole district, he warned, was "redolent with the fumes of putrefaction emanating from privies and gutters," and all conditions known to be essential to the production of a raging epidemic were present. He reported that he had issued an unprecedented number of orders to clean privies, however, and the flushing of the gutters was going tolerably well. On streets at right angles to the river, the pronounced natural fall from levee to backswamp made the work fairly easy, but the irregular gradient of the cross streets rendered it more of a problem. Residents on those streets were being requested to get out and assist with sweeping and raking. The board of health resolved that the purifying effects of flowing water should be "thoroughly tested" and supported the suggestion made the day before by the director of the Water Works Company, that the heavy-duty pumps at the sugar refineries and oil presses along the levee be requisitioned by the city for gutter flushing. The *Picayune* immediately ratified the proposal with an editorial: "The carbolization of the streets has already mitigated the severity of the type; now then, in its weakened condition, let us attack it with long columns of moving water." It pointed out that the running water would have the additional effect of cooling air temperatures in the city, thereby reducing another recognized concomitant in the production or first appearance of the disease.[12]

11. *Ibid.*, August 3, 6–8, 10, 11, 1878.
12. *Ibid.*, August 9, 10, 1878.

Meanwhile, troubling news was trickling in that the disease had jumped the bounds set for it and was widening its range up-country and downriver, breaking out at points far beyond the purlieus of the city. On August 5, the city received news that yellow fever had been roiling for a week ninety miles below at Port Eads, the principal "pass" on the birdsfoot delta of the Mississippi, where a sizable community had grown up based on the work of maintaining the lighthouses, clearing the ship channel, and firming and extending the jetties. No fewer than fifteen cases had developed, work was suspended and the jetties deserted, and the supervisors and all others who could afford to had fled to Mobile. Those left behind were crying to New Orleans for relief in the form of medicine, ice, and fresh meat. On August 12, the river city of Vicksburg, three hundred miles up the Mississippi, reported "a general rush out of town yesterday and today," occasioned by the first evident cases of yellow fever originating in that city—one citizen had just died and three others were hospitalized. Two weeks before, on July 26, a "general excitement" had prevailed in Vicksburg after a New Orleans towboat, the *John Porter*, had dropped back there to bury one crewman dead of yellow fever and place two others in the marine hospital. The vessel was disinfected, the city commenced a general program of cleaning and disinfecting, and when no other cases seemed to follow, confidence was restored and the scare subsided. As to these later, so-called indigenous cases, the members of the Vicksburg Board of Health did not yet all agree on the diagnosis, but this time the state of alarm in the streets could not be quieted. Even worse news came to New Orleans the same day by telegraph dispatches from Grenada, a railroad town in north-central Mississippi where at least one hundred cases and ten deaths had occurred over the previous three days. "Business is entirely suspended, and trains pass by without noticing the place. The distress is truly fearful." The first death from yellow fever at the town of Plaquemine, Louisiana, was reported on August 13. "Could hardly find enough to bury her, everyone seems afraid of it," said a letter from Plaquemine. "I do not care about dying in such an unchristianlike place."[13]

Quarantine regulations in the towns and cities tributary to New Orleans continued to be piled on heavier and clamped down tighter, shutting out not only travelers and their baggage but shipments of most kinds of

13. *Ibid.,* August 7, 13, 14, 1878.

dry goods and groceries as well. Hempen and woolen articles were especially dreaded as fomites—so many little traps bearing the latent germ of
yellow fever. Typical were the regulations published on the twenty-second
by Franklin, Louisiana, which kept out everything coming from the direction of New Orleans except hardware, so long as it was unpacked, and
first-class mail, so long as it was disinfected. Quarantine enforcement in
the country towns was generally in the hands of volunteer pickets and
patrolmen, loosely directed by local boards of health that had been hastily
cobbled together by the citizenry. Penalties against local importers of
banned goods, as well as against trespassers from the outside world, were
commonly in the form of stiff fines and instant banishment—along with
a cudgeling, depending on the humor of the quarantine posse. On August 1, the city council of Vicksburg decreed a chain-gang sentence for
violators of that city's quarantine against New Orleans, and remarks made
by the Vicksburg *Herald* in approving the action illustrate the temper of
the hour: "Such an ordinance cannot be made too strict, or the penalty for
its violation too harsh. If the city had the power, we do not think it would
be unreasonable to visit the death penalty on anyone who would willingly
violate measures adopted to protect the lives of thousands." The Natchitoches *Vindicator* explained another substantial worry in the backcountry:
"Should yellow fever occur in the Red River Valley the cotton crop will
be almost a total loss, for every white person will abandon the river and
go to the hills."[14]

Ouachita Parish totally banned the movement of steamboats within
its boundaries as of August 27. Monroe, seat of the parish and the chief
shipping point on the Ouachita River, reportedly had on standby a force
of thirty-five minutemen equipped with Remington rifles. New Orleans'
major connections upriver were also being sharply constricted or severed
altogether. On the twenty-fourth, the St. Louis-based Anchor Line decided to withdraw all its boats from the lower river. Another St. Louis
company was going to maintain just one packet as far down as Baton
Rouge; only the M.V.T. line intended to keep handling through freights
to New Orleans. As the St. Louis *Republican* observed, not only the northward movement of cotton, but the southward flow of western produce
and northern merchandise as well would have to "await the pleasure of the

14. *Ibid.*, August 3, 23, 31, 1878.

fever." So, in quick succession, the city's working connections with the interior were chopped away, and its industrial and commercial life quickly slumped in consequence. Retail stocks of all kinds were soon reported to be in short supply at nearly all towns in the lower valley, the direct result of having cut themselves off from their natural emporium, while the "baleful effects" of quarantine on the Crescent City were symbolized by the unique sight of twenty-one steamers idled at the foot of Canal Street. "Only our mosquitoes keep up the hum of industry," quipped the *Picayune*'s humor columnist, drollery that seems as wickedly ironic now as it was ruefully apt then. All through the month, the *Picayune* railed vehemently against the quarantine "monomania" and the "hysterical timidity" of its adherents, pointing out the practical futility of local quarantine as a means of fending off yellow fever and using all combinations of ridicule and remonstrance to expose the inconsistencies and inequities of quarantine enforcement.[15] Its editorial scolding of "the burgs and crossroads" on August 2 set forth its basic concern:

> They cannot afford to stop trade and cut off their supply, nor can New Orleans afford to be victimized in her commerce by the whimsical and inflected apprehensions of the people of other cities. Whatever other foolish things they may be permitted to do to their own damage, they must not attempt to shut New Orleans out from intercourse with the world exchange by way of the Gulf, the river, or railroads. With two hundred thousand mouths to feed we are all interested in having access to the sources of supply. Those means cannot be cut off from us for any long period without enormous distress.

The situation was having its effect on other commercial centers in the region. The Mexican state of Tamaulipas declined to quarantine against New Orleans, whereupon authorities at Galveston declared rigid quarantine against all Mexican ports, and for good measure quarantined the border town of Brownsville as well. Commercial navigation through Galveston Bay and the Bolivar Channel was paralyzed, while to the east, quarantine regulators were blocking all railroad traffic into south Texas at Orange on the Louisiana border. A committee of Houston businessmen complained that all their inlets and outlets were stopped up and petitioned

15. *Ibid.*, August 16–18, 20, 22, 27, 28, 1878.

the governor to order some relaxation of the restrictions, but to no effect. Shreveport, Louisiana, had surrounded itself with a circle of armed volunteers, and the board of health was requiring all local merchants to take a solemn oath that no goods from New Orleans or other infected places would be received or distributed. The other Red River towns that had been ravaged by the King of Terrors in 1873 were equally serious about their regulations. Goods illegally landed at Campti by certain storekeepers were seized and burned and the culprits ordered out of town, while the neighboring town of Coushatta embargoed Campti for its negligence in letting the contraband slip in. At Marshall, Texas, an entire railroad car containing cotton sacks and wooden ties from New Orleans was set on fire and destroyed by a posse that had resolved to take no chances. The legality of actions like these was questionable to say the least, but at this point the quarantine bug was as virulent as the germ of yellow fever, and the location of the incidents hardly favored any challenge in the courts. Even a federal supply boat moving up the Red River from New Orleans was intercepted by quarantine regulators below Shreveport and compelled to rest at anchor for twenty days in midchannel, where ice and provisions were floated down to it from a safe distance.[16]

The wholesale stoppage of the mails, another consequence of the fomites doctrine, was becoming particularly irksome, especially to New Orleans' commercial interests. Second- and third-class material was being turned back almost everywhere, for reasons explained by the Vicksburg *Herald:* "A large number of small parcels of dry goods are sent daily through the mails, and these constitute fruitful vehicles for the conveyance of infection." At a great many places across the interior, at insignificant hamlets like Tigerville as well as major centers like Monroe and Natchez, local officials were refusing on their own authority to admit postage of any class. Essential business correspondence between New Orleans and many places in its trade area became impossible. The city's postmaster, along with the heads of its two most prestigious business organizations, the chamber of commerce and the cotton exchange, jointly petitioned Washington to order a halt to this interference by local quarantine regulators, but the postmaster general replied that he had no legal power to intercede, that in fact the national government was enjoined by the recent Quaran-

16. *Ibid.*, August 20, 31, September 5, 7, October 26, November 19, 1878.

tine Act to support and supplement all reasonable health measures enacted by local bodies. On August 17, the surgeon general of the army advised that roasting the mail sacks at a temperature of 325° F should be adequate to destroy any germs and allow free dispatch. The suggestion was gladly endorsed by the post office, since the sulfur fumigation practiced by many places under nominal quarantine had tended to bleach the ink and ruin the letters. In spite of this breakthrough, most rigidly quarantined places held firm in their policy. For a while, New Orleans was able to send mail for Texas and Arkansas upriver to be forwarded down the inland railroads with a St. Louis postmark, but the authorities in those states, scenting the trick, threatened rigid quarantine against St. Louis, and the rerouting was promptly stopped. At Dallas an entire shipment of mail was dumped and burned by the local health officer in a demonstration of resolve. Inside Louisiana it was difficult to get even fumigated letter mail east beyond Lake Charles or north past Red River Junction, and most of that was also retained at New Orleans.[17]

By the fifteenth of August, 794 yellow fever cases had been reported in New Orleans, with 210 deaths. While the board of health was still scanning the daily fever report in hopes of discerning something that would augur a favorable turn, the city's churches were planning a day of united prayer to avert what they feared was an impending disaster. By now the sickness was quite widely distributed in the Second District of the city. Disinfection efforts had begun there with the first recognized case of yellow fever, and altogether, 80 squares and 1,566 premises had been painstakingly treated with a 10-percent solution of carbolic acid. "Notwithstanding the thorough application," the sanitary inspector of the Second District said in his subsequent report, "there was no abatement of the fever, and on August 14th it was discontinued." In the Fourth District, the persistent use of carbolic acid had appeared to be keeping the disease in abeyance as late as August 18, "but after that date it broke out with an uncontrollable fury, and soon raged as an epidemic." Streets embracing 137 squares had been sprinkled with carbolic acid by the tank wagons, and the floors, walls, and yards of 1,367 premises had been "thoroughly carbolized" by hand.[18] In his official report for 1878, the president of the board of health would

17. *Ibid.*, August 7, 9, 10, 18, 31, September 8, 18, 19, 28, 1878.
18. Louisiana Board of Health, *Report for 1878,* 54, 82–83.

eulogize the season's experience with carbolic acid in these terms, so much in contrast with the optimism of previous years:

> It is obvious that the plan of out-door disinfection is applicable only to the beginning of an outbreak, before it has attained wide proportions, because the operation is quite expensive and laborious, even on a limited scale. Besides, at the best there is great uncertainty in its efficacy, even admitting that the germ theory is correct, and that the disinfecting agent is positively destructive to the germs. The uncertainty is due to the fact that we are attacking an invisible foe, sometimes appearing unaccountably, and already occupying an undetermined area, the extent of which must be estimated by a mode of calculation involving several unknown quantities. To these difficulties must be added the impracticability of bringing surface disinfection to anything more than a rather rough approximation of completeness, especially within enclosures occupied by buildings.
>
> Another obstacle to the arrest of the disease by disinfection is the impossibility, with the existing powers of the Board of Health, of preventing people from entering localities presumed to be infected, and carrying away articles liable to convey the infection. It is therefore no wonder that in 1878 an unseen and scarcely suspected enemy should have lurked undiscovered for weeks until, by multiplication in its successive generations, and by gradually spreading, it had attained proportions too vast for control before its presence was actually recognized.[19]

Confidence in the efficacy of carbolic acid flagged markedly as the epidemic gained ground in August, and the board of health began to concentrate its efforts on an extensive liming of the gutters, a much cheaper course of action. On the twenty-second the *Picayune* reported a "Holocaust of Fish" in the New Basin, evidently killed by chloride of lime washed in from the city streets. These innocent casualties of the war on yellow fever shortly began to stink. They had to be seined out by a city crew and hauled to an isolated place down the levee, where they were burned with sulfur. Undaunted, the board of health reported that another ten carloads of the disinfectant were on the way from Chicago. Lime was also to be scattered over the sloughs and bayous around the suburbs, as well as over the "unsightly and unsanitary holes" that existed all along the levee front—dirty

19. *Ibid.,* 11–12.

pools that had long been notorious as the source of noisome exhalations, mostly derived from the garbage and dead animals dumped in them by the market people. On the fifteenth, the city council had granted the mayor emergency powers to raise funds, by special loans or otherwise, for the purchase of disinfectants and labor to apply them.[20] In the interior, town councils and parish grand juries had clothed mayors and boards of health with almost dictatorial authority, and the presumptive destruction of the yellow fever germ's theoretical habitat was being carried out under terms approaching martial law. These were the sanitary measures taken by Bayou Sara, a village on the Mississippi about 160 miles above New Orleans:

> The very efficient and intelligent mayor of Bayou Sara, Mr. J. F. Irvine, being invested with dictatorial powers, on the first day of August, 1878, established a quarantine, removed a large portion of the privies, finding that it would endanger health to cleanse the vaults, put in disinfectants and filled and packed them with earth, had new vaults made and disinfectants constantly used in them, disinfected all houses, yards, stables, every place in fact. Fires were kindled every evening in the houses. Supplies of coal and tar were constantly kept at regular distances throughout the town (part of the time pine tar), and the coal and tar at these stations were fired at sunset and kept burning till sunrise during the whole season. . . . The disinfectants relied on were nitrate of lead, a small quantity, mixed in a solution of chloride of sodium (common salt) in larger quantity. Premises, and especially dwellings and their attachments, were sprinkled with this mixture.[21]

The crisis in urban sanitation spotlighted by the yellow fever invasion was stimulating parallel clean-up efforts in major cities both within and outside the region. The first refugee case at New York City was discovered on August 16—an Irish blacksmith who had fled New Orleans a few days before, finding his way to a boardinghouse at Tenth Avenue and Fifty-third Street. The attending physician called the sanitary condition of the lower west side neighborhood "utterly wretched," full of unclean stables and garbage-strewn lots, and warned that it would "readily germinate and spread the baleful disease unless preventive measures are adopted." The

20. New Orleans *Picayune*, August 16, 18, 22, 1878.
21. D. L. Phares, "Bayou Sara vs. Yellow Fever," in *Transactions of the Mississippi State Medical Association, 1879* (Jackson, 1879), 117–18.

president of the city's board of health assured: "Every possible precaution has been taken by the Health Department to fortify this city against an attack of yellow fever, and I don't think it would be possible in the present sanitary condition for the disease to become widely prevalent, even though it should obtain a foothold in a favorable locality." But a former health commissioner warned: "There is no reason why, if the fresh germs were deposited in a bed of filth, they should not remain and propagate till the frost." The New York *Herald* began devoting long, front-page columns to identifying and condemning the numerous "Pest-Breeding Spots" that could be found all over the city. It was not forgotten that Yellow Jack had claimed over two hundred lives in Brooklyn in 1856, and as recently as 1870, three cases of local origin had been reported in the city, the infection supposedly derived from fomites off a New Orleans vessel.[22]

Three refugee cases had turned up at Washington, D.C., and although the nation's capital had not had a serious brush with yellow fever since 1833, the disinfection of its "bad localities" was being pushed with special interest and vigor. Similar reports came from Norfolk, Philadelphia, and Baltimore, all former haunts of yellow fever, where thousands of bushels of lime were being scattered over the streets. The disease had never been recorded at St. Louis, but precautionary steps were being called for there, too. One St. Louis doctor suggested that in view of the yellow fever germ's known sensitivity to cold, it might be cheaper and more effective to distribute blocks of ice along the gutters, in preference to sprinkling them with disinfectants.[23] The Chicago *Times* speculated that yellow fever might in a larger sense be interpreted as "Nature's scavenger, engaged in the work of cleaning up, and it comes only to those countries which will not do the cleaning up themselves. . . . It does not come where it is not invited, or to any locality where there is not made express provision for its sup-

---

22. New York *Times*, August 19, 1878; New York *Herald*, August 17, September 5, 1878. Although the city papers failed to publicize the fact, one of the docks at the Navy Yard had been seriously infected since early July, forcing the temporary abandonment of four ships lying there. The infection was blamed on ballast recently discharged at the dock by a vessel from Havana, with the effluvia from a nearby channel, into which one of the main Brooklyn sewers emptied, indicated as a contributing influence. See J. G. Ayers, "Yellow Fever at the Navy Yard, New York," in U.S. Navy, Bureau of Medicine and Surgery, *Hygienic and Medical Reports, 1879*, 711–28.

23. Chicago *Tribune*, August 18, 20, 1878; St. Louis *Globe-Democrat*, September 2, 1878.

port." As chief conservator of New Orleans' civic pride, the *Picayune* denounced the idea as "stupidly absurd" and insisted the disease attacked clean and filthy cities impartially, just as at the individual level it was as apt to strike down the temperate, athletic, and cleanly as the dirty and negligent. "The *Times* might as well assert that shipwreck is invited by the mariner and that cyclones are the 'scavengers' of the great sea."[24]

The *Picayune*'s reply to the *Times* was understood to be mere defensive sophistry. The awareness of filth as a causative factor in disease, especially this disease, was keen enough, but the habits of the past were ingrained and much had slipped by unconsciously. In New Orleans, a scandal would break in October that would threaten the tenure of the city's administrator of improvements. Lengthy hearings before a special committee appointed by the mayor gradually established the fact that municipal crews in the spring had fetched as many as four thousand cartloads of refuse from a dump behind the city and spread the stuff in low spots on various back streets. Also, many residents had been resorting to the dump all summer for fill material to "improve their sidewalks." Although most of this refuse consisted of mud and cinders, which were considered innocuous enough, it was found to contain a dangerous admixture of rice chaff, horse manure, and rotten fish. In one neighborhood, it had seemed expedient to drop the bodies of stray dogs that had been killed for their pelts by a local Negro into the potholes before filling them. Hogs had subsequently rooted up most of those carcasses, creating a "terrible stench" and drawing flies in such numbers that they seemed "as thick as bees."

The administrator of improvements was roundly denounced by the sanitary inspector of the Fourth District for allowing such goings-on, but in the end it was impossible to prove any connection between the filling of the streets and yellow fever, and the residents themselves expressed no complaints at all. The people of Liberty Street regarded it as "the best improvement that had been done there in a long time," and were "thankful indeed" when it was completed. "Well, the street I don't believe had anything to do with the yellow fever at all," one of them testified. "I'm not much of a scientist, and don't know much about these things, but seeing Dr. Choppin and the Board of Health discussing about the matter out there, it seemed to me as if it came from along the front of the city." On

24. New Orleans *Picayune*, September 7, 1878.

Dorgenois Street, the citizens had been so anxious to see the filling project carried out that they had gotten together a purse of $35 as a special inducement for the street foreman. One resident declared: "Among the exposed people in the low places and about the vicinity of the dump ground it has been almost nothing, the mortality. . . . I've always, for thirty-five years, considered all persons exempt from epidemic diseases who live in the vicinity of dumps."[25]

After the middle of August, the situation in New Orleans' hinterland began disintegrating in manifold panic and confusion as the fever, seeded far and wide in spite of all quarantine and disinfection measures, started breaking out explosively at numerous places. On August 18, the health officer of Vicksburg telegraphed "at least 100 cases and increasing rapidly," noting that the infection was starting to proliferate in the low, crowded section of town behind the river-front, bidding to make its first and worst inroads among the city's poorest classes. The city council of Vicksburg raised its quarantine against the outside world on the nineteenth, deciding that any restrictions at this point would only hamper the receipt of vital relief shipments. On the seventeenth, New Orleanians were informed through the *Picayune* that Memphis, Tennessee, had suddenly lifted its rigid quarantine sanctions against them, and they also learned details of the pell-mell exodus from that city, as the first yellow fever cases erupted there: "The people are panic-stricken, leaving the city as fast as trains will carry them." That day a special cabinet meeting was called in Washington to discuss the alarming situation unfolding at Memphis and other southern towns and cities. The surgeon general of the Marine Hospital Service advised that yellow fever of apparently unprecedented virulence was spreading up the Mississippi Valley, and that in view of the unusually warm summer, there was a general apprehension among doctors that it could go on to engulf the Ohio Valley and even reach the cities of the Northeast. President Hayes directed the postmaster general and the secretary of war to exercise their authority "within the scope of a liberal construction of law" to check the menace and extend relief to infected cities.[26]

Jackson, the capital of Mississippi, had never put up more than a nominal quarantine against New Orleans and, strangely, had developed no

25. *Ibid.*, October 19, 23, 1878.
26. *Ibid.*, August 17, 20, 1878.

yellow fever cases so far, but the depressing intelligence from Washington, coupled with the fearful reports coming out of Vicksburg, just forty miles to the west, and Canton, only twenty miles north, was apparently enough to unnerve the populace. On August 21, a state of "unparalleled" panic prevailed at Jackson, with state offices closed, business of all kinds suspended, "and nothing thought of except escape from the scourge." "People are fleeing from the pestilence in every direction," according to a communication in the *Picayune*. "The situation is truly horrible." It was estimated that half the city's six thousand people—three-fourths of its white people—either fled or made ready to flee during these anxious days. "We are in hourly expectation of the pestilence in Jackson," the grand secretary of the Mississippi Freemasons explained in an anticipatory appeal for relief to his brethren across the nation. Traffic on the important east-west Vicksburg & Meridian Railroad had to be shut down on the twenty-fourth, as the fever had appeared at stations on both sides of Jackson, but not before rural Rankin County, embracing the countryside around the capital, had been "overrun with refugees from Vicksburg who have gone into all sorts of shanties or cabins or live in tents." These people had flocked to the vicinity in vain hopes of obtaining some kind of relief from the state government. Many others were reported along the dirt roads leading out of Vicksburg, either straggled singly or in camps. Most of them lacked the barest necessities, with more than a few developing the fever after arriving in the country, condemned to go unattended while sick, and uncounted when dead. One Vicksburg man claimed to have seen three or four people lying solitary under trees beside the road, apparently dying: "In trying to get out of reach of the pestilence, they had got out of reach of the city charities."[27]

Jackson evidently managed to shake off its hysteria by August 25 and was reported to be "working with the energy of despair" to hold off the encircling threat. "Every dirt road and the railroads are watched night and day, and the town patrolled. Citizens, both black and white, have constituted themselves detectives, and all strangers unable to give an account of themselves are marched to the city limits and warned not to return. The fire bells ring at 10 P.M. and all persons found on the streets after that hour are arrested." The movement of trains was kept open on the Chicago,

27. *Ibid.*, August 17, 22, 27, 29, 1878.

St. Louis & New Orleans Railroad, the region's crucial north-south artery, though it was subject to a gauntlet of impediments and restrictions imposed by various places along the route. The railroad company managed to placate most of the towns along its line by donating loads of chloride of lime for application to "dangerous spots." The town of Magnolia, on the railroad about midway between New Orleans and Jackson, took the additional protective step of distributing pinewood to its citizens, requiring them to build at least one fire on their premises every night. The town of Summit allowed no persons or merchandise from either direction to be landed by the trains and had on hand a force of twenty pickets by day and thirty by night to guard against violations. Even people from the surrounding farms were being chased off. One "obstreperous negro" was actually shot dead by jumpy sentries. "Such a panic as now exists was hardly known during the most depressing period of the late war," was the word from Osyka, another town on the railroad. Like other stops up and down the line, Osyka deemed itself fever-free so far and was struggling to keep itself safe through resolute quarantine and disinfection; testimony, however, would show later that the stealthy infection had already gotten a solid foothold in the town back in July.[28]

At the close of August, the official "fever report" at New Orleans counted 3,111 cases of yellow fever and 915 deaths, and the number of new cases being reported in the city had surged to between 200 and 300 a day. "A spirit of general uneasiness is for the first time prevalent," the correspondent of the New York *Times* observed on September 3. "There is not a shadow of hope that there will be any abatement this month. On the contrary, the speedy seizure of all unacclimated persons is the only prospect." The First District, where much of the city's susceptible immigrant population was concentrated, had become "intensely infected," and the problem of extending timely relief to these people was threatening to slip out of control. Bodies were found set out on the curb for removal almost every day on almost every square, and more than a few tragic instances of "family annihilation" were being discovered.[29] A letter dated September 8, from a lady in the city to her sister in Chicago, described the situation: "Right opposite our house a young man died last night, and his shrieks

28. *Ibid.*, August 18, 25, 27, 29, October 20, 24, 1878; "The Epidemic in Osyka," Paper 8 in "Report of the Yellow Fever Commission," RG 90, NA.

29. New York *Times*, September 4, 7, 9, 1878.

were horrible. . . . Go where you will, you are sure to see a hearse, and the charity wagons go out loaded to the potter's field. I have seen eight in one wagon; the Irishman driving sitting on top and smoking his pipe apparently as unconcerned as the farmer who rides on top his load of hay on his way to market. However, I suppose these drivers see so much of this sort of misery that they get hardened."[30]

Amid the crush of sickness and death, the board of health was finding it difficult to get disinfectants in the quantities needed. With the chemicals of choice in short supply, the people were advised of a cheaper substitute: "An ordinary wineglassful of turpentine dissolved in a bucket of water will thoroughly deodorize and disinfect any ordinary sink or cesspool." The infection now seemed to be striking a new salient along St. Charles Avenue into the Sixth District, toward the suburbs of Carrollton and Jefferson City. It was remembered that a lady out on Peniston Street had come down with evident yellow fever as early as the sixteenth of July, a few days after going to the funeral of a friend in the First District who had died of supposed "malarial fever." An initial attempt to disinfect the spot with carbolic acid had been foiled "by unknown parties who emptied the tank during the night," showing that at least one citizen's hatred of the obnoxious chemical had not waned in recent years. When it seemed no subsequent cases were going to appear a repeat was not attempted. Other supposedly "sporadic" cases had occurred out past Louisiana Avenue in early August, but all those potential focuses, the sanitary inspector of the Sixth District asserted, had been "virtually suppressed in every instance by timely and efficient disinfection." Now came fresh outbreaks all along that line, "until the multiplicity of cases occurring here and there throughout the district rendered sanitary measures of little or no avail." Soon a solid twelve-square area centering on General Taylor Street was infected, defying carbolic acid even when laid on at 20-percent strength. Public complaint at first blamed the rank effluvia from the many *vacheries*, or stable-dairies, located in this district, but subsequent inquiries showed that yellow fever was really no more malignant in the neighborhood of cowsheds than elsewhere. Instead, the "exciting elements" were believed by the sanitary inspector to have existed in "the miasma arising from foul and stagnant waters in the gutters."[31]

30. Chicago *Tribune*, September 14, 1878.
31. New Orleans *Picayune*, September 6, 1878; Louisiana Board of Health, *Report for 1878*, 115–17.

Some flocks of wild geese were sighted over the city on September 9, flying southeastward. The *Picayune* picked up on this hopeful omen and prayed that it signaled the early onset of frosty weather, with its "speedy sanefying of the poisonous atmosphere." A few days later, a weather front passed over Louisiana, followed by several days of north wind in New Orleans. This breeze drew across the infected First and Fourth districts and carried over to the right bank of the river, where the wafted smell of carbolic acid was strong enough to elicit comment in the industrial suburb of Algiers. After it died down, cases of yellow fever "sprang up in every direction" in Algiers. The sanitary inspector of the Fifth District later wondered if perhaps the wind had not been a factor in conveying the germ across the river, but acknowledged that "at the time there was uninterrupted intercourse with infected districts, this in itself being sufficient to implant the disease among us." As the infection gradually embraced all parts of the city, the quirks and vagaries of its incidence gave ample scope for all kinds of speculation. Later in the month, some of the doctors in New Orleans called attention to the "Peculiar Fact" that cases of yellow fever were considerably more numerous on streets running straight back from the levee to the swamp than on cross streets. The theories put forth to account for this came quite literally from opposite ends of the streets. "One gentleman advanced the idea that the phenomenon was occasioned by the seeds of the disease passing along the gutters with the water from the river. . . . Another gentleman thought that the malaria rising from the swamps to the rear of the city, having a clean sweep through these streets, engenders the disease."[32]

As the disease became more widespread and prevalent, the idea that the problem was in the overlying atmosphere obviously became much more plausible. "The very atmosphere seems impregnated with the infection or poison," noted a September letter from Port Gibson, Mississippi. "The leaves of the China trees, and of garden plants, some of them are withering; the fowls seem affected, and the hogs about the street likewise seem to have imbibed some substance which makes them puny." This was the kind of highly subjective observation that would have been received as positive evidence of a pervasive "epidemic atmosphere" by the Sanitary Commission of New Orleans a quarter of a century before. One idea of

32. New Orleans *Picayune*, September 10, October 4, 1878; Louisiana Board of Health, *Report for 1878*, 105.

the old Sanitary Commission was recalled on September 20, when the board of health sought an injunction against the Water Works Company to prevent the breaking of ground in the Fourth District to lay new feeder pipes. Official statements assured the people that carbolic acid was still being applied efficiently in places where it had some chance of doing good, but in fact the futility of the disinfection campaign had become apparent to everyone by this time. The germ theory seems to have temporarily taken a back bench, while concerns and notions about miasms in the city began to be advanced, especially in the thinking of the lay public. One citizen's letter in the *Picayune* urged the city to suppress the sale of shrimp in the markets because "the water they are washed in is thrown into the gutters and the stench from it is terrible, and bound to cause sickness." Another reminded the people to make a point of eating a heavy breakfast with coffee before venturing out in the morning, to better fortify the system against absorption of the "malaria" that was still afloat at that hour— advice which even at the time might have seemed ludicrous had it not merely repeated one of the recommendations made by the eminent Dr. LaRoche in his famous treatise on yellow fever.[33]

A letter from the president of the board of health of little Magnolia, Mississippi, observed that yellow fever had never prevailed in presidential election years, and thought this might be attributed to the influence of the many bonfires and torchlight parades, the "opening of houses" and general "cheering and hilarity" at night. He suggested the city might produce the same effect by obtaining pine resin and burning it festively in the streets. "You have easy access to the pineries and can no doubt obtain large quantities gratuitously." A letter from "Old Citizen" complained about the fumes of carbolic acid and agreed that burning of pine tar would be more healthful and beneficial, if only because it would put to work "the idlers who are drawing rations who ought to be glad to make themselves useful." Someone else advised cleansing the city's "low, foul, heavy air" by having householders and city officials gather up a huge stock of coal and cord-wood with which to set fires burning in all the streets, hearths, and stoves for a day or two simultaneously, since it was understood by everyone that simple fire is a wonderful purifier of the atmosphere. After all, had not the great cholera epidemic at St. Louis in 1849 died out spontaneously after an accidental conflagration of steamboats lying at the docks?[34]

33. New Orleans *Picayune*, August 24, September 7, 21, 26, 1878.
34. *Ibid.*, September 7, 1878.

An open letter appearing on September 11, claiming to represent "the universal opinion of our old citizens," championed the disinfecting power not of flame but of smoke, and requested everyone to "build fires of anything that will make plenty of smoke. . . . The purifications and disinfecting such as we have had never did or ever will do any good, any more than a man's washing his feet to cleanse his dirty face." The people in their desperation made a surprisingly widespread response to the appeal. The next day, residents of the Second District were trying to smudge out the pestilence by piling windrows of green straw along the principal streets and keeping them smouldering and smoking night and day. Within a week their example was being imitated in neighborhoods all over the city, "at almost every corner." The correspondent of the New York *Herald* reflected on the "strange, wild, unearthly character" the fitful light from these grass fires gave the city at night. We might smile, and remember accounts of the ancient Athenians doing the same thing in time of plague.[35]

Misconceived schemes to alter the state of the atmosphere did not absorb all the city's energy and imagination, however, and the epidemic summoned up a flurry of prophylactic potions and nostrums. In a circular issued at the beginning of the crisis, the New Orleans Board of Health correctly noted that "preventive medicines are useless," and on the question of treatment, the board went no further than to advise a dose of oil to clear the bowels and a hot footbath to induce a mild sweat, followed by strict bedrest. This easygoing policy represented the so-called expectant method or creole cure honored by long experience in south Louisiana, and upon which modern medicine has really improved very little. There is still no curative drug or serum for yellow fever, and careful nursing and supportive therapy is still the only responsible course of treatment for a viral infection that is essentially self-limited and of short duration. But the epidemic of 1878 occurred in the golden age of individualism and laissez faire—of "empiricism" and outright quackery—and the very lack of a sure cure, in the absence of any recognized medical or pharmaceutical authority, encouraged the circulation of preventive and remedial formulas in crazy profusion. "Hundreds of quacks in different parts of the country are trying to introduce their medicines in yellow fever here," observed the *Picayune* on September 5. "Let them come to New Orleans and try it on themselves." At least one of them demonstrated his faith by his actions;

35. *Ibid.*, September 11, 12, 15, 1878.

on the thirtieth, the papers noted the death from yellow fever of a Boston doctor who had been vending his "English Remedy" out of one of the hotels. As one of the Crescent City's own physicians related in a letter to the *Boston Medical and Surgical Journal:*

> Innumerable specifics of infallible efficacy have been suggested in letters to the mayor and Board of Health, by individuals who never saw a case of yellow fever, and probably would not like to see one. Our newspapers teem with advertisements of sure remedies, and I have been called out of bed at night to see one credulous fellow who made himself seriously ill with one of these nostrums, which exhibited the familiar odor of ipecac. Many trust in Holman's liver pad, and others in little bags of assofoetida and camphor suspended to the neck. This mild fetichism affords great comfort to minds which lean on faith in the mysterious, a faith unshaken by failure and disappointment even to themselves; therefore it is not quite useless, and on the whole vastly preferable to those frauds which are palmed off under the guise of great medical discoveries.[36]

Although the Orleans Parish Medical Society had recently decided by an eighteen-to-four vote that quinine was of no value in fending off yellow fever, the drug was still extremely popular and was recommended by many responsible physicians. It was known to be effective in treating malaria, which many still considered a kindred disease. Its specific action on plasmodia in the blood was not yet understood, and it was thought to be useful as an all-around alterative, antipyretic, and germ killer. Others sought to fortify their systems against the dread virus with doses of salicylic acid, hyposulfite of soda, and various other supposed alterative compounds. Sulfur, rolled into pills or stirred into gin or some other agreeable solvent, was the chief reliance of many people. One communication advised rubbing the powder freely into the armpits and groin, to facilitate its full absorption into the system. Various preparations of arsenic were also in fairly common use, in discrete and not-so-discrete doses. Arsenic was popularly employed as a specific against malaria and, like quinine, was therefore supposed to have a protective effect against yellow fever as well. The dangerous fascination earlier generations had with heavy prophylactic

36. S.S.H., "Letter from New Orleans," *Boston Medical and Surgical Journal*, XCIX (1878), 448.

dosing with another mineral poison, the drug calomel (mercurous chloride), had fortunately receded by this time, although calomel was still widely applied in the treatment of developed cases, both for its laxative effect and to encourage the kidneys.

Many believed that congestion of the kidneys and suppression of urine was the deadliest effect of the yellow fever "poison," and to counteract it, people dabbled with all manner of herbal teas and tonics, from the traditional boneset to the newly touted eucalyptus. These infusions were often laced with saltpeter to heighten the diuretic effect. Teaspoon doses of turpentine enjoyed a high degree of favor, partly because of its stimulating effect on the kidneys and partly out of a feeling that the oil would have inwardly the same balmy and health-inspiring effect that the burning of pine tar produced on the atmosphere of the streets. A letter from an Alabama doctor recommended a little kerosene two or three times a day, observing that "employees of gas works are uniformly exempt from fevers." Preventive medicines of more exotic provenance were also in supply. In an August communication to the *Picayune,* a member of the Sociedad Medica of Santiago, Chile, charitably informed New Orleanians that the bark of the Andean balsam tree made an excellent tonic and had saved many from yellow fever at Callao and Guayaquil. Parke-Davis of Detroit acted quickly on this tip and soon had a bottled extract of "boldo" on the market, but with negligible medical results. There was also a broad offering of patent poultices and externally applied "organ regulators," such as a "liver and stomach pad" widely advertised by one New Orleans firm, but all of them, as a Grenada, Mississippi, physician observed that winter, "went down most ingloriously as preventives of yellow fever." [37]

By the first week of September, yellow fever was violently scourging many other towns and cities in Louisiana and Mississippi. The estimated number of cases in Vicksburg had soared to eight hundred by September 1, then to two thousand, and finally to three thousand by the eighth.

37. New Orleans *Picayune,* July 30, August 3, 30, September 21, 24, 29, 1878; Bemiss, "Yellow Fever in Louisiana," 172, 182–83, 188; Mississippi Board of Health, *Report for 1878–79* (Jackson, 1879), 45–46, 51, 74, 153, 159. See also S. M. Bemiss, "Yellow Fever," in *A System of Practical Medicine,* ed. William Pepper (Philadelphia, 1885), 649–55; John M. Keating, *The Yellow Fever Epidemic of 1878 in Memphis, Tenn.* (Memphis, 1879), 46–73; Ezra M. Hunt, "The Prophylactic Treatment of Individuals as a Means of Preventing Epidemics of Yellow Fever," *Medical Record,* XV (1879), 52–56.

The city was being literally decimated, and the scenes of misery and horror were said to "beggar description." "We have the greatest difficulty to obtain labor even to dig graves," a communication to Washington from the president of the local Howard Association said. "God knows when the suffering will stop. Lights are burning in nearly every inhabited house over the dead and dying." Among the past week's victims had been the city's mayor and the president of the board of health. The secretary of war directed a special issue of 40,000 army rations to Vicksburg, but declared that he had neither legal nor moral authority to order military doctors into service in the infected city. The older physicians of Vicksburg declared that the infection was "far more violent and malignant" than in 1853, and unacclimated doctors and nurses interested in relief work were thanked for their good will, but advised to stay away. The Vicksburg & Meridian Railroad, which had resumed train service intermittently after the first wave of panic two weeks before, was now conclusively shut down, except for the transport of emergency supplies. Excitement was running higher than ever in south Mississippi, and at some places there had been threats to fire into the trains.[38]

The epidemic had finally made its debut at Jackson, Mississippi, on August 31, with one death reported. Jackson took encouragement from the fact that most of its unacclimated population had already retreated to the rural districts. Nearly all the city's tradesmen had fled and business was at a standstill, but the local relief organization reported $8,000 on hand, and supplies were thought to be adequate for the present. It was consolingly noted that "our editor, physicians, and clergy are in place." The board of health at Baton Rouge, Louisiana, acknowledged the appearance of the fever there on August 30, and on September 1 a terse report stated that "all business is stopped." It was widely believed that the city had been contaminated by New Orleans people who had been in town earlier in the summer for the state Democratic convention, and it was true that the first cases to appear in Baton Rouge were among the employees of a hotel and restaurant that had catered to the delegates. Up at Memphis, affairs had gone from bad to worse, "surpassing the worst imaginings of

---

38. New Orleans *Picayune*, September 11, 13, 1878; New York *Times*, September 8, 1878. See also Ernest Hardenstein, *The Epidemic of 1878 and Its Homeopathic Treatment* (New Orleans, 1879), 26–33. Hardenstein was a Vicksburg practitioner who served through this epidemic.

misery," and it was disclosed that authorities there had resorted to burying the dead in mass graves. "It has even been suggested to burn the dead if they cannot be buried more promptly, as corpses are known to have lain unburied for 48 hours, burdening the air with foul odor and becoming so revolting that it is with difficulty that men can be hired to haul them to the potter's field."[39]

Port Gibson, Mississippi, had recorded 55 deaths from yellow fever by September 3, and estimated that out of only 550 people remaining in town, 400 were presently down with the fever. "The distress is very great—many dying with no one to give them a drink of water. Help and funds needed." Delhi, Louisiana, telegraphed for aid on the fifth of September, saying that "almost everyone is down with it—it is a terrible sight." On the ninth, the town of Plaquemine, Louisiana, on the Mississippi 100 miles above New Orleans, reported itself "sadly prostrated" and declared that "outside assistance is an imperative necessity." The first two deaths at the ill-fated town of Greenville, Mississippi, were announced on August 31, and the people were said to be "panic-stricken and flying to the country." From that start the sickness swiftly proliferated, and by the fifth of September, there were 75 cases and 20 deaths. The lavish use of disinfectants, including carbolic acid, did nothing whatsoever to stay the progress of the fever. Although located on the Mississippi River, the town of Greenville had never been visited by yellow fever, and so furnished the very conditions where an epidemic could strike with sledgehammer force. The population of Greenville before the epidemic was about 2,500; the final death count, according to the report filed with the Mississippi State Board of Health, was 296, including 101 Negroes. As possible aggravating factors, the reporting physician mentioned the spongy character of the alluvial soil and the town's excessive reliance on privy vaults for disposal of its waste, "which permeates the entire substrata with the germs of pestilential poison."[40]

There was a precipitate stampede out of Osyka, Mississippi, on September 11, two days after the local board of health positively denied the existence of any unusual sickness. A few days later, Osyka acknowledged that "many of the cases that occurred previously were of a mild form of

39. New Orleans *Picayune*, September 2, 5, 1878. See also E. Lloyd Howard, "Baton Rouge," in Bemiss, "Yellow Fever in Louisiana," 167–71.

40. New Orleans *Picayune*, September 1, 3, 5, 6, 10, 1878; R. S. Toombs, "The Epidemic at Greenville," in Mississippi Board of Health, *Report for 1878–79*, 63–65.

yellow fever." This, in fact, was a common pattern during the initial phase of an epidemic. Communities almost always vehemently claimed that they had no trace of yellow fever, even when appearances were decidedly against them. Small towns no less than large cities dreaded the prospect of having personal and commercial contact with the outside world impeded or cut off, and the prevailing conviction that yellow fever implied bad sanitary conditions added a note of embarrassment to their plight, causing them to react to imputations of fever much as an individual might if accused of having a venereal disease. The defensive language of a notice sent out from Crystal Springs, Mississippi, on the twenty-third of the month, over the signatures of twenty-five local businessmen and doctors, was typical in its seriocomic tone of awkward formality and wounded virtue: "To correct false rumors and slanderous reports concerning our town, we beg to state that to our certain knowledge no yellow fever exists here or within ten miles of this place, and we know of no excitement here or in this vicinity." A telegram on September 12 from Meridian, Mississippi, insisted that the town was enjoying perfect health despite all rumors to the contrary; but on the sixteenth it was disclosed that Meridian was sending its women and children out to the country.[41]

The pestilence was also beginning to sweep into the creole communities along Bayou Lafourche immediately west of New Orleans. On the fourth of September, Labadieville reported thirty cases. On the same day, Thibodaux declared the appearance of fever in town and on at least one plantation outside town. "The citizens are fumigating the town by burning sulphur every evening in front of their houses, and pine tar in various places." The disease had also manifested itself at many of the watering places along the Mississippi coast, little beach towns where many people of means from the Crescent City had taken refuge in July. One of the resorts that had become infected was Bay St. Louis, where an estimated two thousand New Orleanians were summering and where hardly a week before, the mood had been secure and carefree enough for a regatta. It was recalled that in the early days of August, a New Orleans vacationer had been attended through a sickness "which was not known at the time to be yellow fever." His flannels were subsequently given to a needy family living nearby, and from them, it was supposed, the epidemic had spread.

41. New Orleans *Picayune*, September 10, 12, 17, 24, 1878.

By October, Bay St. Louis would record over five hundred cases and seventy-eight deaths, many of them children from the city.[42]

At the village of Lake, Mississippi, on the Vicksburg & Meridian Railroad one hundred miles east of Vicksburg, rigid quarantine had been declared on August 22 after the health officer of Vicksburg disclosed two hundred cases of yellow fever and admitted that the infection had gotten completely out of hand. Here, as elsewhere, it proved impossible to enforce the policy with sufficient rigor and surveillance. That very evening a young man fleeing Vicksburg was let into Lake by the town's quarantine guards, by virtue of the fact that he was the mayor's son-in-law. The next morning he was sick with what was thought at the time to be "a very slight attack of malarial remittent fever." The house where he convalesced was later a focus of unusually fatal yellow fever. By the time a doctor from Jackson arrived on September 7 to organize medical relief, there were at least thirty persons down with the disease, which seemed, however, to be abating. Soon thereafter, the epidemic took a malignant turn, apparently gaining fresh impulse from a number of peculiar atmospheric influences.

> Deceived, therefore, by the appearance of safety, in consequence of the rapid decrease in the number of cases, some parties, whose names it is unnecessary to mention, in utter disregard of my orders, opened up one of the infected rooms and placed the mattresses and bedding on the front fence, on the main thoroughfare. Other parties afterward did the same, and in a very few days there were some twenty persons attacked in rapid succession. . . . By the 22nd September there had been some twenty or more deaths. The corpses were interred in the burying ground, north of the town, and very near, say half a mile, from the center. On the night of the 22nd there was a heavy rain storm, which continued part of next day. The newly made graves, dug in the light sandy soil, sank, and within twenty-four hours the half-exposed, putrifying corpses emitted a most offensive and deadly stench. Of course, the graves were promptly refilled and packed down, and lime and carbolic acid were freely used. The number of attacks then became very great, and in rapid succession, reaching at one time nine deaths in twenty-four hours. . . . The family living nearest the graveyard (widow and children, and mother-in-law and sister-in-law of Capt. McFarland), after having been some two weeks previously exposed to the case of Capt. McFarland, who died on the 10th Septem-

42. *Ibid.*, September 5, October 23, 1878.

ber, and who continued to occupy adjoining rooms to his (which, however, had been made air-tight and fumigated), and who, up to this time,
about 26th September, had remained in perfect health, were all, seven in
number, attacked within twenty-four hours of each other, most of them
throwing up black vomit, and in thirty-six hours all were dead, save the
youngest and feeblest child. . . . The house is large, airy, well-built, and
is one of the most comfortable residences in the place. The premises were
scrupulously clean and the family were well-to-do, refined, and educated
people. Furthermore, the house occupies a high elevation, removed from
and overlooking the village, and there is therefore scarcely room for a
doubt in my mind that the inmates were directly poisoned from the gases
arising from the graveyard, which was scarcely two hundred yards back
of the house.[43]

A community of about 350 people, only a few of whom managed to
flee in time, Lake suffered 330 well-marked attacks of yellow fever, entailing 78 deaths. A description of the phenomenon of extrinsic incubation
was embedded, unconsciously, in the above account of yellow fever at
Lake. Similar valuable observations were made elsewhere in 1878, but recognition of their significance was shunted aside in every instance by the
preoccupation with modes of transmission other than personal contagion.
The origin and progress of the epidemic in a number of Louisiana towns
were studied by the Baltimore expert Dr. E. Lloyd Howard, who came in
November as a member of a special Yellow Fever Commission organized
under the auspices of the American Public Health Association. At the
town of Thibodaux, Howard appears to have succeeded in identifying two
original focuses of infection. One was at a nunnery on the outskirts of
town, where a sister came down with yellow fever on July 30, one day after
arriving from New Orleans. The first two secondary cases among the residents here appeared on August 17 and 18. On the twenty-sixth, a little girl
from the town was stricken. She had been accustomed to play around the
convent grounds, "almost under the windows." From her the virus spread
to her family and neighbors. Another focus of infection developed on
Crazy Street around the house of a member of the town's quarantine
guard, who had been boarding and inspecting the coaches on trains com-

43. F. E. Daniel, "Epidemic at Lake, Miss.," in Mississippi Board of Health, *Report for
1878–79*, 53–59.

ing from New Orleans. This man fell sick on August 8 and died a few days later. "In from 10 to 15 days after Mr. Marange's death there occurred nine other cases in his house." From those focuses (and, no doubt, a number of others), the fever spread until the whole town was involved. Although most of Thibodaux' 2,800 people were of acclimated creole stock, the epidemic there produced at least 750 cases and 65 deaths.[44]

At most localities it was altogether impossible to pinpoint infecting cases, making the spread of infection from personal contagion appear to be the exception rather than the rule. Despite the most earnest efforts to enforce their local quarantines, these towns were in fact never more than illusorily guarded against infection from the metropolis or each other, and obviously were visited and infected by mild or incipient cases that went unrecognized at the time. When local people began falling sick in large numbers two or three weeks thereafter, the mosquitoes still held their secret. At the town of Plaquemine, Professor Howard attributed the introduction of the fever to fomites, since neither of the first two local cases (who happened to live across the street from each other) had visited New Orleans or knowingly been exposed to any sick people, but both happened to have received packages from the city a few days before falling sick; one had opened a parcel of ladies' lingerie, the other a box of window shades. Plaquemine was a town of some 1,500 inhabitants. Yellow fever, which began raging there toward the end of August, struck down more than 1,100 people before the season was over, killing 125.[45] At Canton, Mississippi, where 150 died, the source of infection was so obscure that even the fomites theory could not be invoked, and the reporting physician, A. T. Semmes, was inclined to favor the possibility that the fever had originated spontaneously from local causes. Semmes, obviously an older doctor who clung to outmoded ideas about the origin and propagation of yellow fever, took particular note of "a very filthy lagoon that had been festering all the summer, filling the neighborhood every evening with a horrible stench." He recalled the similarities to 1855, the last time yellow fever had come to Canton:

As early as June the unusual heat had begun to produce much sooner than common, serious spells of remittent fever, and as the month of July

44. E. Lloyd Howard, "Thibodaux," in Bemiss, "Yellow Fever in Louisiana," 162–64.
45. E. Lloyd Howard, "Plaquemine," *ibid.*, 164–67.

came, filling each successive day with a heavier roll call of fever for all the physicians in the surrounding country, suspicions of the yellow scourge began to excite the fears of all who had any recollections of 1855.

Noticing closely, day by day, the features of our bilious fever patients showing a constantly increasing shading off into many symptoms of yellow fever, I expressed my honest belief that without some marked improvement in our climatic conditions, we should certainly drift into a visitation of the dreaded scourge. The pointings of the thermometer and barometer, the excessive luxuriance of vegetation, the oppressive odors from the bayous, all brought back to the minds of the older citizens the similar circumstances of 1855.

On the 20th of July I attended a young man who had no communication with any persons or goods of any sort by which he could be infected; still his case had every feature and symptom of the cases of yellow fever which I had nursed in the epidemics of 1853 in New Orleans and 1855 in Canton.[46]

How yellow fever's complex etiology could elude a comparatively thorough and critical investigation by the highest medical authority in the land can be illustrated by the case of Morgan City, Louisiana, which was visited in January, 1879, by the surgeon general of the U.S. Marine Hospital Service, Dr. John M. Woodworth, working in connection with the Yellow Fever Commission. Morgan City, a sugar port at the head of the Atchafalaya estuary 80 miles west of New Orleans, represented the westward limit of epidemic yellow fever in Louisiana in 1878, and its vicinity was one of the worst ravaged. The town's normal population of about 3,000 was reduced to an estimated 1,200 when people fled after yellow fever broke out. At least half of those who stayed behind fell sick, and 109 died. Carried from there to the nearby community of Pattersonville, population 500, the disease took another 75 lives. Spreading out to Lagonda and the other big sugar plantations along Bayou Teche—sizeable towns in their own right—the epidemic produced at least another 1,000 cases and took more than 100 lives, ravaging a contingent of recently arrived Polish laborers and also killing an unusual number of Negroes. Woodworth took down much testimony at Morgan City and sifted the evidence. He considered and ruled out several possible sources of infection the people told him

46. A. T. Semmes, "History of the Yellow Fever Epidemic in Canton, Mississippi, in 1878," *New Orleans Medical and Surgical Journal,* n.s., VII (1879), 600–606.

about, including a Mexican circus troupe that had passed through town in June—by way of Texas, where there was no suspicion of infection—and a ship from Cuba that had arrived in August—but had been sent away by the quarantine guards without landing any people or goods.

Woodworth determined that the town's first case of yellow fever had occurred in the person of a laid-off sailor who was taken sick on August 17, three days after he had dodged the Morgan City quarantine guards and slipped back into town from New Orleans, where he had gone to visit a house of prostitution. The man threw up black vomit and died on the twenty-second. From August 24 to 31, ten more well-defined cases appeared in town, six in the same rooming house where the first victim had lived and the others in lodgings close by. In retrospect, we can say it is quite possible that the sailor contracted the disease in New Orleans, possible too that he carried the virus back to Morgan City, but that he was not the original case or primary source of the epidemic in Morgan City is plain when we remember the necessary period of extrinsic incubation. An interval of at least two weeks would have been required for Morgan City mosquitoes, having bitten the man, to have become capable of transmitting the disease and for secondary cases to have begun appearing. Dr. Woodworth, unaware of this hitch in the evidence, was reasonably satisfied that he had ascertained the infecting case and established the right connection. He did note one additional fact: earlier in August, seventeen days before the sailor's death and the general eruption of yellow fever in the place, the woman who operated the rooming house had come home sick from Bayou Boeuf and had taken to bed for several days with fever and headache. Woodworth wondered, as might we, if that could have been a mild case of yellow fever—but the information was complicated by her statement that she thought she had already suffered an attack of the disease as a girl twenty years earlier.

Woodworth included in his report a number of observations that serve to illustrate the bewildering complexity of evidence facing the pioneer epidemiologist and which show how, without the concept of an intermediate vector to guide the investigator, the evidence for personal contagion inevitably fell short, while all discoverable facts tended to point back to the fomites doctrine. He was informed that in the summer of 1877, a yellow fever case off a Cuban boat had been nursed in the room later rented by the sailor, the first victim of 1878. This was one of those coincidences that gave credibility to the fomites theory, the vision of disease germs lurking in the environment like dry seeds and erupting from dormancy when suitable conditions presented themselves. Among the fever's earliest victims in Morgan City were two little children, daughters of the town's postmaster, who lived just down the street from the rooming house but had not been permitted to visit it. Woodworth recorded the poor father's belief that his girls had been stricken because he had negligently let them play trampoline on the mailbag from New Orleans a few days before. Plotting the town's first thirty-six cases on a map, the surgeon general observed that the infection had at first spread exclusively along streets south of the New Orleans railroad. On September 14, however, the disease leaped suddenly and unaccountably to a house four blocks north of the tracks, striking down a little girl who had not been allowed out of her yard. Woodworth could not explain this by any means of contagion or infection, except to note that the girl's father owned a coffeehouse in the infected district and had visited his place of business not long before, and so might have brought germs home on his clothing. The man developed yellow fever and died shortly after his daughter. After this extension, the epidemic spread rapidly over the whole town, and any further effort to reconstruct its development became impracticable.[47]

At the close of September, the New Orleans Board of Health enumerated 9,385 yellow fever cases in the city up to that date, with 2,845 deaths. By then, however, it was freely admitted by the authorities that all proper count had been lost. Not all the deaths and probably less than half the yellow fever cases were being reported, as many of the sick were going unattended and most doctors, in the haste and urgency of the hour, were neglecting to turn in statements. The board of health could do little more than remind doctors of an ordinance requiring them, as well as ship captains, hotel keepers, and others in positions of oversight, to promptly report all cases of febrile or otherwise suspicious sickness. The board's president, Dr. Samuel Choppin, had briefly held out hope of a therapeutic breakthrough when he set aside a ward in Charity Hospital for experiments with a new medical invention, a special rubber cot on which fever-burned sufferers would recline naked while being subjected to a continu-

---

47. John M. Woodworth, "Morgan City, La.," in Bemiss, "Yellow Fever in Louisiana," 174–82.

ous spray of cold water. The unfortunate New York physician who had patented the device caught the fever a few days after arriving in the city to conduct a demonstration, and died, strapped to his contraption, on September 23. Dr. Choppin acknowledged that he and the faculty could endorse no new therapy or cure, but said responsible experiments should be encouraged. Some of the city's prominent physicians were advocating severe sweating to drive out the "poison," others were applying heavier doses of quinine and calomel, but as a visiting journalist observed, "The mortality is great enough under both systems."[48]

The epidemic was now setting in "with great virulence" in the Third District and was spreading to the low-lying back streets of the First and Fourth districts, including the so-called Congo section, where many of the city's blacks were coming down with the sickness. The Second District was reported to be thoroughly infected, "from the river to the swamp." On some blocks, notably along Euterpe, the fever had become so prevalent that the residents of neighboring squares had thrown up barricades in the streets and sealed them off with revolver-packing volunteer guards. Most of these barriers the administrator of improvements declined to order removed. Elsewhere, as a courtesy to the sick, wood shavings were being spread over the streets to keep down the clatter of hoofs and wagon wheels on the cobblestones. On September 20, the mayor requested the Chief of Police to cease the customary tolling of the curfew bells, supposing the noise might be prejudicial to the thousands of sick in the city. Previous orders had halted night work at various mills and foundries and compelled the streetcar company to remove the bells from its mules. Noise abatement had become a matter of serious concern and general comment in view of the fever situation. One complaining citizen asked why, when ice-cream vendors were forbidden to tinkle their bells, express wagons were suffered to rumble through the streets at full tilt. When those vehicles rolled over the iron bridges, he said, "a noise almost equal in intensity to thunder is produced." A black congregation on Laurel Street that had been "in the habit of making night hideous by the boisterous manner of conducting their religious ceremonies" was warned by the police to moderate the tone of its evening services.[49]

48. New Orleans *Picayune*, August 30, September 20, 25, 1878.
49. *Ibid.*, August 31, September 8, 12, October 4, 1878.

The cordon of quarantines against New Orleans was bearing down on the life of the city at least as hard as the disease itself. Merchandise from the Crescent City was interdicted over most of its usual trade area, and the normal inflow of commodities from the tributary region was blocked and diverted by the spread of yellow fever or by the thick web of inland quarantines. Docks and railroads were substantially hushed, and enterprise of all kinds in the city slowed down or closed up. The stifled movement of even so vital a commodity as flour expresses the situation well: receipts declared by New Orleans wholesale houses in September totaled just 24,119 barrels, contrasting with the 66,145 barrels moved in September, 1877. Local demand was quoted at about 2,000 barrels a day. Transshipments to the interior were almost completely closed off, and the loss of this handling trade cut deeply into the city's normal volume of commercial activity. The situation had thrown the nationwide market for provisions—meat and meal, sugar and coffee, and so forth—into a state of collapse. Locally disruptive as they were, the evacuations, dispersals, quarantines, and general paralysis of communication in the Mississippi Valley could not have removed more than a few hundred thousand people from the overall market, which in a nation of 45 million people should not have had more than a minor impact on the overall trade in provisions. The problem was vastly magnified and multiplied, however, as the familiar mercantile phenomenon of "discounting the probabilities" came into play. The financial editor of the Louisville *Courier-Journal* explained:

> It was inferred, of course, that only a hand-to-mouth trade could exist in the Southwest. The dealers in other parts of the South reasoned that this check upon demand from that quarter would probably incline the market in their favor, and besides they were apprehensive of the safety of their own sections; hence they also held back. The dealers of the North reasoned that if the whole southern demand were reduced to a hand-to-mouth basis, the whole market would be sensibly depressed. The speculative element, seeing in all this one of those opportunities for which it is ever watchful, went in and "burst the thing wide open," and so instead of a decline of a fraction of one percent we have a decline of fifteen to twenty-five percent.[50]

A New York commercial circular complained that the fever and attendant quarantines had cut off the markets and exchanges of the lower Mis-

50. Louisville *Courier-Journal,* September 11, 1878.

sissippi Valley as effectively as "a high wall, or an unnavigable sea." A Liverpool newsletter reported that receipts of raw cotton at English docks were materially diminished by the yellow fever situation and expressed the hope that American shippers would quickly establish new channels of export through East Coast ports. Trying its best to keep a hopeful light on the situation, the *Picayune* quoted a Boston paper to the effect that the trading season was not lost, merely retarded and delayed. The regional business crisis stemming from the yellow fever invasion in fact weighed heaviest on the lower stratum of New Orleans' working class, as families living from one payday to the next in normal times now found themselves stranded, with little or nothing in the way of savings and no options for relocation or escape. The board of health's considered estimate at the end of the season was that at least half the industrial population of the city, no fewer than twenty thousand men, had been turned out of employment by shutdowns and stoppages occasioned by the epidemic, with a loss of wages over the ninety-day period approaching four million dollars. There was only charity to stand in the gap, for the principle of public relief assistance, of government's material responsibility to the jobless and stricken, was still quite remote. While the New Orleans Police Department remained the largest single administrator of relief rations, purchased with the private contributions coming to the city from across the nation, the great bulk of the aid was handled by an assortment of benevolent societies and public service clubs, chief of which were the Howard Association, the YMCA, and the Peabody Association. By the first week of September, relief requisitions amounting to more than fifteen thousand rations a day were being filled by those organizations, working in concert through a Committee of Arrangements, and the task of distribution at the main commissary on Magazine Street was said to engage a corps of thirty clerks along with "a strong body of police."[51]

By the first week of October, as the crisis deepened, over 40,000 rations a day were being distributed in the city. Louisiana's congressional delegation had been able to secure a special issue of 200,000 rations of pork, flour, rice, sugar, and coffee from U.S. Army stores on September 4, but—so alien and uncomfortable then was the notion of federal involvement in welfare matters—a second issue scheduled for early Octo-

51. New Orleans *Picayune,* September 4–6, 10, 17, 1878; Louisiana Board of Health, *Report for 1878,* 13.

ber was canceled by the secretary of war. He agreed with the attorney general that it technically would be "an unlawful diversion of supplies voted for use by the army" and reasoned that private charity would be sufficient to tide New Orleans through the remainder of the crisis. The collector of customs, the ranking federal official in the city, cabled the secretary of the treasury in appeal: "There is more need of aid than ever. The wharves are bare, industrial enterprises closed up, and nearly every laboring man out of employment." A joint manifesto by thirty charitable organizations engaged in rations distribution in New Orleans emphasized the "state of complete destitution" existing in the city. The New York *Herald* called it a "painful dilemma" and editorialized: "One of the consequences of the great freedom of the people of this country from the interference and control of authority is an equivalent absolution of authority from any responsibility for the welfare of the people." "Labor prostrate at the feet of Capital begs for bread," cried an anonymous letter to the *Picayune.* "Who will lead the way to a larger and more comprehensive charity?" The yellow fever crisis exposed some other serious tensions in the community. A series of letters in the *Picayune* over the suggestive signatures "Reformer" and "Battle Axe" damned landlords for their allegedly harsh and exacting treatment of poor tenants in arrears for rent because of sickness or unemployment.[52]

On top of having to cope with its own affliction, New Orleans found fever-stricken towns for hundreds of miles around looking to the metropolis to extend relief of all sorts. Often the city's first knowledge of a yellow fever outbreak at some interior point was by way of distress telegrams crying for crackers and canned meat, for ice and medicine, and for volunteer doctors and nurses. Somewhat typical was the communication received on October 12 from the village of Tangipahoa, sixty miles north of the city, which found itself entirely cut off and badly in need of everything, the country people refusing to approach the settlement with supplies. The parish rustics had excellent reason to be afraid. Yellow fever had already killed forty of Tangipahoa's two hundred people. Another common predicament was illustrated on September 19, when the town of Labadieville on Bayou Lafourche requested donations of crackers and rice because its people were too distracted by sickness to shift for themselves, and New

52. New Orleans *Picayune*, September 5, 7, October 3–5, 1878.

Orleans grocers declined to forward foodstuffs on credit for fear the consignees would die, leaving no one to pay off their notes. "The amount of distress, poverty, and want (in some cases not made known in time, starvation) in consequence of this curse—or affliction of Heaven shall I say?—may be imagined but not realized until seen," declared a September letter from Port Gibson, Mississippi.[53]

Perhaps the season's most anguished appeal was a telegraphed message from St. Louis on September 19 by the captain of the steamer *Ben Allen*, one of the very few boats still working the lower river. When it was flagged over to the landing at Greenville, Mississippi, on its upriver trip, this is what it encountered: "Situation is horrible. 400 remain and cannot get away; 200 sick; nearly 100 deaths. No boats running; telegraph line down for about ten days; cannot make their wants known; are shut out from the world. For God's sake get nurses, supplies, and money on other boats." It transpired that shotgun-toting posses of farmers were resolutely scouring the roads and footpaths around the infected town, barring exit and entry and forbidding repair crews from getting at the downed telegraph line. The closest point by a railroad was 80 miles to the east. Over the next few days, poignant scribbled messages ("Fever raging. Deaths terrible.") were smuggled out to the nearest telegraph stations and relayed over the wires to New Orleans, along with anxious cries for champagne, mustard, and orange leaves—rather an odd shopping list for a place in such desperate straits, we might say, but each of those items had an important place in popular yellow fever treatment at the time. The packet *Kate Dickson* was loaded with supplies and dispatched from New Orleans, and a U.S. marshal followed by a strong posse went up from Vicksburg to oversee repair of the Greenville telegraph. On September 27, the captain of the *Dickson* reported back that the Greenville death toll had mounted to 237 and only 15 of the 450 whites trapped in the town had not had the fever. A few parties of despairing townspeople had managed to break out and had been picked up along the riverbank, where they were camped out under the most wretched conditions.[54]

Observations and conjectures about miasms, relayed from all points of the geographical and theoretical compass, continued to be batted about

53. *Ibid.*, September 24, 26, October 16, 1878.
54. *Ibid.*, September 20, 21, 29, October 4, 1878.

in the daily press at New Orleans. A communication from Mandeville, on the other side of Lake Pontchartrain, groped for a reason why the town should be afflicted this year, when it had entirely escaped infection in the great epidemic of 1853. Local people apparently favored the idea that the recent breach in the Mississippi levee at Bonnet Carré had rendered the lake "brackish instead of salt," giving rise to an unusual malaria. "If the crevasse were closed the salubrious waters of the Gulf would fill the Lake." A diametric view came from a seasoned American resident of Tabasco, Mexico, who wondered if the variations recently observed in the flow of the Gulf Stream could have had the effect of sweeping up "columns of infected air" from the tropics. "Have we not many proofs of the continuous existence of infection over those currents when running in the tropical regions?" An imaginative doctor residing at Hot Springs, Arkansas, wrote to the *Picayune* to suggest that a series of air samples be collected for spectrum analysis, which ought to turn up some conclusive information about "the vitiated state of the atmosphere. . . . The spectroscope should reveal to the scientist all important marginal changes in the atmosphere." On its own initiative, the *Picayune* sent a reporter around the city to interrogate the managers of a tallow works, a soap-boiling establishment, and three places handling green hides, out of a longstanding concern that the gases and odors arising from industries of that sort could be aggravating factors in yellow fever. These businesses employed a total of fifty-seven men, continuously exposed to the often very foul vapors and effluvia of their raw material, but declared that so far not a single case of fever had occurred in any of their crews. One year later in Havana, Cuba, Dr. Carlos Finlay would follow a similar investigation to a similar finding, whereupon he abandoned his former miasmatist beliefs and gradually turned his attention to the offbeat notion that the fever was actually propagated by mosquitoes.[55]

More immediate and widely shared concerns had to do with the supposed danger posed by exhalations from the numerous cemeteries inside city limits. On September 28, the *Picayune* complained editorially of the "intolerable bad odor" emanating at night from the shallow burials in the corporation graveyard on Metairie Ridge, and on October 17, it passed along as a "Pertinent Suggestion" a citizen's letter denouncing the condi-

55. *Ibid.*, September 28, 29, October 1, 9, 10, 1878.

tion of the old town cemeteries, especially one on Claiborne Street where the dilapidated crypts were described as little more than "crumbling ovens, through whose disjointed roofs may be seen the ghastly and decomposing remains of mortality lying exposed to view, from the upper to the lower tier of vaults, and exhaling their pestiferous gases out into the open air." A real tempest threatened to blow up in local politics over this general problem a few days later, when witnesses summoned before the city council confirmed that in neglect of a standing ordinance, the city sextons had been "reopening vaults of yellow fever corpses for the accommodation of the more recent dead, and the putrefying masses have been exposed to the atmosphere to spread disease and death." The *Picayune,* weary by now of further sanitary scandal and wary of its potential damage to the city's Democratic administration in a critical election year, tried its best to minimize the revelation, but it was given full play in out-of-town papers. The stench released on one occasion was described in the St. Louis *Globe-Democrat* as "positively crazing, and its effect on the funeral procession escorting to the grave the later corpse in the highest degree nauseating."[56]

Certainly, if bad smells were to be admitted as any factor in causing the disease, then the fumes from its festering victims should have been especially distressing. The embarrassed board of health ordered that the vaults in question be fumigated with burning sulfur and carefully resealed with cement. The bad condition of the city's intramural burying grounds remained a live issue for the rest of the year, however. All the sanitary inspectors addressed the problem in their official reports for 1878 and admitted that the situation of the graveyards was a reproach to the city that demanded speedy correction, yet none of them could say that the incidence of yellow fever had actually been worse around the cemeteries than elsewhere in their districts. The report by the sanitary inspector of the Fourth District on the state of affairs at the potter's field at Sixth and Locust puts us in touch with the just apprehensions of New Orleanians on this matter:

> I myself, making an inspection, witnessed the burial of a corpse. The grave was prepared by uncovering a coffin, opening it, raking the bones together and throwing them out, breaking up and prizing out the old

56. *Ibid.,* September 28, October 17, 1878; St. Louis *Globe-Democrat,* October 22, 1878; Bemiss, "Yellow Fever in Louisiana," 98–99.

coffin and depositing the new in the mould of the former. When laid in its uncertain resting place the lid of the box, like that of the one preceding, was two inches below the surface of the earth. To hide it, the earth formerly removed was piled upon the coffin in a mound about two feet high. In this covering I counted the skulls of three former occupants, besides observing other bones innumerable. So filled with bones was the earth as to make the use of the spade extremely difficult. Another coffin lid, warped by the sun, displayed in hideous reality the body of a poor wretch who had died a few months before; the stench was disgustingly perceptible. The whole surface of the ground was strewn with ribs and small bones, like pebbles upon the hills. Here and there huge thigh bones served as head and foot stones to the unknown dead.

The citizens living in the vicinity set forth . . . how in the summer season the stench from human bodies pervaded their homes; how, whether eating or sleeping, they were ever in an atmosphere heavy with exhalations from the dead. They pictured the disgusting sights forced upon the gaze of themselves and their children. They referred to their pitiable condition during epidemics, when the putrefying dead were piled in heaps under a blazing sun awaiting burial, and the overburdened earth reeked with rotting human flesh, while clouds of flies swarmed back and forth upon the graves, *and upon their tables!* . . .

The neighbors assured me that hogs repeatedly made their way through the picketed fence, and even declared to me that they had been known to root up the dead out of their graves and revel in their carcasses the livelong night, filling themselves with human flesh to fatten on it. Whether this statement be true or not, it is certain that they were frequently in the graveyard, and the coffins, sometimes not below the level of the surface, were often made bare by the rains. Adding danger to the disgusting features of this horrible picture, the boards of coffins broken up as described were in constant demand to be used as firewood for cooking and for the construction of yard fences by certain degraded whites and negroes living in the district.[57]

In September it was bruited in the Associated Press that the actual "sporae" of yellow fever had been "discovered" by Dr. Joseph Jones of New Orleans. Jones, professor of chemistry and clinical medicine at the University of Louisiana, was one of the country's most reputable pathologists and, unlike many later hunters of the yellow fever germ, was too

57. Louisiana Board of Health, *Report for 1878,* 90–92.

cautious to advance any such claim himself. He had, however, been making investigations into the microbial contents of the "yellow fever atmosphere" during the course of this epidemic, and had made some intriguing observations that tended to support the prevailing views of yellow fever's etiology. Jones described his experiments in a series of long articles published in the *New Orleans Medical and Surgical Journal* in 1879. Using a bellows to force air through tubes immersed in crushed ice, he had condensed samples of the atmosphere inside certain houses in New Orleans where especially violent cases of yellow fever had occurred. He viewed the milky water under his microscope and saw that it abounded with a great variety of forms. He observed large, colored cells that he recognized as resting spores of certain common gutter algae. Some of the smaller shapes he could make out as various spirilla, micrococci, and rod-shaped bacteria; others he could identify as fungi, mainly torulae and penicillia. He saw tiny, threadlike filaments that he supposed were "the mycelia of some singular delicate fungus," and he also noted "minute particles of vibrating matter which could not be resolved into specific shapes under the highest powers." He observed that all these cells and particles had an affinity for the minute wool and cotton fibers that were floating in the condensate. Jones also condensed samples of air collected directly over foul gutters in infected localities, and was able to describe the same set of microorganisms. When condensate from either source was injected into the shoulders of rabbits, it produced a local infection, with inflammation and fever. Dr. Jones found the tissue at the site of injection marked by "acute fatty degeneration" after a few days. He drew samples of blood from yellow fever patients into clean stoppered bottles and watched it putrefy over the course of a few hours, by which time it was swarming with spores and bacteria "similar in all respects to those of the yellow fever air, previously described." This fluid produced a similar toxic reaction when injected into his rabbits, as did specimens of the urine and vomit of fever victims. Joseph Jones was one of those who were still inclined to the theory that yellow fever was of spontaneous origin, evolved locally from certain combinations of heat, dampness, and decomposition. But regardless of whether the germ was of local or imported origin, or whether any of the microbes his experiments revealed really was the causative germ, he believed that he had found something that harmonized with the observed facts of the disease's etiology. His observation indicated the actual mechanism by which the infection contaminated whole localities, propagating in filthy gutters and the stagnant air of houses, and how it was carried from one place to another in fomites:

> The demonstration by the microscope of numerous living organisms (spores of plants, bacteria, and animalculae), and of minute animal and vegetable particles in the yellow fever atmosphere, and the fact also that these minute bodies are found in greatest abundance in the meshes of the particles of wool and cotton floating in the sick room, is important as it illustrates the mode in which the contagium of the disease may be propagated and wafted from house to house, and across considerable spaces. In this view it is not necessary to regard the micrococci and criptococci, bacteria and spores, and minute particles, as the essential causes of this disease, although under the circumstances in which yellow fever prevails they are the necessary companions of the yellow fever contagion, *and may take part in its elaboration,* during certain putrefactive changes, and may be the vehicles of its propagation through the atmosphere and of its preservation and concentration in spongy fabrics as cotton and woolen clothing. . . .
>
> However the poison may have originated, whether from a "foreign imported germ," or from the decomposing masses of filth in the city itself, or from human beings, in whom a specific disease was excited by the chemical and physical conditions of the surrounding atmosphere, it will be admitted that the lower forms of animal and vegetable life, active in the phenomena of putrefaction and fermentation, abounded in the atmosphere, and that it is not unreasonable to regard them as active agents in the propagation and spread of the *Pestilence.*[58]

A few rivulets of commerce began to revive after the middle of September, as cane, cotton, and rice harvests got under way in the uninfected parts of Louisiana. On the twenty-fifth, for example, Iberia Parish, to the west of the city, along with the parishes of West Feliciana and Pointe Coupee to the north, reported that the gathering of crops was going on "steadily" and "without drawbacks" behind their high quarantine walls. The *Picayune* gratefully reported that those districts were not backward

---

58. New Orleans *Picayune,* October 6, 1878; Joseph Jones, "Yellow Fever Epidemic of 1878 in New Orleans: Extracts from Clinical Lectures," *New Orleans Medical and Surgical Journal,* n.s. VI (1879), 711–15, 764–80, 852–72.

about forwarding their crops to New Orleans factors, but lamented that mercantile shipments to the interior were still stopped up by the quarantines, and the larger packets had to carry cargo both ways to make a paying trip. The season was so late, and the need to reprovision was so acute, that some places were persuaded to part their iron curtains slightly. In the third week of September, some of the upper Red River parishes declared their willingness to accept boats from as far down as Alexandria, and those along the Ouachita relaxed their blockade enough to allow through passage of St. Louis freights to Monroe, where the scarcity of some supplies was said to be getting serious. Emboldened by that news, the owners of the big New Orleans–based steamer *Pargoud* announced plans to send their vessel out on a circuit of "the usual bend landings." But they desisted when they were confronted with a telegram from the sheriff of Issaquena County, Mississippi: "Learn you will come up. Your trip will cost you money; officers of boat will be arrested; therefore stay away until frost. This is the wish of the community, merchants, and planters."[59]

Louisiana's cotton crop that summer had been reduced by the appearance of army worm in most parishes, but the growth of cane had been excellent, causing many to recall the heavy sugar harvest of 1853, another dreadful year for yellow fever. The Thibodaux *Sentinel* wondered: "Does sugar cane fatten on the poison of yellow fever? Or is it the effect of the mild winter and the extraordinarily long and hot summer bringing it to such fine condition?"[60] The question reflected an old Louisiana aphorism, that the best years agriculturally, with particular reference to the sugar crop, were the worst in terms of health and mortality, especially with regard to yellow fever visitations. Stanford Chaillé, a medical professor at the University of Louisiana committed to demolishing the last vestiges of miasmatism, checked this particular bit of folklore against the record a few years later. He found that in the sixty-year period from 1822 to 1882, New Orleans had suffered thirteen major yellow fever epidemics, but the sugar crop had been unusually good in only six of those years, and in two of the years it had been quite poor. He also showed that exceptionally good crops had occurred in six healthy, nonepidemic years. Dr. Chaillé sensibly concluded:

59. New Orleans, *Picayune,* September 18, 22, 26, 27, 29, 1878.
60. *Ibid.,* September 11, October 10, 1878.

Yellow fever originates from one kind of germ, sugar from quite another, and an epidemic requires abundant unacclimated material which the sugar crop does not require, and as long as these and other such different causes characterize each, the two cannot always coexist. If all causes peculiar to each happen to coexist, and if the causes common to both should at the same time occur, only then would both an epidemic and a good sugar crop result. Now, prolonged warmth and moisture are common causes which promote the growth not only of yellow fever and of sugar, but also of plants generally, hence it is not singular that all these should not infrequently grow vigorously in seasons of prolonged warmth and moisture. In such a conclusion there is nothing either novel or surprising.[61]

Yellow fever is essentially a plague of cities, not the countryside, and over most of the region its effects on agriculture tended to be circumambient rather than direct, though still producing considerable obstruction and inconvenience. Quarantine nuisances were everywhere and posed trouble in many ways. Several times during the season, the *Picayune*'s financial editor observed that cotton picking was seriously hampered at many places in the interior by a shortage of sacks—bagging, of course, ranking high on the list of dreaded fomites. Local relief administration at Vicksburg, Baton Rouge, and other inland cities was undergoing a strain similar to that being felt at New Orleans, as thousands of seasonal laborers were compelled to lie over in the stricken cities and draw rations. At Jackson there were unsympathetic comments about "the armies of idle negroes who hang about town," but the rule of shotgun quarantine prevailed on country roads all around, and planters of the surrounding farm counties either would not or could not receive field hands coming by way of infected places. At the same time, the city was keeping up the formality of its own quarantine line, with the aim of excluding any additional "idlers" from the surrounding country, who in apparently troublesome numbers were willing to risk infection for the sake of free issues of food. The unemployment, destitution, and demoralization resulting from the epidemic tended to cover a wide radius, even where the virus did not.[62]

61. Stanford E. Chaillé, "Our Yellow Fever, Sugar, and Cotton Crops," *New Orleans Medical and Surgical Journal*, n.s., IX (1882), 683–90.
62. New Orleans *Picayune*, August 22, September 29, October 2, 13, 1878.

In the vicinity of the smaller towns where the King of Terrors held court, late-season farm operations were completely disarranged, and picking and ginning of the all-important cotton crop had fallen to a state of near-limbo. A letter from Lebanon Church in Hinds County, Mississippi, on October 19, exemplified the predicament of many stricken rural places: "All business is suspended, crops are standing in the fields, the negroes and still-surviving whites are panic-stricken, and no one seems to think of anything but the fever." The disruption of receiving and shipping at key points along the railways was an effect of the epidemic that became especially hurtful to agriculture in the fall. The loss was particularly severe at Meridian in Lauderdale County, an important railroad center and forwarding point for a considerable share of the Mississippi cotton crop. Most of the town's four thousand people had scattered in panic when the fever broke out in September; among the five or six hundred who remained, there had been four hundred cases and one hundred deaths. Meridian cotton shippers were not in a position to receive the first bales from the countryside until the second week of November. Sporadic cases of yellow fever were still being reported in the town at that time, but the local newspaper decided to take no further note of them, rationalizing that the reports stemmed mainly from "hearsay," and by keeping the people from coming back were hurting the revival of business. Meridian later estimated commercial losses of $300,000 from this epidemic, owing to suspension of business and diversion of trade.[63]

The last week of September found the movement of people and crops almost totally paralyzed in Warren County, Mississippi, embracing the country around Vicksburg. Fever or rumors of fever were breaking out at "all points" and spreading with a "fearful rapidity." Bovina, a hamlet of only seventy-five people ten miles outside Vicksburg, suffered six deaths from yellow fever on a single day, the thirty-first. In dismay, and against official advice, many of the refugees who had established themselves in the small towns or in camps outside Vicksburg earlier in the summer began drifting back into the infected city, where at least rations and medical attention were available. Uncompromising shotgun quarantines along the Big Black River prevented them from going out to more distant havens.

63. *Ibid.*, October 10, 25, November 12, 1878; P. H. Griffin, "Epidemic at Meridian, 1878," in Mississippi Board of Health, *Report for 1878–79*, 155–59.

Of the twelve fever deaths reported in the city on the first of October, three were identified as recent returnees. The relief committees of Vicksburg not only had to accommodate this added burden but were being called upon to forward material assistance to the surrounding country at a cost of over $4,000 a day. Most rural stores were closed up, since purveyors were refusing further advances of supplies, and many of the plantations already idled by sickness were now "suffering for the actual necessities of life." There was a similar extensive spread of the fever to rural places in adjoining Claiborne County, where people were completely dependent for their day-to-day necessities on relief forwarded through Port Gibson, itself sorely stricken. By mid-October, the cotton fields of that whole section were reported to be white with open, overripe bolls. Early storms had already blown much of the cotton onto the muddy ground, and the fear was that only half the standing crop could be gathered before heavy weather set in.[64]

It was announced on October 1 that the pride of the river fleet, the still-legendary *Robert E. Lee,* was coming out of enforced idleness and would resume its regular Vicksburg run. In the ensuing week, the other large steamers based in New Orleans followed the *Lee*'s initiative and began putting out again, with reasonably full freight lists. By the thirteenth, a "decided improvement" could be reported in business at the docks in New Orleans. New cotton was coming in quite freely by then. In fact, the 24,765 bales brought into New Orleans in the first half of October represented a pace virtually abreast of the 29,230 bales received in the same period in 1877. Thousands of people had been prostrated by yellow fever at Vicksburg, and at least 1,200 of its 12,000 citizens were dead, but the outbreak of new cases was finally slacking off: "Avenues of trade are opening and trade reviving in consequence." The crisis had passed at Morgan City, and already talk on the streets was turning to the splendid cane crop and the upcoming fall elections, even though "more deaths occurred in a single day last week than usually occur in an entire year!" In New Orleans, the correspondent of the St. Louis *Globe-Democrat* reflected on "the grotesque combination of an active political struggle coupled with streets blockaded by funerals and fluttering crape upon nearly every square."[65] At

64. New Orleans *Picayune,* September 28, October 2, 13, 1878.
65. *Ibid.,* October 1, 13, 1878.

Osyka, Mississippi, the pestilence finally seemed to be on the wane, after causing over 200 cases and 33 deaths, a heavy blow for a village of only 500 people. The turgid but unquestionably sincere sentiments of a letter posted from Osyka on October 17 could have expressed the feelings of the whole region:

> The frequency of death, the wide-spreading and increasing sickness, and all standing in jeopardy of life, seem in a measure to dull the sympathies of friends, but when this "King of Terrors" shall have taken his final leave, and when health again smiles around, then to bereaved hearts will come the full realization of their losses, then the anguish of the surviving be fully known. But not until the revelations of the last day, when the records of the earth will be all unrolled, will the aggregate of privations, sufferings, heart-rendings, and all the accumulation of woes which have followed in the trail of the destroyer be fully understood.[66]

As long as the weather continued warm, mosquitoes remained active and the fever could keep "spreading and feeding" in other places, where there were still plenty of unacclimated humans. Fifty to one hundred new cases a day were reported at Baton Rouge, as the infection spread gradually from the upper to the lower part of town, a curious reversal of the usual pattern. At this point, the second city of Louisiana was "little more than a hospital," and relief committees were struggling to meet a "growing and incessant" demand for rations and other supplies. "The epidemic although not fatal to colored people is prostrating them by hundreds. When striken they are found in need of everything." Almost every day for the first three weeks of October, word came of the fever's appearance at yet another town in the interior, with the usual stories of hubbub and flight, and of grief and misery among those who tarried. It had broken out at the village of Hayne's Bluff, Arkansas, and the panic was "worse than that of a routed army. . . . So great has been the terror that two well authenticated cases have occurred where the parents of dying children abandoned them to the mercies of strangers." It had appeared at Clinton, Louisiana—introduced, it was thought, by means of some new blotters the parish clerk had lately gotten from a New Orleans printer—and straightaway the town was "nearly depopulated and business entirely suspended." There were

66. *Ibid.*, October 19, 1878.

suspected cases at Crystal Springs, Mississippi, where "great and increasing uneasiness prevails, and people are preparing to fly." The nearby settlement of Dry Grove was in the grip of a malignant fever that local doctors were either unable or unwilling to call by name, but which was, regardless of nomenclature, "extremely fatal and very unattractable to treatment," in the words of a lay correspondent. The city of Mobile, Alabama, had become infected, and on the seventeenth admitted to a total of seventy-three cases and twenty-three deaths. Authorities there were applying the usual psychological salve: "Although it is plainly evident that the fever is spreading, it is also evident that it is not spreading to the extent that some alarmists have reported."[67]

Closer to New Orleans, the sickness was sweeping the suburb of Gretna, on the opposite bank of Mississippi, and was "alarmingly on the increase" in the scattered settlements on both sides of the river above and below the city, in the parishes of St. Bernard and St. John the Baptist. Cases of black vomit were being reported at Logtown, Mulatto Bayou, and various other places along the Pearl River just east of the city. The town of Pearlington said it had no fever as yet but was nevertheless "in a state of perfect dread and awe-stricken. . . . Every day or two we see a cart loaded with the necessary goods for camp life moving out of town back into the country, in order to avoid the prevailing scourge. Every vacant house five miles out of town is engaged, and every old hut is repaired and held in readiness for a retreat." To the west of New Orleans, in Assumption and Lafourche parishes, yellow fever was said to be spreading "all over" and the ravages were "fearful." It was reported on October 9 that fully half the people of the village of Paincourtville were prostrated by the fever, and at many little places on both sides of the bayou below Lafourche Crossing, the disease was making similar "sad havoc." A special call went out from those places for French-speaking nurses. Farther out, in the parishes of Vermilion and St. Landry, the towns of Abbeville and Opelousas reported that they were rigidly quarantined and still healthy; nevertheless, parish offices were closed, courts had been adjourned, and many families were getting ready to move out to the country. Mercifully, the season was not too long in breaking, and the arrival of cold weather not long delayed. Light frosts were falling in central Mississippi by October 18, and in Louisiana as far south as the Teche country, by the twenty-third.[68]

67. *Ibid.,* October 3, 6, 15, 20, 1878.
68. *Ibid.,* October 9, 11, 12, 15, 16, 19, 24, 26, 27, 1878.

The *Picayune* immediately resumed its editorial preachments on the hated quarantines. "They all want our supplies, and we want their cotton. There are large orders pending here which cannot be filled from the present limited offerings and unsatisfactory assortments, and stall from the detentions caused by the epidemic and the quarantines. It is high time for the cotton movement to resume its usual course, and for trade to flow through its natural channels, but the great obstacle is these interior quarantines, and the sooner they are abolished the better for the common interest." Small-town merchants were accused of keeping up the sham of quarantine merely to have an excuse for continued price gouging. The St. Louis *Journal of Commerce* crowed that the wholesale merchants of that city had enjoyed their "taste of new territory," profiting by hundreds of thousands of dollars on orders diverted from New Orleans because of the fever blockade. Daily train service between Jackson and Vicksburg was reestablished at the end of October, and at both cities it was said that business of every kind was rapidly turning back into its accustomed channels. At Jackson the epidemic's toll had come to only 428 recognized cases and 69 deaths. By any standard of comparison, the Mississippi capital had come through much better than the nearby town of Canton, only one-third the size of Jackson, which had suffered over 1,100 cases and 150 deaths. In the river counties above Vicksburg, it was reported that the air of "demoralization" was gone and the cotton pickers were working "as well or better than they ever did." "Demoralization" was explained as "the reluctance of negroes to work while they could obtain rations free of cost."[69]

At the close of October, the official "fever report" for New Orleans counted 13,083 cases and 3,929 deaths for the season, figures that were later reevaluated by the authorities and upped, in round numbers, to "not less than 27,000" sick and "not less than 4,600" dead. The *Medical Times and Gazette*, a British journal, observed that the loss of even 3,000 lives in a city the size of New Orleans was equivalent, in proportional terms, to 60,000 deaths in London. The first of November was All Saints' Day, normally a red-letter observance on the New Orleanian calendar, but this year the *Picayune* followed local doctors in discouraging people from the traditional decking of graves and crypts. "Owing to the unusual number of burials that have taken place during the past few months, and the sometimes hasty and imperfect inhumation that has been performed, the air in

69. *Ibid.*, October 25, 27, 30, 31, 1878.

some of our public cemeteries cannot be entirely pure and wholesome." The ceremonies were nevertheless very well attended by all classes of the community. An occasion of greater moment to those still fretting in the flesh was just four days off—the first general elections in the state since the withdrawal of federal forces and the end of Reconstruction. Fairly or unfairly, some northern papers were accusing the city's Democratic bosses of recklessly urging their refugee constituents to come home so they would be on hand for the big day. From some of the parishes came reports that armed gangs operating under the pretext of quarantine enforcement were preparing to "bulldoze" black voters.[70]

The first frost in New Orleans was recorded on November 2. The city of Mobile immediately lifted its rigid quarantine and Galveston was expected to follow soon, and the *Picayune* was pleased to report a "general abatement and almost complete cessation of yellow fever in every direction." Local quarantines were being raised all along the Red and Ouachita rivers, and from Natchez, notorious for the sternness of its quarantine even in a season of harsh policies, came welcome word that packets would be able to put in sometime the following week to take on cotton, though armed guards would still be posted around the wharf to keep any people or fomites from being landed. Many places, in fact, would keep mattresses, jute bagging, woolen goods, and similar articles under ban until well into December. The board of health in New Orleans issued a bulletin advising that, as final safety measures, living quarters should be fumigated with burning sulfur, and commercial buildings and crated merchandise should be opened up and exposed to the purifying action of the cold air. Meanwhile, the city's months-long depression was rapidly lifting, the hotels were reopening and filling up as a result of the revival of railroad and steamboat traffic, and as the city's leading daily summarized: "The political cauldron is boiling, the organ grinder and the tramp have reappeared, and New Orleans is once more herself again."[71]

70. *Ibid.*, November 1, 1878; Bemiss, "Yellow Fever in Louisiana," 91–94; *Medical Times and Gazette*, October 26, 1878, p. 498.

71. New Orleans *Picayune*, October 30, 31, November 1, 3, 1878.

FOUR

The Disaster at Memphis

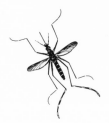

The most aberrant and surprising feature of the 1878 epidemic was Yellow Jack's deep reach into the interior—to many places in Mississippi, Tennessee, and Kentucky it had never visited or even remotely threatened in the past. The tragedy of the epidemic was vastly augmented by its diffusion to scores of virgin communities whose populations were almost entirely non-immune. Yellow fever would touch down with the most desolating effects in those very towns that had no history of the disease. The long, warm spring had obviously served to foster unusually numerous and lively populations of *A. aegypti* at these up-country locations, where in previous years the yellow fever mosquito had never managed to develop more than a feeble presence. The malignant outbreak at the town of Grenada in the heart of Mississippi, three hundred miles north of New Orleans, epitomized the deadly results of that combination of factors. The heavy mortality of the epidemic, the suddenness of its onset, and its bomblike effect on an astonished community focused national attention on this obscure country town for a few weeks in August, until events at Grenada were overshadowed by even more disastrous developments at the city of Memphis.

Like the other towns in the area, Grenada had no prior acquaintance with yellow fever in epidemic form. The town had taken in refugee cases from Memphis as recently as 1873 with no ill consequence to itself, and as Dr. H. J. Ray, president of the Grenada County Board of Health, recalled: "This lulled our people into a state of apathy, and they hugged the delusive idea that the death-dealing poison never would spread here." After yellow fever was proclaimed at New Orleans, the town enforced a nominal quarantine, to the extent of banning a few goods thought liable to carry infection. Trains were allowed to stop, although "suspicious characters" (presumably meaning those known to have come from infected neighborhoods in New Orleans) were not allowed to remain. Dr. Ray acknowledged that "these rules were not strictly enforced, and simply amounted to no quarantine." "Notwithstanding this, however," as it was later recognized, "the terrible malady which stealthily insinuated itself into an unsuspecting community had been scattering the seeds of poison for two weeks or more before quarantine was even talked of, which later brought forth a harvest of suffering and death."[1]

On the evening of July 24, the day yellow fever at New Orleans was first disclosed in the newspapers, two ladies were suddenly taken with chills at a residence on Depot Street in Grenada. One shortly recovered, but the other, a Mrs. Field, died on the thirty-first. "She had black vomit, suppression of urine, skin very yellow, and the body after death very much discolored, swelled rapidly and very offensive." These were all classic tokens of yellow fever, but her case was recorded by the unsuspecting doctors as one of "congestive fever." There was a brief lull, then on August 5 two more fatal cases cropped up farther down the street—a clerk at a variety store and a mulatto woman who dwelled at the county jail. These deaths were tentatively diagnosed as "malignant bilious fever." From those apparent "points of infection," the disease proceeded to "spread like wildfire over ‚the town." "Her physicians were so completely dazed that they could not realize what they had to deal with. The people, panic-stricken, began to flee into the adjoining country and to distant cities." On the eleventh, a group of expert diagnosticians called up from New Orleans identified the mysterious plague as "yellow fever of the most aggravated type," whereupon citizens remaining in town attempted a frantic cleanup in imitation of the Crescent City, emptying and disinfecting privies and cellars, and removing and burning all sorts of rotten debris. "The town was strewn with lime from one end to the other, carbolic acid was freely used, and tar smokes were kept up night and day, almost to suffocation, to the great annoyance of both well and sick." "All this availed nothing,"

1. H. J. Ray, "The Epidemic at Grenada, 1878," in Mississippi Board of Health, *Report for 1878–79* (Jackson, 1879), 41–42.

Dr. Ray's subsequent report to the Mississippi State Board of Health observed, "but seemingly served as pabulum for the all-conquering disease." The atmosphere over the stricken town had meanwhile taken on a "yellow saffron appearance . . . quite prominent," we are assured in the same document, "because it was noted by the physicians and others," but attributable, in retrospect, not to any miasmatic condition but to the mind-bending effects of high anxiety.[2] Dispatches from Grenada printed in the *Picayune* on the sixteenth suggest the volcanic suddenness with which yellow fever had overtaken the community and the nightmarish situation it engendered:

> Oh sir it is heart-rending every morning to learn that some relative or dear friend died during the night. About twenty-five died up to sundown yesterday. Five died last night and this morning up to nine o'clock. We have 150 to 200 sick and new cases every hour or two. What is to become of us God only knows. Many are yet without nurses or provisions. [August 14]
>
> Last night was fearful on the yellow fever victims. The death list— fourteen—was the largest since its appearance. There was great excitement during the day, many more flying the town. The population is now reduced to not over 300 whites. Total deaths 55; number of cases down estimated at 150. The New Orleans physicians pronounce it the most virulent type. The distress is too fearful to contemplate. [August 15]

"There is a wild panic throughout Mississippi," the St. Louis *Globe-Democrat* reported on August 13, as news of the unprecedented outbreak at Grenada sent a shock wave of fright and surprise through the threatened region. Surrounding towns and counties were promulgating rigid quarantine restrictions and barricading lines of travel, but the sudden scattering of Grenada's citizens earlier in the week had already carried the virus to many nearby communities. The town of Water Valley, thirty miles northeast of Grenada, had been in direct daily contact by railroad with its infected neighbor, had already taken a number of fugitives from there into its midst, and had time to make only a feeble gesture at organizing a quarantine before hysteria took the upper hand. A letter to the *Picayune* posted from Water Valley on August 15 described the panicky flight to wherever

2. *Ibid.,* 42–46.

of most of the town's white inhabitants, a strange parade of wheelbarrows, dray carts, rockaways, buckboards, "in fact every conceivable style of conveyance is pressed into service to help the exit. . . . Everyone who can get away from Water Valley is getting. They stand not on the order of their going." Another communication on the twentieth from the same correspondent offered fuller details. "A citizen of this place at work in Grenada came home a few days ago and said he had eaten two watermelons and drank more whiskey than was good for him, and went to bed sick. His case has since been pronounced to be a well-developed case of yellow fever, and then the exodus from this point began. His house has been so barricaded with boxes and barrels that a rocky mountain goat could not get over them." "The fear of the fever at this point and at villages situated off from the railroad is unbounded," the writer emphasized. Water Valley people trying to obtain board out in the Yalobusha County countryside were being met by reception committees packing loaded shotguns, and it was said some of the bridges outside town had been burned in an effort to turn away the efflux of refugees.[3]

Communications from Grenada indicated a rapidly disintegrating situation. The town was cut off from all its sources of supply, and provisions for both sick and well were running out. "The negroes are demoralized. Stores are being robbed," a telegram from the desolate town cried on August 23: "Not over twenty active men in town. The agony and suffering of the sick is beyond description." The infection, pursuing a rapid east-to-west course over the town, had invaded the Negro section, and most of the blacks, terror-stricken, had scattered into the nearby hills, where they were reported to be fashioning huts for themselves from mud and branches and living off the land. The town was consequently left in its emergency without a work force. It appeared that Grenada's sick were being left to die, and the dead left unburied. "The burial corps has disbanded, leaving those who are well to bury the dead in the nearest soil," wrote the Associated Press agent in the area. "The only hope for Grenada is for a corps of men to go there and remove the population, sick and well, to the hills south of the town and put them in tents." At the direction of the secretary of war, the U.S. Army Quartermaster at Louisville dis-

---

3. New Orleans *Picayune*, August 17, 22, 1878. See also H. A. Gant, "The Epidemic in Water Valley, 1878," in Mississippi Board of Health, *Report for 1878–79*, 69–72.

patched volunteers with tents and 15,000 rations of pork, beans, sugar, and coffee to the Grenada vicinity on August 26.[4]

The rations were distributed and the chaotic situation was somewhat relieved, but it was not practicable to thoroughly depopulate the town, and the infection continued its relentless "feeding." "The most fearful war could not have produced a greater desolation," remarked a correspondent of the St. Louis *Globe-Democrat,* who came through in the first week of September aboard a train to New Orleans. Trains would not consider stopping at the accursed spot but would roll through only as slowly as safety dictated, but never at less than 20 miles an hour and with their whistles blowing and doors and windows shut tight. "Grenada, passed in the night, contained a single light, illuminating the yellow face of a corpse lying on the railway platform." "Tonight the air is filled with bad odors," a letter from the helpless town said on the 4th. "The disease has accumulated to where there is no safety anywhere, so far as the infection is concerned. The end is near and the victory to the demon of plague." A definite abatement in the Grenada fever was not reported until two weeks later, and then travelers were warned it was not because the pestilence had grown less malignant but only because it was feeling "a want of material to feed upon"—which was a way of saying that the epidemic was finally running out of nonimmune subjects. The seemingly histrionic newspaper accounts of yellow fever's virulence at Grenada were not at all exaggerated, as it turned out. Grenada had been a community of about 2,500 people, almost evenly divided between blacks and whites. According to H. J. Ray's final estimate, 1,050 severe cases in the ordeal left not fewer than 260 whites and 90 blacks dead. "Only four persons escaped who remained through the epidemic."[5]

The first professional appraisal of what was happening at Grenada came from W. R. Mandeville, an experienced physician and autopsist who had been among the first to answer the call to the stricken town, and then returned to New Orleans on the nineteenth of August. Although a veteran of several severe epidemics in the Crescent City, as well as at Shreveport, Dr. Mandeville declared that he "never saw anything that could begin to compare with it, it is fearful beyond description." He said that although

4. New Orleans *Picayune,* August 23, 24, 31, 1878.

5. St. Louis *Globe-Democrat,* September 6, 1878; New Orleans *Picayune,* September 6, 25, 26, 1878; Ray, "Epidemic at Grenada," 45.

the fever was of an extraordinarily malignant type, black vomit did not seem to be frequent in the fatal cases. "The disease seems to attack the kidneys more violently than is generally observed in yellow fever, and sometimes the patients die from effusion of blood in the brain." He discussed some of the ideas that had emerged concerning the genesis of the Grenada fever, the favorite theory being that it was traceable to some evil-smelling debris that had been exposed when a "sewer" was dug up for repairs back in June:

> Several causes are assigned by the people of Grenada for the origin of the fever. According to one theory it was produced by the opening of a sewer which runs through one of the principal streets. In this sewer were found many carcasses of hogs, dogs, cats, and other animals, which were in a condition of putrefaction, and under the torrid heat of the sun were shortly decomposed, giving off gases of a nature most deleterious to health. A Mrs. Field, who lived near this sewer, which was left open for weeks, was taken ill and died. Other cases of a similar character followed, and in a few days about thirty-five persons were down. . . . Another hypothesis which has been put forward to account for the appearance of the fever was that Mrs. Field, shortly before her illness, had received a dress from New Orleans, and had been infected by the garment.[6]

A local-causationist from an earlier period would unhesitatingly have fixed upon the "sewer" as the source of the fever epidemic, but H. J. Ray was not inclined to give any weight to the theory in this instance. In his report to the Mississippi State Board of Health, he explained that "the famous sewer" was in fact nothing but an ordinary street culvert, and the section that had been opened had been no more than twenty feet long and perhaps three feet deep. "Visitors would be astonished at its almost insignificance, and it would never be discovered unless pointed out to them." While admitting that the emanations could have exercised a certain "noxious influence," he flatly declared that "I do not believe it had anything to do with generating the yellow fever poison." Dr. Ray observed that many families had lived closer to the drain and to the filthy part of town than Mrs. Field. He was unable to confirm the rumor about the mail-order

6. New Orleans *Picayune,* August 23, 1878.

dress, however, and so the mystery of how the "poison" came to Grenada and why it singled out Mrs. Field for its first target remained unsolved.[7]

The infection's derivation was somewhat clearer at the town of Holly Springs, 80 miles northeast of Grenada, where the first imported case of yellow fever—a Grenada man—was in evidence by August 19. By the twenty-fifth, six cases of yellow fever had appeared at Holly Springs—all Grenada refugees—and other communities in the state, including Jackson, saw reason to put Holly Springs under quarantine and began to refuse mail from it. "As the fever is confined altogether to refugees," a letter from the town protested, "this cannot be rightfully called an infected place." Holly Springs was situated in healthy pine-hill country, boasting an elevation of over six hundred feet, and its officials continued to insist that its atmosphere was "too pure for yellow fever to spread." Subsequent events soon demonstrated the contrary. A telegram from the town on the second of September admitted "considerable sickness among our people the past few days." The prevailing indisposition was supposed to be a type of "congestion," which was blamed on "the recent change in the weather," another hot spell having set in. On the fourth, the *Picayune* reported fifty people stricken down at Holly Springs, with two deaths, and what was in progress was described as "a grand hurrying out of town by railroad and private conveyance." The malady in question was described as "a hard chill, followed by a fever of the most obstinate character. . . . The physicians say it is not yellow fever, but it threatens life just the same." Of course it really was yellow fever, and this cry of distress was telegraphed the following day: "The stores are all closed and all the people gone away who can. . . . Physicians are broken down. . . . Many cases will die today. . . . Gloom, despair, and death rule the hour, and the situation is simply appalling. The outside world are appealed to for help."[8]

The banks and post office at Holly Springs were shut down, business of all sorts was paralyzed, and the general situation, according to one dispatch, was like nothing so much as "a terrible dream." "I served through the Peninsula campaign with McClellan, and there became accustomed to scenes of excitement and death," wrote a Chicago doctor who had rushed

7. Ray, "Epidemic at Grenada," 41–42, 45.
8. New Orleans *Picayune,* August 25, September 3, 4, 5, 1878.

to the town to volunteer his services, "but what I witnessed yesterday and today in this town, in the way of black vomit, fever, and delirium, by far surpasses all former experience." "The best feature is," a communication on the eighth said, "most of the population is gone." But this obviously referred only to those fortunate enough to have places to go and money to carry them. Three weeks later, on the twenty-sixth, Holly Springs reported "affairs fearful" and said at least 500 were down with the disease. Indeed, at few places were the effects of the epidemic so traumatic as here. At the end of October, more than a week after the first hard frost, all the stores were still closed and no business was being transacted. Holly Springs, a community of 3,500 when the epidemic commenced, had been reduced to 1,500 people during the peak of the outbreak, of whom only 300 or so were whites. Only a few dozen escaped the fever, and 215 whites and 89 blacks had perished.[9]

The town of Winona, 20 miles south of Grenada, was in a position to learn from Holly Springs' grievous example and emptied itself so thoroughly in a stampede on September 20 that it was said only 150 of its 1,500 people remained. Among the first to run were the town's three doctors, along with the sheriff and all his deputies. The wisdom of prompt evacuation was apparent at the end of the season, when Winona counted only 31 cases and 10 deaths.[10] The panicky abandonment of communities that had fallen into the fever's grasp had a counterpart in the desperate efforts of uninfected towns to ward off the disease. The dead-serious policy of "shotgun quarantine" became, for a season, the overriding consideration in all aspects of Mississippi life in both town and country. "Without leave, license, or law, trade was embargoed and travel prohibited," J. M. Keating would write. "For the sake of humanity, men became inhuman. For the sake of saving those out of the fever's reach from its touch or taint, they denied a refuge to those who were fleeing from it. Law was everywhere suspended, but order was maintained."[11] Wagon roads leading into settle-

9. Chicago *Tribune*, September 11, 1878; New Orleans *Picayune*, September 6, 8, 26, 27, October 29, 1878; F. W. Dancy, "The Epidemic at Holly Springs, Miss., in 1878," in Mississippi Board of Health, *Report for 1878–79*, 59–63.

10. B. F. Ward, "Epidemic at Winona, 1878," in Mississippi Board of Health, *Report for 1878–79*, 151–55.

11. John M. Keating, *The Yellow Fever Epidemic of 1878 in Memphis, Tenn.* (Memphis, 1879), 109.

ments were placarded with no-entry notices, and armed pickets were posted outside town limits. According to the regulations in force at most places, strangers were allowed to pass only if they could show papers demonstrating "indubitable proof of freedom from infection." Physicians around the state were said to be doing a brisk business supplying these affidavits. The documentation necessary to get into Aberdeen, a county seat of some 2,300 inhabitants situated 80 miles east of Grenada, was spelled out as follows: "To let none pass or repass except such as were duly qualified by having a certificate from a practising doctor of medicine, with an oath before a Justice of the Peace avowing its correctness, etc., and the impressed seal of a county official. The certificate to certify that the bearer had not been in a yellow fever infected district nor exposed in any way to yellow fever for twenty-five days past. Goods of no description were allowed from infected places." [12]

The railroads were recognized as the main couriers of infection and were subjected to a particularly close watch. A relief physician from New Orleans, who took the train up through central Mississippi to Winona in September, described scenes "perhaps the most remarkable of any previously recorded in any epidemic which has preceded this." Tracksides and depot platforms were snowy with scattered quicklime; streets fronting on the tracks were roped off and guarded by men with shotguns; bonfires burned in the intersections—a tribute of sorts to the widespread acceptance by this time of the germ theory of yellow fever.[13] Of course, these quarantines were much more effective in choking off commercial intercourse and the flow of goods than they were in preventing the infiltration of people—a result not really unanticipated or undesired, since fomites, after all, were perceived as the main danger. Retail business in most country towns was brought to a dead standstill, but the net consequences were open to different interpretations. No town suffered actual starvation, and it could be argued that what the merchants lost in sales and profits was just that much saved by the farmers and laborers, a retrenchment especially to be appreciated when the cotton crop came short that fall. Oxford, like most towns, estimated business losses in the thousands of dollars and bemoaned its hardships, but a few of the deeper thinkers, like a doctor in

12. Mississippi Board of Health, *Report for 1878–79*, 139.
13. New Orleans *Picayune,* September 26, 1878.

the nearby town of Pope, saw the forced economy brought about by the quarantine situation as a real benefit, "as it stopped to a great extent so much credit trade, which is a curse to any community."[14] As the summer dragged on, the towns inevitably found themselves having to balance the necessity of keeping infection out against that of bringing mail and vital supplies in, and quarantine rules were modified accordingly. The experience of Sardis, a town on the Mississippi & Tennessee Railroad midway between Memphis and Grenada, was typical:

> We quarantined against Grenada, New Orleans, and other points south on the day the fever was declared to exist in Grenada. This saved us, as we learned next day that the train would have brought us a number of refugees from that city, but for our prompt action. Two or three days afterwards, the fever having been declared at Memphis, we quarantined against that city and all other infected points. First we permitted no trains to stop, but exchanged mails as the trains ran slowly through. After a few days we permitted trains to stop at the depot, but did not permit passengers to land or mingle with citizens, nor any baggage or freight to be unloaded, except ice, medicines, disinfectants, and certain kinds of provisions. No one was allowed to come in contact with the men running the trains except those whose duties required them to do so, such as depot agent, telegraph operator, and mail carrier. Trains were stopped at designated points out of town and boarded by an officer who notified passengers of these regulations. On the 4th of September we quarantined against all mail matter except first class. On the 9th of September, finding it impracticable to keep citizens away from trains when they stopped, we prohibited the stopping of trains inside the corporate limits, and established a station outside where mails were exchanged and freights not prohibited received and shipped. October 7th it was ordered that no goods or freights of any kind should be permitted to come in except drugs, and those only from points not infected, and to be unpacked outside of town and the packing burned.
> When the fever broke out at Senatobia, thirteen miles distant, and was raging at Hernando, Holly Springs, Water Valley, and other towns around us, the roads leading into town were picketed to prevent persons coming in from infected places. A volunteer police force patrolled the town at night for the same purpose. All quarantine regulations were abolished about the 11th of November.[15]

14. Mississippi Board of Health, *Report for 1878–79*, 111, 129.
15. *Ibid.*, 116.

We can readily see that even Sardis' rigid quarantine left open plenty of opportunities for introduction of the infection, and yet, owing to a lack of *A. aegypti,* or some other fortuitous circumstance, the epidemic never appeared there. In fact, many towns like Sardis were passed over and like Sardis would attribute their escape "altogether to quarantine, so far as any human agency was concerned." Places where yellow fever broke out in spite of comparably strict measures tended to conclude it was because their quarantines were "inefficiently conducted." "While many of our towns became infected," the delegation from the Mississippi State Board of Health would tell the American Public Health Association in Richmond in November, "still most of them entirely escaped through the efficiency of quarantines, and instances are not wanting where entire counties occupying exposed positions thus escaped." The health officer of Adams County expressed the idea more forcefully, if less politely: "Vigilance, activity, fearlessness, and the double-barrel shotgun will give a community entire immunity from yellow fever."[16]

The germ theory and the danger of yellow fever's importation were uppermost in the minds of responsible officials at Memphis, Tennessee, and there was great concern in Memphis on July 27 when the telegraph brought warning that the *John Porter,* the New Orleans towboat that had just put off two "sunstroke" cases at Vicksburg that turned out to be yellow fever, had passed Helena, Arkansas, and was continuing up the river. "That it exists in New Orleans at this time cannot now be doubted, and that it may be brought here by river communication is equally unquestioned," the mayor of Memphis admonished the city's board of health that evening. "We owe it to the public to diminish the possibilities of the visitation of this dreadful scourge, and so I must urge upon you the adoption of any means to secure this end." The board commenced hasty arrangements to hedge the city about with quarantine stations at all major points of access. All inbound railroad freights were ordered to be immediately offloaded at points several miles outside the city for ten days' detainment and disinfection. Starting August 3, all freight originating in New Orleans or Vicksburg was to be embargoed completely and sent back to where it came from. Examining physicians and squads of "detectives" were also stationed at these checkpoints to scrutinize passengers headed for Memphis. Anyone whose condition appeared "suspicious" was to be escorted

16. *Ibid.,* 32, 91.

directly to the city hospital for further observation. All baggage was to be intercepted and impounded. River traffic was subjected to the same general regulations. A quarantine and detention facility was set up at the lower end of President's Island, six miles below the city, and furnished with a twelve-pound cannon to underscore its authority.[17]

Property owners in the city were meanwhile enjoined to remove garbage, empty privies, and otherwise clean up their premises, and police were directed to double as sanitary inspectors on their patrols, looking for accumulations of filth and issuing orders to remove nuisances. On August 1, the last of the city's contingency fund was drained to hire 125 laborers to rake out gutters in the downtown section and cart away the debris. A citizens' committee resolved to raise more money by subscription to further the work. Hogs and cattle, which normally enjoyed the freedom of the city, were to be rounded up by their owners and driven outside the corporation limits by the sixth. The *Avalanche* helpfully suggested that those who kept stables should sprinkle them well with carbolic acid. The *Appeal* offered that, in spite of the close weather, people should keep wood or resin fires burning in their houses at night. On their own initiative, householders around the city had begun burning substances like camphor and pine tar around their yards, along with such other things as charcoal soaked in turpentine, and coal oil mixed with sawdust. The board of health confidently asserted that Memphis would be put in excellent sanitary order within a week, and it was reported abroad that "there seems no possibility of the fever's reaching Memphis this year."[18]

Memphis' early preparations were followed by a fortnight of high tension and suspense as the board's quarantine program had to be defended on several fronts. On August 2, a deputation of merchants protested that a thirty-car train carrying $40,000 worth of sugar, coffee, and hardware from New Orleans had been sidetracked at Whitehaven by the management of the Mississippi & Tennessee Railroad in view of the impending Memphis embargo, and the people there were making threats to burn it all up if it were not moved on. An implied lawsuit was obviously an effective pry to use on a nearly bankrupt city government that had just had

17. Memphis *Avalanche*, July 28, 31, 1878; Mildred Hicks, ed., *Yellow Fever and the Board of Health: Memphis 1878* (Memphis, 1964), 8–9.

18. Memphis *Avalanche*, August 1, 1878; New Orleans *Picayune*, August 1, 1878; Memphis *Appeal*, August 6, 1878.

difficulty scraping up even $8,000 for emergency sanitary work. The train was given special permission to proceed to Memphis. Leaks in the quarantine against persons were a great worry also, and it was widely known that unprincipled skiffmen from over on the Arkansas shore were ferrying parties across under cover of darkness and landing them at isolated places under the bluff. On the seventh, the board of health finally prevailed on authorities in neighboring Hopefield, Arkansas, to cooperate in policing out travelers from downriver. All the same, on the evening of the ninth, the Memphis night watch had to head off five boats that approached "with muffled oars" and tried to effect a landing at the foot of Beale Street.[19]

The tempo of events quickened after August 12, when a flurry of distress telegrams from Grenada, one hundred miles away, confirmed the worst about the nature of the sickness that had broken out there. Grenada, which just a few days before had denounced as a "canard" the suggestion that the "bilious fever" making such rapid strides in the town was really yellow fever, sent Memphis this description of the state of affairs on the twelfth: "All are panic-stricken. The mayor is down. The sheriff and all the city officers have left, the jail thrown open and the prisoners gone. New cases are developing all the time." At least half of Grenada's whites had fled; more than one hundred were already sick with the fever; banks were shut down; merchants had closed shop; and because farmers were not coming to town, chickens, milk, and other necessities could not be had. The Memphis Board of Health immediately posted armed guards at all stations on the railroad between Grenada and home and with reassuring bulletins tried to quiet the "extravagant rumors" circulating in the city. "There is considerable uneasiness in Memphis," observed the *Avalanche*. "Frightened people repeat frightful stories of cases all over the city, and men who ought to have better sense, and more manliness, are giving currency to wild reports. . . . As a matter of fact Memphis was never in summer freer from disease of all kinds than now." As a matter of fact it later transpired that fever cases of a malignant character had been occurring sporadically around the city since at least July 21, but the symptoms had been too unclear (or the doctors too intimidated) to make the diagnosis of yellow fever. The season's symbolic first bale of new cotton was brought

19. Hicks, ed. *Yellow Fever and the Board of Health*, 11–15; Memphis *Avalanche*, August 9, 10, 1878; Memphis *Appeal*, August 11, 1878.

up from Bolivar County, Mississippi, on the twelfth, a good two weeks ahead of the 1877 schedule. Memphis newspapers discussed the fine prospects this signaled for the city's fall trade, a rebuke to the "alarmists on the street corners" who threatened to spoil the cheerful outlook with their continued talk about yellow fever.[20]

The same hot weather that made the cotton precocious had given encouragement to Memphis' mosquitoes, making the city a virtual yellow fever powder house—into which live embers had already floated unobserved. On the morning of August 13, the death of a woman who kept a waterfront eating stand was disclosed—an unmistakable case of yellow fever—and the reaction was immediate. The *Avalanche* described the vigorous effort being made to check the disease. The whole block of Adams and Front was cordoned off by the police, and the infected site was surrounded by barrels of coal oil and carbolic acid, "from which men were filling buckets and sprinklers, and with speed sprinkling walls, streets, and pavements. . . . The sidewalk was black with carbolic acid, and from streets and walls arose the smell of tar and lime almost stifling." The city's health officer analyzed the snack house: "A bad dwelling place, redolent with the odor of fish. There the woman, an habitual and very hard drinker, lived, right in among the fumes of her food and its debris and its trash. A boatman from New Orleans, had he carried in his clothes to that spot the smallest amount of contagion, it would have found a soil in which the seed of disease could not but germinate." Local residents pointed out that a shipment of sugar lately brought in from New Orleans was warehoused nearby, suggesting another likely source of "contagion." The woman's body was coffined up tightly and taken out and buried that afternoon, and the contents of her shop were burned in the street out front. The attention directed at this case tended to obscure the simultaneous death from yellow fever of a policeman living on Poplar Avenue.[21]

The next day another nineteen cases of yellow fever were identified in Memphis and there were three more deaths; the long-brewing crisis was unquestionably at hand. "The terrible plague that is so rapidly spreading

20. Memphis *Avalanche*, August 13, 1878. See also Tennessee Board of Health, *First Report, April 1887 to October 1880* (Nashville, 1880), 82–84, 87–92; "The Epidemic in Memphis: Histories of Early Cases," Paper 2 in "Report of the Yellow Fever Commission on the Epidemic of 1878," Record Group 90, National Archives.

21. Memphis *Avalanche*, August 14, 1878; Memphis *Appeal*, August 14, 1878.

in our midst requires prompt and continued action," cried the newspapers. The board of health reported only twelve barrels of carbolic acid in inventory and requested the city to order thirty more by express. Some of the barrels on hand were forwarded to the police department for free distribution in the slums. The board resolved that all persons dying of "any suspicious character of fever" should be coffined and buried within six hours and advised the public against attending their funerals. It received complaints from a group of citizens about the "offensive odors" emanating from the huge talus of excrement that had piled up at "the slide and dump at the foot of Webster Street," the point on the bluff where Memphis householders had been discharging the contents of their privy vaults in compliance with the board's clean-up order of two weeks before. The board directed that all such dumping be stopped and asked that people begin treating their privies with disinfectants instead. It also decided to call a halt to the city crews' scraping and stirring of the gutters, holding that the activity only aggravated the foulness of the town's atmosphere.[22]

The city's chief of police was alarmed to find out that for the past two weeks travelers off the river had been slipping freely into South Memphis at night by way of the unguarded yard of the gas works at Fort Pickering. Spontaneous departures from the city had meanwhile commenced "with a terrible rush. . . . The trains on the Memphis & Charleston and Memphis & Louisville railroads leaving the city yesterday and last night were jammed and packed to the very last degree, and hundreds upon hundreds of our very best citizens left for the East and North." General evacuation of the city was already being counseled by the city's doctors and newspapers, but intelligent Memphians had gotten sufficient taste of yellow fever five years before and really needed no special prompting. The "camping scheme" suggested in 1873 was remembered, and tentative provisions were being made for orderly removal of the city's poor. On August 15, the Memphis postmaster requested the loan of one thousand tents from the U.S. Army arsenal at Louisville. The request was granted immediately but somewhat awkwardly, Secretary of War McCrary remarking that there was "no law for such proceedings other than the law of humanity."[23]

For the next three days, observers marveled at the "unparalleled stam-

22. Memphis *Avalanche,* August 15, 1878; Hicks, ed., *Yellow Fever and the Board of Health,*17–20.

23. Memphis *Appeal,* August 16, 1878.

pede" and "mighty outpouring" taking place at Memphis. "The trains leaving the city continue to be jammed and crowded by frightened citizens." It was said at least 20,000 people took off by rail, and a single line reported ticket sales in excess of $35,000—no small sum when a dollar a day was considered a not-unreasonable wage. The hurry and anxiety about getting out of town was heightened by the girdle of rigid quarantines closing down around Memphis on all sides. The city council of Little Rock, capital of the neighboring state of Arkansas, stretched its charter powers to the limit in commanding—and enforcing—a total shutdown of traffic on the 140-mile Little Rock & Memphis Railroad on August 16. Evansville, Indiana, completely embargoed all traffic from points south of the Ohio River. Cincinnati, Ohio, was refusing all baggage from the south and was granting admission to refugees only after they had been certified as fever-free by the city's own sanitary officers. Though it was admittedly acting "without a shadow of a law to sustain it," the health department of Cincinnati reached into adjoining states and establishing halting stations on the railroads 30 miles out, at Lawrenceburg, Indiana, and Walton, Kentucky. Physicians and policemen rode the passenger trains in from those points, and if they detected "any persons suffering from suspicious symptoms," they had orders to see to it that the parties in question passed through Cincinnati without ever stepping out of the coaches. All boats ascending the Ohio River were being hauled over to the Kentucky shore for similar scrutiny.[24]

Although it was condemned for its laxness and even threatened with rigid quarantine by Cincinnati, the city of Louisville, Kentucky, declined to enforce any restrictions at all and stood as the main beacon of escape for Memphis refugees. Public opinion in Louisville was fortified by the published statements of the faculty of its medical college, who maintained that the city's latitude, altitude, and improved sanitary condition rendered it "plague-proof." In a newspaper interview, one of them went so far as to

---

24. Memphis *Avalanche,* August 17, 18, 1878; R. G. Jennings, "The Quarantine at Little Rock, Arkansas, during August, September, and October 1878, against the Yellow Fever Epidemic in Memphis and the Mississippi Valley," *Reports and Papers, American Public Health Association,* IV (1878), 223–27; Thomas C. Minor, *Report on Yellow Fever in Ohio as It Appeared during the Summer of 1878* (Cincinnati, 1878), 40–45. See also "Shot-Gun Quarantines," *Boston Medical and Surgical Journal,* C (1879), 338–42, for a good account of the travails of a Memphis businessman and his family, who sought refuge in the Arkansas countryside at this time.

declare that the yellow fever refugees presented no more of a threat to the safety of Louisville than "the securely-caged wild beasts in a zoological garden." Louisville's liberality was quite the exception, however. Pittsburgh, Pennsylvania, three hundred miles beyond Louisville, and over seven hundred miles from Memphis, was alarmed to the point of establishing quarantine stations outside its city limits. Illinois was turning back all freight from the south, while the city of Cairo, the most exposed point in the state, went a step further and established a rigid personal quarantine that prohibited trains from stopping and steamboats from landing if they came from anywhere below. On August 19, Cairo extended its ban to include all vessels bound up or down, after discovering that wily refugees had been crossing up the system by transferring at places upriver and coming back down on other boats. Memphis, like New Orleans, found the smaller towns of its immediate neighborhood falling in behind the larger and more distant centers in imposing quarantines and embargoes against it. On the fifteenth, the burg of Collierville, twenty miles out on the Charleston Road, served notice in the typical way: "Memphians had better hunt homes elsewhere, as they may subject themselves to heavy fines by stopping here. Our own citizens will not be allowed to return without a permit, if they go to Memphis on business. Trains will not be allowed to put off a sick passenger here. The railroad and dirt roads will be thoroughly patrolled. Conductors of trains would do well to notice the fines for bringing any sick or complaining to town." Collierville apologetically went on to say that there had been no fear of yellow fever and no lack of hospitality to refugees in 1873, but in view of the alarming developments at Grenada, "we are having to stir ourselves." Lots and yards in Collierville were meanwhile being cleaned up, the streets were white with lime, and "the carbolic acid smells to Heaven." By the eighteenth, the Memphis & Louisville, Memphis & Paducah, and Mississippi & Tennessee railroads were terminating regular service to Memphis for the season, though the Memphis & Charleston line advertised, with sublime euphemism indeed, that its road through Somerville to points east would be open a few days more to accommodate "those who wish to free themselves of the heat and mosquitoes of the city."[25]

The great exodus by train was substantially over by August 18, and

25. Memphis *Avalanche,* August 15, 1878.

what remained of Memphis' population settled down to wait out the course of events. Just one hundred cases had been brought to light in the city so far, but in the excited public mind it might as well have been ten thousand. "Never, perhaps, in all history, certainly not in modern times, was there ever so complete a panic and so nearly a complete evacuation of a civilized city as has taken place in Memphis during the last few days," said the *Avalanche*. "Those who remember the hasty desertion of cities threatened by investing armies declare that nothing they have ever seen could compare with what has just transpired here. . . . A sad, weird kind of silence has fallen on the whole city and enveloped it in a mantle so strange and new as to make it appear ghostlike and supernatural to the last degree." There had been a final spurt in large-order business as the plantations below Memphis hastily and liberally stocked up on provisions, "enough to last them until after frost," but that, as well as ordinary retail trade in the city, was utterly dead by now. In the downtown area could be seen "an occasional desolate-looking streetcar passing along Main," and yet "along whole squares stores are closed, the windows are nailed and barred, and a placard here and there alone tell the tale of the absent owners." The flocks of pigeons had the intersections mostly to themselves, undisturbed. In residential parts of the city there was "a quietness surpassing that of a Sabbath in a New England village. . . . The windows are closed, the curtains down, the doors locked. . . . All is still, absolutely still. Occasionally a little negro passes by, but he seems affrighted at the noise of his own stick rattling against the paling, and moves quickly along in a subdued way."[26]

A citizens' meeting at the Opera House on the morning of August 16 had come to grips with a perplexing situation, after it was seen that most of the elected members of the city council had followed the policy of the rest of Memphis' "better class" and abandoned the city in the general stampede. The instincts of self-government came to the fore, and a "Citizens' Relief Committee" was promptly formed to take care of relief arrangements and organize basic municipal services. Property protection was uppermost in mind: police salaries were four months in arrears as it was, and many of the force had already deserted. The committee directed the mayor (who, to his credit, had stayed at his post) to raise $30,000 immediately

26. *Ibid.*, August 18, 1878.

and to pledge the next year's tax receipts as preferred security, and they proposed to force the issue with a writ of mandamus if he balked. Appeals for relief assistance were simultaneously telegraphed to the president in Washington and to the mayors of various northern cities.[27]

Evacuating the poor of the city loomed as the next critical problem. After the wealthy of Memphis had sped away by coach and rail to Newport and Niagara, and the middle class to intermediate resorts in the mountains of Tennessee and Kentucky, the people of few means or no means at all, leaving the city on foot or in wagons, had to hunt for places of refuge much closer at hand—whatever shelter could be cheaply reached and cheaply held. In the countryside all around Memphis, old slave cabins and even many chicken houses had been appropriated by city refugees, while at the Shelby County Fairgrounds, "every booth, every stall, to say nothing of the larger buildings, have been made the homes of people having fled for their lives." The government tents arrived from Louisville with an issue of 100,000 rations on the nineteenth, and the county militia, overriding the armed protests of farmers in the neighborhood, effected the establishment of a campground on a low, wooded rise five miles south of the city, a few hundred yards off the line of the Mississippi & Tennessee Railroad. About 100 Memphis people were located there immediately, and accommodations were readied for a total of 3,000. Ultimately, however, the municipal camp seems never to have attracted more than 600 or 700 of the city's people. Most preferred the more independent course of camping by themselves, as families or in small groups, which was not discouraged by the authorities, since it tended to save on rations and supplies. If a family would post bond for a tent, it was given to them to be carried to any point in the country they desired. On August 21, for example, 25 families had met together at the courthouse square and constituted themselves a typical "colony." They had located a place 6 miles out on the Cuba Road and intended to settle there directly. By the end of the week, it could be observed that "the flutter of private canvas is to be seen in every grove around Memphis." A letter from "Countryman" on the twenty-third complained about the widespread plundering of gardens and fruit trees in the suburbs by these people.[28]

27. *Ibid.*, August 17, 1878.
28. *Ibid.*, August 20, 21, 1878.

By August 22, the "equatorial" temperatures of the preceding week, when the mercury hovered around 100° F, had subsided into the eighties, yet the skies over Memphis were cloudy and oppressive by day, and the nights were "intensely warm"—ideal conditions for the activity of *A. aegypti*. At first it had been hoped that the fever could be confined to a certain infected district between High Street and the river, north of Jefferson Street and south of the Louisville railroad. The authorities were applying carbolic acid around infected houses and doing their best to collar "stray" cases for removal to the city hospital for isolation. The apparent geographic concentration of early cases was soon complicated by the breaking out of new cases on Alabama Street near the bayou; on certain blocks along Poplar, Washington, and Commerce; on Main near Washington; and on Linden past Lauderdale. Contemplating these "sorties" of the fever, the *Avalanche* concluded that "there is no doubt but what it has begun to defy the limits placed upon it." By August 23, new infected spots had been discovered on Monroe east of Wellington, at several places along Madison Street, and on Linden near Causey. Fifty-one new cases and ten deaths were reported that day, and the Memphis Board of Health was impelled to declare officially: "The increase in the number of yellow fever cases throughout the city has been so large, the Board feels it their duty to declare it epidemic, and urge all who can to leave the city forthwith." [29]

The depopulation of Memphis was not nearly so thorough as had been wished. Nearly all of the city's 15,000 blacks remained, believing (mistakenly, as it turned out) that they were inherently secure from yellow fever. Of the whites, an estimated 5,000 to 10,000 still lingered. Many stayed because they were apprehensive about leaving their property to the rather skimpy security that a makeshift police force could provide; a few because they had designs on the valuables others left behind; some because they were honor-bound to sick or dying friends or family; and others because of a larger sense of duty to the community. Perhaps a large percentage tarried because they were reckless, fatalistic, or simply stupid, but undoubtedly the greatest number stayed because they were destitute and convinced that they had no place to go. Efforts to get the people out of town were redoubled. "Depopulation is the forlorn hope," the *Avalanche* editorialized, "and to that end all the influences of begging, persuasion, and

29. *Ibid.*, August 22–24, 1878; Hicks, ed. *Yellow Fever and the Board of Health*, 26.

even compulsion must be turned on together. . . . These people must be gotten out of the city, must be, and the fever stamped out through lack of material for its ravages." Another 500 Army tents were forwarded to the city. The Memphis & Charleston Railroad was prevailed upon to offer free rides out of town to the indigent. Special police details and squads of volunteer relief workers ("visitors," they were called) began canvassing the infected neighborhoods, looking for unremoved dead and unreported sick, and urging all others to go out to the camps. These parties declared their astonishment at the terrible headway the epidemic had already made in the poor-white rookeries of the lower wards, as they came upon miserable scenes like this in a tenement room off Commerce Street: "Upon the bed lay the living and the dead—a husband cold and stiff, a wife in the agony of dissolution. On the floor, tossing in delirium, were two children of this pair, and beside them their little cousins, two little girls, themselves sick. To complete the repulsiveness of the scene and give it a touch of disgusting horror, a drunken man and a drunken woman, parents of the little fever-baked girls, were reeling and cursing, and stumbling over the dying and the dead."[30]

Out at the municipal camp, meanwhile, all was reported to be going well. Carbolic acid was being sprinkled over the ground, and the trunks of all the trees were being whitewashed. Nineteen refugee cases had appeared, but all of them had been promptly hospitalized, and it was earnestly hoped that the fever "can not spread in the pure air of those hills." Assurance was given that every comfort was provided at the municipal camp, and provided free, and that Negroes were welcomed with perfectly equal treatment—though all facilities, of course, were kept rigidly segregated.

The muggy weather broke with a rainstorm on the morning of August 26, and "vapors warm, oppressive, and foul" rose from the city's wooden pavements. The *Avalanche* reflected on the incongruity of a hot, bright sun overhead while below "the unseen shadow of disease and death is stalking streets and alleys." No fewer than 52 deaths from yellow fever had occurred over the weekend of August 25 to 26, 161 new cases had been reported, and it was understood that the latter figure approximated just a fraction of the real number. "The fever shows no abatement. On the con-

30. Memphis *Avalanche*, August 27, 1878.

trary, it has appeared in so many portions of the city, attacking so many persons who have not been exposed to the infection of the 'fever district,' that we are forced to the conclusion that the whole air is impregnated with the poison." The *Avalanche* dutifully continued to point out nuisances to the city authorities, as if the puny sanitary efforts still in progress could make a difference at this point: a stagnant, scummy gutter on New Madison Street badly in need of liming; rumors of new cases farther out on Poplar; and the crowded cabins of "Charleston Hill," a Negro slum at the head of Monroe Street, which would require "a curry comb to clean it out." As yet there was no great concern that the city's blacks were themselves seriously menaced by the epidemic, but their poor hovels were perceived as "foul nests of disease," where the ferment of yellow fever would soon be "germinating rapidly." The paper discussed a dominant mood of gloom and "individual fatality" in the city, with many taking to heavy doses of gin and whiskey, others to overloads of drugs. Public intoxication had become a serious problem, partly because of the prevailing demoralization and partly because of a belief cherished by many that to "get drunk and stay drunk" was good prophylaxis against yellow fever. At the concluding sessions of the police court, "drunk after drunk was brought in, tried, and mercifully discharged. . . . Keep your head," the paper pleaded, warning against intoxication as well as the spreading of rumors that could lead to panic or riot. Reports of widespread debauchery and housebreaking in the city, it assured its readers, were false.[31]

The isolation of the city was emphasized when it became known that the Vicksburg & Meridian Railroad had halted its trains the week before. "This cuts Memphis entirely off from Vicksburg, there being no river service below Friar's Point, Mississippi." Regular railroad service in and out of Memphis was now entirely suspended, though the Memphis & Louisville line had agreed to run short trains into the city with basic supplies as the call arose. On the river, cargo rates had been boosted prohibitively high and packet arrivals had largely ceased because of the quarantines, but it was expected that the departure of several boats from St. Louis would relieve the impending shortage of flour and cornmeal. Local-supply articles like milk and eggs had become extremely scarce, and for those there was no recourse. In commercial circles: "Three-fourths of the stores and

31. *Ibid.*, August 27, 28, 1878

business firms of the city are closed and the other fourth are doing nothing but a small order and retail business. Stocks are running very short and the market is bare of several articles of prime necessity. At present there is no talk of replenishing." The city's banks had not entirely closed their doors, but business was reduced to essential checking and depositing—all dealing in scrips and securities and the like was of course moribund—and hours were trimmed to just two a day, "short forces keeping short hours, and doing the little there is to do in short order." No shortage of funds seems to have developed, however, and despite the exodus of people, the volume of currency on hand was reported to be at its usual level.[32]

Every morning saw hundreds of people wheeling into the infected city in buggies and wagons. The motley parade was led by employees of the business houses that remained open, together with many others going in to shop, loaf, get rations, or get drunk. When evening approached, they all hurried back to their camps a few miles out in the country, safely away from "the noxious night air of the city." "The influx from the dusty roads begins about nine in the forenoon, and at six they are all scampering off again." Neither doctors nor police ever cautioned against this strange commute. Here we see in operation one of the most widespread, long-held, and dangerous of the fallacies about yellow fever—namely, that "daylight communication" with an infected place was "safe." Apparently, the notion was first advanced by Pliny the Elder with reference to malaria. It was reiterated centuries later by Lancisi and became entrenched in malaria folklore, and after settlement of the New World, it gradually became incorporated into the accepted wisdom about yellow fever as well. Its rationale depended on the classical concept of "miasma" as a toxic vapor that rose up from the ground after sundown and floated low in the night air, inducing "malarial" sickness in those who were out and exposed to it. We might speculate that it was an indirect recognition of the fact that the anopheline mosquitoes that transmit malaria are most active after dusk. The theory and practice of "daylight communication" could not have reflected any unconscious grasp of the circadian cycle of the yellow fever mosquito, however, for *A. aegypti* is, in fact, a daytime feeder and tends to be most active in the afternoon hours. If there was any truth in the theory as applied to yellow fever, it probably had to do with the fact that the

32. *Ibid.*, August 28, 29, 1878

destination of most daytime visitors to an infected city would have been the business and industrial districts, where *A. aegypti* was generally less abundant.[33]

Temperatures mounted back into the nineties in the first week of September, and the city embarked on a month of the utmost tribulation. The infection was rapidly gravitating to the suburbs, and appeals for everyone to clear out of all sections of Memphis were repeated: "The Plague's course is surely and directly toward the south. The old infected district having been burned black and bare, the fever's fires are striking human blood in South Memphis and burning it up. In the suburbs cases have appeared in every avenue almost, in many places deemed spots of perfect security." This development was particularly disturbing, since the higher and supposedly cleaner southern parts of the city had entirely escaped infection in 1873. This year, when the fever first appeared downtown, many residents of the "infected district" had rented rooms in these neighborhoods, thinking that they would be quite safe there, without the inconvenience of going out to the camps or away to northern cities. There had been at least 137 yellow fever deaths over the weekend of September 1, and the board of health no longer bothered trying to keep a tally on the myriads of new cases. "Fort Pickering is full of it; the Seventh Ward, including all of Beale, Vance, and adjacent cross-streets, are also thick with fever-stricken people; while Chelsea is covered with sick people. There is now no part of the corporate limits of the city not thoroughly infected with the fever poison." All through the weekend, all over the city, private hearses had "followed each other at a trot, carrying cases to the grave unattended by any but the hearse drivers." Some considered the absence of funeral processions to be a good thing, since they had formed one of the most depressing aspects of the plague in 1873. Nevertheless, according to the *Avalanche:* "Even this was not fast enough, and corpses accumulated in various parts of the city

33. *Ibid.,* August 22, 25, 1878. On the circadian cycle of *A. aegypti,* see S. R. Christophers, *Aedes aegypti (L.), the Yellow Fever Mosquito: Its Life History, Bionomics, and Structure* (Cambridge, Eng., 1960), 472–74; Leland O. Howard, Harrison G. Dyar, and Frederick Knab, *The Mosquitoes of North and Central American and the West Indies* (4 vols.; Washington, D.C., 1912), I, 262–70. On the theory of "daylight communication," see René LaRoche, *Yellow Fever, Considered in Its Historical, Pathological, Etiological, and Therapeutical Relations* (2 vols.; Philadelphia, 1855), II, 553–56; Henry Rose Carter, *Yellow Fever: An Historical and Epidemiological Study of Its Place of Origin* (Baltimore, 1931), 256.

until the fearful stench became alarmingly offensive. . . . Much confusion and disorder naturally follows this state of things."[34]

Even the official tally of deaths in the city lagged well behind the awful reality. Tracking "the scent of dissolution," police and citizens were making scores of grisly discoveries in all out-of-the-way places, even theater lofts and business offices, where delirious sufferers had closeted themselves and died. "One peculiarity manifested among many of the sick is a desire to seclude themselves, while among the poor there is unreasonable dread of being sent to the infirmary." The rotting bodies of three unknown tramps found crumpled between the book stacks at the deserted county library; a comatose wretch discovered in his room "alone, stark naked, and literally covered with flies"; a poor Negro woman dead in a hovel off Commerce Street, her still-living baby tugging a putrid breast; the corpse of "a well-known gentleman" discovered in the back office of a cotton brokerage, face eaten away by mice—these are a few specimens of the "Horrors of Memphis" retold lushly and luridly in newspapers across the country, but which originally appeared as matter-of-fact brevities in the columns of the Memphis half-sheets. "It is this that makes the situation so horrible," the New York *Herald* commented: "These decomposed bodies would cause sickness even in a more healthy atmosphere, but when the air is as poisoned as at present the fact of so many bodies remaining unburied for so long a time causes the best workers to despair of successfully fighting the fever." On September 4, the Citizens' Relief Committee threatened the county undertaker with prosecution if recovery of the dead were not expedited. Four big furniture wagons were pressed into service, which shuttled through the streets piled as high as possible with cheap, pine coffins. Burials at the potters' field were put under the direct supervision of the police department. An extra shift of diggers was hired to take advantage of the waxing moon, and the grim work of excavating the anonymous trenches and interring the city's fast-accumulating indigent dead was carried on around-the-clock, "among the weird shadows of night."[35]

34. Memphis *Appeal,* September 1, 1878; Memphis *Avalanche,* September 3, 1878.

35. Memphis *Avalanche,* September 5, 6, 1878; New Orleans *Picayune,* September 5, 1878; New York *Herald,* September 5, 1878. Interesting incidents and anecdotes, mostly gleaned from Memphis newspapers, are compiled in Keating, *Epidemic of 1878 in Memphis,* 145–94, and J. P. Dromgoole, *Yellow Fever Heroes, Honors, and Horrors of 1878* (Louisville, 1879), 61–106.

Officials hoped that these measures would bring the situation under control and that "the revolting discoveries of the past few days" would be over with, but daily mortality from the disease kept surging forward: 101 dead were listed on September 6, 112 on the ninth, 127 on the fourteenth, and the number of dead that eluded the official count was anyone's guess. With a macabre perfunctoriness, the *Avalanche* was pointing out "nuisances" of this character: "Yesterday on the corner of Vance and Avery Streets the horrible sight of three corpses three days dead met the eye of the visitor. Two had swollen to bursting, and all lay in a state of putrefaction. This does not look as if burial arrangements have attained to that boasted system and promptness." "Memphis," the Associated Press aptly declared at the height of the crisis, "is a charnel house torn open." The special correspondent of the Louisville *Courier-Journal* roamed avenues and alleys and sent the outside world strange word-pictures of the extremity to which an essentially modern American city had been reduced by pestilence: the "graveyard gloom and stillness" of the streets; the unattended sick crouched nodding and delirious in doorways; the hot humid atmosphere "heavy with the stench of dead bodies." "We read the history of the London Plague and it reads like romance, yet many parallel incidents are reproduced in this Southern Plague, and they are to us frightful realities."[36] The Chicago *Tribune* also had a reporter at the scene of destruction, and the impressions he recorded rival the most appalling passages in Defoe's history:

> Everything about the city bears the impress of calamity, dissolution, and forgetfulness. This is as true of Vance, Shelby, and Poplar Streets, where in time of health the beauty and chivalry of Memphis reign supreme, as it is of "Happy Hollow" and "Hell's Half-Acre," devoted to thieves, prostitutes, and the incubation and commission of crime. Robeson Street has been completely wiped out.
>
> The air is filled with the stench arising from burning and decaying matter, from the disinfecting mediums employed, vainly as some believe, and with the peculiar odor of the disease itself, which cannot be likened to anything in the arcana of Nature, but which can never be forgotten by those who have inhaled the poison. . . .

36. Memphis *Avalanche*, September 7, 1878; Louisville *Courier-Journal*, August 27, September 4, 7, 13, 1878.

As I write this evening the air is filled with poisonous gases from the body of a negress, "Jenny," who was employed as a cook at a boarding-house at the corner of Third and Madison Streets. Her remains are sup-posed to have lain where they were found—in a shed abutting on an alley to the rear of the *Appeal* office—for nearly ten days, as that was the last time she was seen alive. The body, bloated, and eaten by rats, pre-sented a hideously repulsive appearance, and the sickening stench is only partially dissipated by a lump of camphor in front of me. . . .

A short time back the house occupied by a respectable resident of the northern portion of the city was noticed as "smelling." Upon enter-ing the house the wife and mother was found occupying a chair at the center of the room, with her infant child, its lips fastened in a death-grasp to the mother's nipple, dead and decomposing. The husband and father, on his back in the bed, had been dead for some time, with the vomito glued to the wall in black masses, as it came from his stomach. The son lay dead on the floor. . . .

Last Sunday evening the household of H. W. Blew, publisher of the Methodist paper in this city, and residing on Pontotoc Street, developed another of those terrible secrets which are hourly brought to light. Him-self, his mother-in-law, and three children were found dead in their beds, awaiting the call of the undertaker and their consignment to the grave.[37]

On September 9, the surviving members of the Citizens' Relief Com-mittee, along with the acting mayor (the elected mayor was down with the fever) and the Shelby County Sheriff (who would himself be dead of yellow fever in a few weeks), jointly addressed a desperate bulletin to the people of Memphis, beseeching them to "leave the city as the only hope for saving them from entire destruction." A force of forty physicians and seven hundred nurses organized by the Howard Association could not begin to relieve the sick and dying, who by this time were figured to num-ber at least four thousand. An attempt to set up a system of neighborhood infirmaries had quickly broken down under the weight of cases, and relief physicians were reduced to making rounds as best they could in buggies, or sometimes on horseback or even on foot, carrying not only medicines but rations, blankets, and other articles for afflicted households. "The hor-ribly depressing influences that surround the physician engaged in a strug-gle with pestilence can be estimated only by those who have passed

37. Chicago *Tribune*, September 24, 1878.

through it," related one. "Coming from a house where he had just seen six or eight cases, he was frequently besought by some almost crazed parent or child to come immediately to his dying kindred. A known Memphis physician would have his carriage stopped in the street by a group of panic-stricken people begging him to tell them what to do for their friends. In these circumstances it was impossible to write prescriptions, or to give extended directions; he could only say to one do this, to another do that." The worst instances of suffering resulted from want of any attendance at all, even that of friends. The situation was deteriorating in all respects: estimates were that less than half the sick were being located and properly nursed; fresh meat, bread, and other perishables had become nearly impossible to find; and the Citizens' Relief Committee was urgently soliciting donations of fuelwood from the countryside for the city's destitute. The *Avalanche* explained: "The people in the country are afraid to send in their wagons with chickens, etc., from a fear of having their wagons pressed to bury the dead, and that their chickens will be taken without pay." Officials assured that this was not the case, and rumors that authorities had taken to burning the dead in heaps were also refuted.[38]

Contrary to expectations, the blacks of Memphis were proving to be painfully liable to this epidemic. Of the 99 yellow fever interments officially recorded on September 10, 35 were blacks. Repeating the conventional wisdom about yellow fever, the director of the Howard Association's medical corps had remarked, "The negroes are easily treated. Unlike white men, they sleep through the fever period, and need no medicine beyond purging and sweating." The *Avalanche* pointed out that at least 60 Negro corpses had accumulated at the county undertaker's over the previous two days, and the newspaper gallantly reminded authorities of the destitution, medical and otherwise, of that section of the citizenry.[39] Exerpts from "Pathological Discussions" at the New Orleans Board of Health meeting on the evening of August 30 depict the confessed bafflement of medical science in the face of this unprecedented scourge. "I do not think," said Dr. Taney, "that men engaged in the practice of medicine will ever arrive at any conclusion in reference to the true nature and treatment of yellow fever. It will be the physicist who will determine these

38. Memphis *Avalanche,* September 8, 10, 1878; W., "Letter from Memphis," *Boston Medical and Surgical Journal,* XCIX (1878), 669–73.

39. Memphis *Avalanche,* September 6, 11, 1878.

questions. In my opinion the physicists have committed an error in confining their investigations principally to the air and neglecting the earth. They should examine the subsoil." But Dr. Albrecht added, "If the germ were a tangible, or perceptible thing, the microscope of the physicist could detect it, but the physicists have not discovered it." And according to Dr. Choppin, "The effect of the poison on the nervous system is unknown; it is incapacitated from directing the repair of the tissues of the body and the muscular fiber; instead of the hepatic cells being repaired in the normal manner they are replaced by fatty matter; in a similar manner the kidneys fail."[40]

A comment by Sir Robert Lyons about the Lisbon epidemic twenty-one years earlier aptly applied to the situation: "Disease, in one of its most appalling forms, held sway, while Art stood helpless by." As of September 8, carbolic acid was still being sprinkled along Main Street in Memphis, but this measure seemed quite pointless in view of how far the fever had ranged by then, and the money was redirected toward relief supplies. A suggestion that five hundred barrels of lime be dumped in Bayou Gayoso, the mephitic slough that ran through the middle of town, was "not deemed advisable" by the board of health. As at New Orleans, hopes and conjectures began looking backward to the old ideas about miasms and the "epidemic constitution of the atmosphere." At one point, a plan was considered to dispel the city's germ-laden air with gunpowder explosions. As a communication to the New York *Herald* explained, sections of artillery could be deployed along the streets of Memphis and fired through the night, which would "have the effect of keeping the air warm, while the concussion and release of sulphuric acid would kill the germs of the disease. . . . The air is so light in the day that the germ remains upon the ground, but is taken up in the heavier atmosphere at night and thus breathed through the nostrils and through the lungs poisons the system. This is the reason more people are taken in the night than in the day. It is a well known fact that more of the animal kingdom die at night than in the day." (Here, under a germ-theory veneer, was miasmatism that could have been taken straight out of Pliny.) It was also proposed to "have cannon fired in the bayous and powder exploded as rapidly as possible along the streets," and to send all the refugees back into the city equipped with

40. New Orleans *Picayune*, August 31, 1878.

muskets and powder to enter enclosed places and make the treatment really thorough. After forty-eight hours of this, it was calculated, yellow fever would be evicted from Memphis.[41]

Briefly, until the realization of the expense and general impracticality began to sink in, the so-called bombarding treatment actually had the endorsement of the governor of Tennessee. The Dupont Company was solicited for the powder, and the Western Union Company offered free use of its wires for making the necessary arrangements. Officials recalled that at New Orleans in August, 1853, cannon had been fired constantly for two days and nights with no perceptible effect on the yellow fever, and the noisy experiment had finally been silenced by the mayor as too upsetting to the sick. Another plan, not quite so dramatic but every bit as useless, was put into operation in Memphis after September 4. The board of health purchased one hundred kegs of pine tar to be blended with equal quantities of raw sulfur and burned at strategic locations around the city. A line of blazing barrels was set along the whole length of Railroad Avenue, from Chelsea into South Memphis, and fires of the same substance were lit at key intersections elsewhere. "Sulphur fires burned throughout the city last night," reported the *Avalanche* on September 12, reflecting on the strange effect of the tar and brimstone's lambent light in the dark deserted streets: "The ghosts of Galen and Hippocrates are walking on the Chickasaw Bluffs," the paper said, with learned reference to ancient miasmatists, "and they gaze with curious eyes." The infection raged on, quite heedless of the fumes, and yet as a doctor from Nashville observed: "It was, however, a source of comfort to know that efforts of some sort were being made on the part of those in authority to stay the hand of the destroyer, and especially upon the minds of the lower classes was this effect produced."[42]

The Memphis papers still gave a little space to letters from the public, and here, as elsewhere, observations, speculations, and recommendations about the "Prevailing Topic" were rife. "I believe enough yellow fever germ can be produced in a room to give the disease to a cow," one local

41. New York *Herald,* September 16, 1878. See also T. Tabbs, "Regarding the Bombarding Treatment of Yellow Fever—New and Brilliant Discovery," *Cincinnati Lancet and Observer,* XXI (1878), 124–35—an amusing, cynical account.

42. Hicks, ed. *Yellow Fever and the Board of Health,* 31, 36; Memphis *Appeal,* August 28, 1878; Memphis *Avalanche,* September 8, 12, 1878; Thomas O. Summers, *Yellow Fever* (Nashville, 1879), 68–69.

doctor wrote in a typical epistle. "There are localities, buildings, and rooms that seem almost too full of the germ for anything to live in. It is not difficult to detect by the odor. Could we have powder burned in rooms, buildings, and on the streets it would save a great many from the disease, and all this talk about the firing of guns is all right, but the noise amounts to nothing, as it is the sulphur and saltpetre that do the work of disinfecting." From amateur chemists came endless prescriptions for the internal and external treatment of yellow fever. One letter explained how table salt and sugar of lead stirred together in hot water would evolve chloride of lead, which in turn "will create ozone and absorb all fetid matter in the air." Another suggestion, that powerful disinfectants like iodine and carbolic acid be inhaled directly with the help of a steam vaporizer, possibly added to the burdens of nurses and gravediggers. A country magus revealed his herbal formula, which consisted of aloes, saffron, rhubarb, agaric, zedoary root, gentian, thorias, and angelica root, steeped in muriatic acid and blended with whiskey. The editor of the *Avalanche* archly commented that at least it had the whiskey to recommend it.

Later on, some communications took a decidedly odd cast, perhaps reflecting the accumulated strain and despondency of the prolonged crisis. One lost soul, who claimed to be in contact with the departed spirit of Josiah Nott, the legendary fever-doctor of Mobile, disclosed that Mobile was free from yellow fever this year because of recent plantings there of Pride of India trees and other malaria-defeating plants. He revealed that for the present, Memphis could save itself by burning pine tar in iron kettles. Another letter urged that the pestilence fell with special severity on New Orleans and Memphis as condign punishment for the "heathenish displays" of their Mardi Gras celebrations. Evidently, this point of view was not so eccentric as we might suppose: an editorial a year later in the *Presbyterian*, a mainstream church journal published in St. Louis, expounded on the same theme.[43]

With current events at Memphis a case in point, prominent clergymen north and south preached on sympathy and charity, on the unsearchable relationship of natural and spiritual laws, on mortal tribulation and human chastening.[44] Here, as in the sweeping plagues of medieval times, or in any

43. Memphis *Avalanche,* September 21, 25, 27, October 1, 1878.
44. See, for example, "The Mission of Epidemics," St. Louis *Globe-Democrat,* September 9, 1878; "The Uses of Adversity," Chicago *Tribune,* September 30, 1878.

period of intense human crisis, religious forms were widely taken up to give articulation to the profoundest feelings of helplessness, fear, and despair. Protestant denominations across the country joined in calling for special days of humiliation and prayer for yellow fever sufferers and persuaded the governors of some states to make official proclamations to that effect. These proclamations involved more than mere words, for they generally obliged a closing of all business houses.[45] Novenas were ordered in Roman Catholic churches, and Cardinal McCloskey of New York personally led the daily prayer for aversion of mortal sickness. There was a commotion on St. Martin's Street in Memphis when a voodoo priestess had herself propped up in an open casket before her followers, to await with incantations her personal appointment with the fever-demon. (Instead she was promptly carted to jail on a disturbing-the-peace warrant from the Citizens' Relief Committee.) There were other, uglier reminders of the Middle Ages: in September, rumor circulated in at least one Mississippi town that the fever had spread so disastrously because the Jewish merchants, trying to hold off the scattering of their indebted customers, had bribed local doctors to withhold news of the first cases.[46]

By September 13, only four of the original twenty-four members of the Citizens' Relief Committee were still on duty in Memphis—three had fled the city and all the rest were either sick or dead. This rump, compelled by circumstances to function as the virtual government of Memphis, resolved that day to try to force the people who remained in the city out to the camps by terminating distribution of relief rations in the city. The plan

45. Editor E. L. Youmans of *Popular Science Monthly* criticized one such proclamation by Governor Bishop of Ohio from the enlightened secular standpoint. "Prayer is efficacious just in proportion as it reacts upon the supplicant to inspire a higher activity," said Youmans, submitting that any appeal from the people to the Almighty should first of all contritely address "their sins of neglect and omission, their ignorance, carelessness, and culpable apathy in regard to all sanitary matters. . . . Yellow fever may not now be wholly preventable, but nobody denies that it is partially so, and nobody knows to what degree it may be repressed and escaped when far more vigilant, efficient, and comprehensive measures of precaution are resorted to. . . . There may be many things about the providential government of the world that we cannot explain, but it is not difficult to see the large benignity of severe and inexorable punishment for violated laws" ("Yellow Fever, and What to Do About It," *Popular Science Monthly*, XIII [1878], 747–48).

46. St. Louis *Globe-Democrat*, September 22, 1878; Louisville *Courier-Journal*, October 4, 1878.

was tabled almost as soon as it was announced, as alarming news of the extent of the fever in outlying areas began filtering back to Memphis. Mason's Depot, thirty miles out on the Louisville Road, was "almost deserted" after the disease had broken out in several homes near the station. In Rossville, thirty miles away on the line of the Memphis & Charleston Railroad, two of the locals had developed symptoms of yellow fever, and their fellow citizens had promptly "stampeded and scattered." Hernando, Mississippi, twenty miles south on the New Orleans Road, had several residents who had suddenly taken the fever and died, and the people were "moving out in all directions." "Reports from the country bring the painful intelligence that the fever is spreading to an alarming extent behind our citizens who fled with their families to the interior. The disease has followed them." The thousands of people who had swarmed out a little less than a month before had all passed through these country towns and stations along the railway lines radiating out of the city. Many of them had been taken in as guests and boarders in towns without declared quarantines, and elsewhere, there had been many surreptitious drop-offs and stopovers in defiance of local regulations. More than a few incipient cases of yellow fever had been carried along unnoticed in the stream of refugees. Small-town mosquitoes had obviously taken the virus from those emigrants, had undergone the necessary period of extrinsic incubation, and were now actively transmitting the disease and establishing new circles of infection in outlying communities.[47]

By the end of the month, the telegraphed appeals for help and stories of panic and distress being received at Nashville and Louisville had swollen to a "truly startling" volume, as yellow fever took hold at literally dozens of towns and villages in the lower Tennessee Valley. A dispatch on the sixteenth from Paris, Tennessee, a railroad town of 1,500 people 140 miles northeast of Memphis, was typical of these reports:

Paris was thrown into a fever of excitement this morning, and everybody seems to be moving. Dock Lewis, a native, and who has not been out of Paris, died of a genuine case of yellow fever. The fever was contracted

47. Memphis *Avalanche,* September 14, 15, 17, 1878; Memphis *Appeal,* September 6, 7, 13, 18, 1878; Tennessee Board of Health, *First Report,* 526–38; "The Epidemic in Several Small Towns in the Vicinity of Memphis," Paper 3 in "Report of the Yellow Fever Commission," RG 90, NA.

here. There are two other undoubted cases of yellow fever among our people, with four or five prostrated at the depot. Physicians have pronounced it yellow fever, have declared it of an epidemic character, and have advised citizens to flee the town, which they are now doing as fast as they can move out.

The town is demoralized. The stampede commenced yesterday, forty families leaving the town.

Every precaution has been taken against the spread of the disease, and the town has been whitened with disinfectants. Business has been almost suspended. . . . An unknown man was found on the railroad last Thursday, four miles north of Paris, and it was not until Saturday that anyone could be gotten to bury him for fear he had died of yellow fever. . . .

The depot sits near a cesspool. The larger portion of the town has quarantined against that portion around the depot.[48]

Brownsville, an important cotton town of 4,000 inhabitants, situated 60 miles northeast of Memphis on the Louisville railroad, reported 90 cases on September 18, and despite a lack of tents, relief doctors endeavored to get the people, blacks included, to move out into the countryside. The community was said to be completely paralyzed, abandoned to the unsure keeping of its "poorer class and negroes"; even the post office and gas works were shut down. The infection proceeded to sweep Brownsville "like a besom of destruction," producing more than 800 severe cases and 212 deaths in a population reduced by flight to no more than 1,000. "We are here in the midst of desolation and death," cried one cable from Brownsville: "We ask the prayers of all Christian people that a merciful God may interpose His arm to arrest and save us from total destruction." The same state of commotion and distress existed in other railroad towns where the fever passed over or touched but lightly. At Stevenson, Alabama, a Memphis refugee died, unattended, in a railroad car parked at the outskirts of town: "His grave was dug within a few feet of the box car in anticipation of his death, and he hardly had time to cool before he was buried." Shortly thereafter, it was said that only eight families remained out of a population of 500. At the town of Milan, Tennessee, 100 miles northeast of Memphis, the "climax of fear" was reached on September 24,

48. Chicago *Tribune,* September 17, 1878.

culminating in what was described as "a perfect hegira," with four-fifths of Milan's families deserting. Although no more than a handful of cases actually developed in the town, all confined to an area along the tracks of the Louisville railroad, it was observed in October that only 100 of Milan's 2,000 people remained. As for the others: "They are camped out in the woods and will let no one come near them."[49]

"The fever has embraced in its death fold almost every place within a radius of twelve miles, and the end is not yet," the *Avalanche* solemnly noted on October 2. "It has branched off and followed the lines of the railroads running out of the city, until it has extended for fully fifty miles to the North, East, and South. Only the West has escaped and not altogether, for there are several cases of fever at Hopefield." A typically deplorable situation was reported on October 4 from Collierville, where the infection had found its way in spite of the rigid quarantine measures announced there earlier in the season. Of the town's 1,100 people, all but 120 had stampeded away, and this little remnant reported 80 cases on hand and 35 deaths up to that date. Ultimately, there were 48 deaths from yellow fever in Collierville. Wherever it effected a lodgment, the fever was showing the same harrowing virulence it had exhibited at Memphis. At Germantown, on the Charleston Road 10 miles from Memphis, somewhat less than 100 of the town's 300 people made the mistake of remaining after the disease broke out. Among these, 81 cases and 45 deaths were eventually recorded. Twenty miles farther out, at the village of Moscow, population 200, 75 cases and 33 deaths were recorded among the estimated 100 who stayed in town. It was also reported that yellow fever was breaking out among many of the people camped outside Memphis, even to a distance of eight miles from the city limits. Buzzards were guiding the police to corpses fallen in cornfields and weed patches on the outskirts of town, and there was worried speculation that the whole of Shelby County, town and country alike, was to become "one vast graveyard." All those attacked were later identified as having been among the people who indulged in the hazardous practice of day-tripping into the infected city. In the epidemic of 1879, state and city authorities would take stricter measures to curb the folly of "daylight communication."[50]

49. Memphis *Appeal,* September 19, 20, 21, 25, 1878; Chicago *Tribune,* September 14, 1878.

50. Memphis *Avalanche,* October 2, 9, 1878.

Inside Memphis, the scourge continued to hold high carnival, steadily penetrating, it seemed, every street and almost every house. Even the city hospital had become more a center of hazard than of help, as Dr. Gustavus Thornton of the board of health would recall: "It seemed that the City Hospital was one grand focus for the yellow fever poison, and yet the sanitary condition of the place was as good, apparently, as it could be."[51] The municipal camp for the poor, meanwhile, was providing an interesting experiment in the noncommunicability of yellow fever in a "pure atmosphere." The depopulation of Memphis went on slowly, so that newcomers continued to arrive from pestilential parts of the city almost every day. "Very many reached camp with the fever on them so that as many as seventeen persons fell victims in one night." Communication with Memphis, daylight or otherwise, by those already in camp presented another big problem. Deputy marshals were on hand to maintain a state of "flexible discipline"—work that consisted primarily in driving off liquor peddlers—but with no specific state quarantine law on the books, it was impossible to restrain the people from going into the infected city at whim. "The inhabitants entered the jaws of almost certain death rather than forego the pleasure of a drunken debauch, plunder, or the like," wrote J. F. Cameron, the hardbitten former Union Army colonel put in charge of the camp. He summed up the unruly character of the inhabitants in these supercilious terms: "mechanics, tradesmen, laborers, women of *industrious* habits, of indifferent morality, Catholics in faith, and in very many instances, paupers and indigents of both sexes. . . . Very few worthy people inhabited the tents of Camp Williams."

In a camp whose maximum population was estimated at about 650, 186 cases of yellow fever were treated over the course of the season and there were 58 deaths; nevertheless, "no instance showing infection from contact in camp appeared." Whenever a case of fever appeared at Camp Williams, it became the practice to destroy the person's tent and its contents with fire, because no one could be found willing to reoccupy such tents even after disinfection. The sick were removed to a field hospital, where a huge fire-pit was kept continuously burning and into which all refuse matter and contaminated bedding was cast and consumed. Since the people remained nervous about the danger of infection spreading from

51. "Experiences in the Yellow Fever," *Medical and Surgical Reporter,* XXXIX (1878), 436.

this source, Cameron pitched his headquarters just a few yards from the hospital. "It was found necessary that the officer in authority should set an example of indifference to attack, in order to appease so far as possible the constant anxiety of the population under his charge." Colonel Cameron, along with the surgeon-in-charge and the dispensary clerk, later moved into a shed that had been used earlier in the season as the camp's deadhouse, and they all pulled through in good health. Cameron also related this curious incident: "Four grave-diggers on constant duty at the hospital, carrying the sick, washing the bodies, sleeping on infected bedding in tents, wearing clothing stripped from the bodies of the deceased, remained on said duty seven weeks, with perfect immunity from attack. All went into the city; became intoxicated; remained so three days. On their return, one fell in the woods and died; two others were treated in the hospital at camp and died; one escaped."[52] These experiences outside Memphis in 1878 do not seem to have moved anyone to question the fomites doctrine at that time, yet they distinctly foreshadowed the demonstrations that would be undertaken 22 years later in Cuba by Walter Reed, which finally proved the noninfectiousness of fomites.

The alarm and anxiety excited by the soaring mortality at Memphis was intensified as the fever broke out at places farther and farther up the valley. At the town of Hickman, Kentucky, on the Mississippi River 120 miles north of Memphis, 30 cases of what was at first regarded as a "low malarial" affection were finally recognized as yellow fever on September 2, and the people were reported to be "panic-stricken and flying in every direction to the country." The town was immediately cut off by rigid quarantines, and travel and business in surrounding counties came to a standstill. While the fever decimated Hickman, the inhabitants of Paducah, a city of 10,000 situated only 60 miles to the northeast, were reported to be "ready to fly to the Mountains of Hepsidam at a moment's notice."[53] "A great excitement and exodus" was reported on September 13 at Cairo, Illinois, 160 miles north of Memphis. Yellow fever that would eventually claim 49 lives had broken out in two separate neighborhoods up from the river. Ripples from the alarm at Cairo registered as far away as Vincennes, Indiana, where citizens were demanding immediate imposition of rigid

---

52. John F. Cameron, "Camps: Depopulation of Memphis, Epidemics of 1878 and 1879," *Reports and Papers, American Public Health Association*, V (1879), 152–56.

53. Louisville *Courier-Journal*, September 3, 5, 6, 1878.

quarantine measures. Quarantines on railroad intercourse actually were declared at Carbondale, Harrisburg, and other points in southern Illinois, but cool weather intervened after a day or two, and what would have been the unprecedented phenomenon of a yellow fever epidemic on the prairies of the midwest never materialized.[54] On September 25, the Associated Press agent at Cincinnati floated a sensational report about yellow fever at Louisville, Kentucky. The initial story said that at least 250 cases were under treatment and that the city of 160,000 was on the verge of a stampede. Official releases by the mayor and the board of health of Louisville instantly denounced the rumors as "highly exciting and prejudicial to our city," said they were not only "false" but "unchristian," and insisted that the city's condition was "never so healthy." A revelation of this nature at this time was potentially disastrous to the city's peace and obviously had to be handled with extreme diplomacy: "As public custodians of the health of the City of Louisville, and with a conscientious sense of the weight of responsibility, we affirm sacredly that, while there may have been several instances of yellow fever of an indigenous character, even upon this there has been the greatest diversity of opinion among our most prominent and able physicians. Nor have there been any new cases since Monday last."[55]

It was the extraordinary invasiveness of the disease this season that astounded the experts and set the general public on the edge of hysteria. A Kentucky doctor lamented "the violence of the prevailing scourge, and its steady and ruthless advance up the Mississippi Valley, overleaping all its former boundaries, and reaching points higher up the valley than ever known before." Early writers on yellow fever had recognized the existence of infectible and noninfectible places and territories and had speculated about the natural latitudinal and altitudinal limits of the disease—limits, we now understand, that would have significance only so far as they affect the occurrence of summer temperatures suitable for *A. aegypti*. In 1850, the influential medical scholar Dr. Daniel Drake had suggested that the disease could not occur in epidemic form in the Mississippi Valley at elevations above 400 feet. In 1873, no less an authority than the president of the American Medical Association published a paper that seemed to substan-

54. Chicago *Tribune,* September 14, 15, 17, 1878; R. Waldo, H. M. Keyes, and J. H. O'Reilly, "History of Yellow Fever at Cairo, Ill.," in U.S. Marine Hospital Service, *Report for 1878 and 1879,* 149–51.

55. Louisville *Courier-Journal,* September 28, 1878.

tiate Drake's earlier surmise. After carefully locating on topographic maps all yellow fever outbreaks recorded in North America since 1668, this doctor found that 460 feet was the highest point at which the disease had ever prevailed as an epidemic. "This fact suggests that the stratum of air in which the infection peculiar to yellow fever exists is heavier than air free from the poison, and therefore seeks the lowest and dampest localities." He thought that 500 feet might safely be regarded as the upper limit of the disease, and that people threatened by yellow fever could thus retreat to higher ground and save themselves with no danger of spreading the infection behind them.[56]

At the commencement of this epidemic, a Chicago wag had written the mayor of New Orleans to suggest that the metropolis could invest its energy in no better way than by building a great pavilion 600 feet high, which could serve as a hospital for its yellow fever sick and a safe haven for the unacclimated. No doubt the writer's tongue was crowding his cheek pretty closely when he submitted that idea, but it did reflect what had become a common belief about the disease. "Yellow fever has never been known to spread to elevations 500 feet above the level of the sea," the Memphis *Avalanche* editorialized on August 22, by way of urging the towns of the hinterland to relax their quarantine barriers and allow unhindered passage to the city's refugees: "This fact is proved by official data." The conviction effectively dissolved in the first week of September, as yellow fever overspread the town of Holly Springs, Mississippi, 625 feet above sea level, and the lid came off all former notions about a fixed "yellow fever zone." A Memphis refugee riding an express train to San Francisco came down with premonitory chills, and her coach was immediately sidetracked and quarantined in the Nevada desert outside Reno. Despite assurances that the casket was hermetically sealed, a Westchester County, New York, mob estimated in the hundreds opposed the interment of the remains of a New Orleans refugee who had sickened and died enroute to the North. The Local Government Board for Ireland, meanwhile, had established "intercepting hospitals" and declared quarantine restrictions on all American vessels approaching Cork, Dublin, and other ports of entry. The sensa-

56. J. M. Toner, "The Distribution and Natural History of Yellow Fever as It Has Appeared at Different Times in the United States," *Reports and Papers, American Public Health Association,* I (1873), 359–84, reprinted in U.S. Marine Hospital Service, *Report for 1874,* 63–96.

tional "Horrors of Memphis" were headline news from coast to coast and across the Atlantic as well, and clearly no amount of caution could be too extreme.[57]

As yellow fever was carried farther into the interior, the incidence of the disease became increasingly quirky and mystifying, reflecting the increasingly spotty and irregular distribution of *A. aegypti*. Here, just as in more southerly regions where the epidemic prevailed more extensively, infection by fomites seemed to be the theory best adapted to accounting for the vagaries of yellow fever, and the most improbable connections were traced out and elucidated with all the gravity and certitude of sober science. The disease skipped over the town of Humboldt, Tennessee, ninety miles northeast of Memphis, but broke out violently and inexplicably two miles beyond the town, at an isolated farmhouse about fifty yards off the railroad. Four of the family were attacked, and three of them died. The doctor reporting on this strange outbreak to the Tennessee State Board of Health resolved it this way:

> The cause of the fever at Dunlaps is rather strange and covered up. The family deny knowing any cause, say they had been nowhere, and not having any communication with anyone who had been where the fever was. But I learn that about a week or ten days before the old man was taken there was a blanket thrown out of a car window from around a lady who had the fever; the passengers complained about the blanket and the sick woman's father threw it out to satisfy them. It was described to me as a gray blanket, and I think I remember seeing one suiting the description in the room where the fever first made its appearance. This being the case, the family picked the blanket up, and from it came the contagion.[58]

57. New Orleans *Picayune,* August 13, September 18, 1878; New York *Herald,* October 2, 1878; *Medical Times and Gazette,* October 5, 1878, p. 418. "A good deal of apprehension is beginning to be felt in unscientific circles, lest yellow fever should be imported into England," the *British Medical Journal* editorialized on September 21. "While the European experience with yellow fever, which is essentially a tropical disease, has shown that it does not spread except under very special conditions, the present outbreak appears to be of so malignant a character that no care should be wanting on the part of port sanitary authorities to meet the possible contingency of the introduction of the disease into this country" ("Yellow Fever," *British Medical Journal,* September 21, 1878, p. 440).

58. J. E. D. Scott, "Yellow Fever in Humboldt," in Tennessee Board of Health, *First Report,* 526–28.

At Jackson, Tennessee, one hundred miles from Memphis, there were only thirteen cases, half of them connected to a single household. The president of the local board of health reconstructed the history of the infection, explaining it to his own and others' satisfaction in a manner characteristic of those embracing the fomites theory:

> About the 1st of September Mr. M. M. Bright of this city in company with Judge Hortrecht of Memphis went to Memphis on some legal business and remained only a few hours in the day time. Mr. Bright came home, arrived here on the 4th of September, went to his father's house, changed his clothes, took a bath and left his clothes in the house. He was arrested and compelled to leave the city and remain away ten days. The clothes remained in the house for a week when his mother sent to wash his linen; his pants she sent to a lady nearby to have them mended. On the 16th of September his mother was taken with yellow fever and died on the 21st. The family states that she had only been out of the yard but once in a month, and that was to do some shopping. There had been none staying there but the family. On the 10th of October the lady to whom the pants had been taken to mend was taken with the fever and died on the 14th. Her father was taken about the same time and died on the 15th. Two little boys lived there at the time, but escaped. The lady who mended the pants lived just across the street from Dr. Bright's. On the 16th Dr. Bright took the fever and died on the 21st; his son M. M. Bright, the one who had been to Memphis and returned, took the fever about the same time and died on the 24th. His wife and brother had the fever but both recovered.[59]

The fact that there were six other cases in different parts of town at the same time was mentioned only in passing, without comment. The fact that the woman who mended the infected pants was stricken and died a week before the young man who wore them to town was apparently thought to be insignificant.

At more distant places, doctors either strained at similar tenuities or frankly admitted their puzzlement. In Bowling Green, Kentucky, 190 miles northeast of Memphis, a series of "imported" cases beginning in August finally brought on a localized outbreak in October, causing 13 deaths. The street where these "indigenous" cases occurred ran along a sidetrack of the

59. Frank B. Hamilton, "Yellow Fever in Jackson," *ibid.*, 530–31.

Memphis & Louisville Railroad, and the infected houses were located almost directly across from the town depot. But if anything, it appeared to be in better than average sanitary condition, and disinfectants had been used in the neighborhood all summer. Another, poorer locality bordering on a foul swale where the town's sewage accumulated and stagnated—where, it was recalled, "cholera and other zymotic diseases" had been most severe in past years—had remained strangely free from yellow fever. "Contagion" seemed out of the question, for indigenous cases had not appeared in any of the houses where imported cases had been nursed. As a member of the Kentucky State Board of Health interpreted matters, the central question was "whether the cases of yellow fever we had were from original germs set afloat by the trains, they coming in contact with the mucus membranes of the respiratory systems of those persons who were affected?—or did the germs or spores set afloat from the cars, acted on by the surroundings, reproduce and develop the poison which affected those residing in this district?" On taking a closer look, he concluded that the atmosphere of the infected district in Bowling Green was not, after all, entirely free of the "noxious exhalations" and "decomposing effluvia" that fed and fostered the yellow fever germ. Defective privies were discovered seeping their contents into the limestone soil, "where it was acted on by the extreme heat, generating an effluvia that polluted the atmosphere in this vicinity." Slops and wastewater from the houses were incautiously allowed to puddle in the alley, "where hogs congregated and were accustomed to wallow." Sufficient "telluric conditions" were there to support it, he decided, and the imported "ferment" had finally taken hold when the dry heat of summer gave way to the sultry days of fall.[60]

Out of a population of 1,500, the river town of Hickman, Kentucky, lost 149 to yellow fever. The fact that the town's first victims, a little boy and his sister, had been peddling apples on steamboats at the landing pretty clearly indicated where the infection had come from. The epidemic's subsequent behavior in Hickman was more problematic. The part of town first attacked and most intensely infected was the old section under the bluff, while only a scattering of cases developed in neighborhoods situated on the hills above. It is significant that the governor of Kentucky detailed

---

60. R. C. Thomas, "A History of the Outbreak of Yellow Fever in Bowling Green, Ky., in 1878," in Kentucky Board of Health, *Report for 1878–79* (Frankfort, 1879), xxxvii–xlvi.

not a medical doctor but the assistant state geologist, John Proctor, to report on the facts and circumstances of the Hickman epidemic. Professor Proctor had no difficulty pinpointing all the usual sanitary transgressions—decayed floors, unclean cisterns, foul privies. He also observed that lower Hickman was built over a stratum of "plastic clay," which made for poor surface drainage conditions, and he submitted suggestions for an improved sewerage system. But while Proctor acknowledged that "the abstract proposition that bad sanitary conditions exaggerate most epidemic diseases may be true," he concluded that "there are facts connected with this visitation of fever at Hickman which render arguments based upon the aggravation of the disease by these conditions somewhat hazardous." On one street, "as clean and well drained as could be desired," every last person remaining had the fever and many died, while the hygienic condition of the single house in lower Hickman to escape infection was "exceptionally bad." The less destructive character of the fever above the bluff Proctor attributed to causes other than superior cleanliness—to the fact that the houses were farther apart and the population more scattered than in the lower part of town and to the fact that most of the people living up there fled before the infection reached them.[61]

Any suggestion of yellow fever's "contagiousness," of its transmission apart from some contingent environmental influence, seemed as inadmissible as ever. An estimated 200,000 southern refugees fled across the Ohio River in the summer of 1878, with "imported" cases turning up everywhere from Providence to Indianapolis to Detroit, but no serious outbreaks of the disease occurred anywhere in the North. At least 8,000 of the refugees had lodged at Cincinnati, and while the health officer was reasonably sure that "no absolutely sick person entered the city without being detected," he also realized that "the period of incubation of the fever being so indefinite, it was expected that some at least of the refugees coming to this city would develop cases after their arrival." To meet this problem a vigilant "stamping-out programme" was put in operation inside the city. "With the exception of five patients found in a dying condition, every case of yellow fever, native or imported, was placed in a hospital. Few mistakes were made regarding suspicious cases." Altogether, 35 definite cases were

61. John R. Proctor, "Notes on the Yellow Fever Epidemic at Hickman, Kentucky, 1878," *ibid.*, lxxiii–c.

tracked down and isolated by Cincinnati's sanitary police over the course of the season. Yet in spite of the massive exposure from refugees and the intensive hunt for suspicious cases, only two "native" victims ever came to light in the city. One was a girl who lived near the waterfront, the other a drayman who had handled rag bales from the South. Exposure to fomites was indicated in both cases, but we must assume the two had been bitten by infected mosquitoes that had somehow strayed off steamboats.[62]

The city of St. Louis also took in a heavy influx of refugees from Memphis and other afflicted places down the Mississippi. Here, also, special health wardens were put to work ferreting out suspicious cases, sending them *nolens volens* to a quarantine hospital established on the bank of the river 10 miles below the city. A total of 129 cases were forwarded to the facility over the course of the season, of which 88 were finally confirmed as yellow fever, with 42 cases ending fatally. By mid-September, the quarantine hospital itself was infected. Eventually, 13 of its employees were stricken and 9 died. This was said to be the one and only confirmed instance of indigenous yellow fever in St. Louis, although the city had been fighting rumors of infection since August. "The Rocky Mountain locust can go so far and no farther," one of the city's leading doctors assured: "Each insect life has its home and its sphere—the yellow fever germ cannot migrate to us, neither is it able to live with us." At the end of September, a St. Louis undertaker was actually hauled into court on a charge of criminal libel filed by the president of the St. Louis Fair Association and two other "prominent citizens" after he alleged the existence of virulent yellow fever in the city in remarks that subsequently appeared in a Chicago newspaper. On October 22, however, a local boy died in the suburb of Carondelet, on the city's south side behind the riverfront. The attending physician deemed the cause of death to be yellow fever, and neighbors testified that at least 10 deaths with similar symptoms had recently occurred in the area. The Carondelet outbreak became the subject of warm dispute among the city's doctors. A panel of investigators for the St. Louis Medical Society concluded the sickness was in no way distinguishable from yellow fever, while a local ad hoc committee insisted it was nothing but "malarial poisoning of a very pernicious type." Both sides agreed that the summer and autumn weather had been unusually hot and that Carondelet was full

62. Minor, *Yellow Fever in Ohio*, 3–79.

of "putrescent miasms of animal origin," the district having many vacant lots that its residents used as cow corrals and hog wallows.[63]

At Louisville, Kentucky, where as many as 20,000 people from the south had taken refuge, there was a small but intense outbreak, 50 cases or so, producing 28 deaths, limited to a single block south of Broadway across from the Great Southern depot. "The infected district is, in my opinion, as clean and healthy as any other part of Louisville, indeed both its alleys and streets are, and were at the time of the outbreak of the fever, freer from stagnant gutter-water and filth than most of the streets and alleys of Louisville," wrote Dr. L. P. Yandell, editor of the *Louisville Medical News*, a judgment in which the city engineer, the city physician, and the Louisville Board of Health concurred. Yandell continued:

> The heat of the summer was more intense and prolonged, and we had among us more cases of yellow fever, and more refugees from the infected regions south of us, than ever before. . . . But as to how yellow fever came into and remained confined to the circumscribed district, it is impossible for me to form any positive opinion. That the yellow fever was imported to Louisville is most probable; that it found in the circumscribed district something in the soil or water or air that enabled it to propagate also seems probable; but as to what this something was, I believe that is beyond human ken.[64]

One of Yandell's colleagues at the University of Louisville struggled heroically to reconcile this outbreak with the conventional formula of "an imported factor plus a local miasm." He observed that while the infected district's superficial hygienic condition was not exceptionally bad, closer inspection revealed "many small and crowded tenements, each of which has its own cess-pit." He singled out the hundreds of undisinfected railroad cars and coaches that had been coming in all summer from points south, and theorized that "sections of the infected atmosphere" at Mem-

63. Chicago *Tribune*, October 1, 1878; Walter Wyman, "Notes upon Yellow Fever Epidemic of 1878 in St. Louis and at St. Louis Quarantine," in U.S. Marine Hospital Service, *Report for 1878 and 1879*, 143–46; "The Relations of Yellow Fever to St. Louis," *St. Louis Medical and Surgical Journal*, XXXVII (1879), 131–62.

64. L. P. Yandell, "The Late Yellow Fever Outbreak in Louisville," *Louisville Medical News*, VI (1878), 275–78; see also "The Board of Health's Report on the Yellow Fever in Louisville," *ibid.* 239–41.

phis, Grenada, and other "pestilential centers" had been effectively boxed up and transported thither. When released in downtown Louisville, the "specific poison" had been briefly supported by the not entirely wholesome local atmosphere before being diluted and dissipated, and finally dying out for lack of sufficient nourishment.[65]

On September 12, there was a report of "a general scare" in the neighborhood of Gallipolis, Ohio, a river town about midway between Cincinnati and Pittsburgh. "All the public schools were closed yesterday. Fires of coal tar have been burning for the last 24 hours at the terminus of every street opening on the river. Many citizens are leaving and business and travel is almost suspended." What actually transpired at Gallipolis was the interesting phenomenon of a "floating epidemic," when a boat thoroughly infested with infected *A. aegypti* created a temporary focus of yellow fever infection at a place where the mosquitoes and the disease would never otherwise be found. Similar occurrences had been recorded previously, at St. Nazaire in northern France in 1861 and at Swansea, Wales, in 1865. The vessel involved in this case was the *John Porter,* the New Orleans towboat that was blamed for bringing the fever to Vicksburg and several other places on its upriver voyage. A fresh crew was engaged at Louisville in the expectation that the infection would die out as the boat moved north; instead, it intensified. Proceeding on its way to Pittsburgh, the *Porter* broke some of its machinery above Gallipolis on August 18 and dropped back to a point just below town for repairs. After a few days, the exasperated crew threw the last of their dead overboard and abandoned the boat, which then stayed tied up at the place until retrieved by its owner on September 12. Scattered cases of yellow fever began appearing in Gallipolis on August 28. By September 18, the disease had claimed eighteen lives in the town. The outbreak was as intriguing as it was worrisome, and was investigated and reported by doctors from both the Cincinnati Health Department and the U.S. Marine Hospital Service. Gradually, it was established that all the victims had been on board the infected boat at one time or another and for one reason or another. Some had been among the men sent out by the town authorities to scrub and disinfect the *Porter* after it had been deserted by its crew. Quite a few others, it was ascertained,

65. J. W. Holland, "Nature and Source of the Yellow Fever Epidemic at Louisville, Kentucky, in 1878," *American Practitioner,* XX (1879), 352–58.

had sneaked out to the unattended boat to pilfer rugs, chairs, tableware, and other movables. A lady went out to rescue some caged birds she had heard were starving, and lost her life through her kindness.[66]

On September 20, officials confirmed that the fever had taken hold epidemically in the city of Chattanooga, Tennessee, 320 miles east of Memphis and 750 feet above sea level. The disclosure sparked one of the season's most sensational stampedes, and by September 30 about 8,000 of the city's 12,000 people had fled. Not only were freights and passengers on the railroads out of Chattanooga confronted with a line of rigid quarantines reaching from Montgomery to Knoxville, but the city itself was tightly blockaded by the surrounding country. Whether authentic or not, stories like the following at least indicated the degree of anxiety to which people had been wrought: "Last night a woman refugee from this city died from yellow fever a few miles in the country. The neighbors attempted to burn the house with the corpse and two children in it, but were prevented. They at last buried the woman and sent the children back to the city and burned the house. It is only another instance of the inhumanity and cowardice of many people in the country."[67]

Night riders were harassing refugees who had taken to camps outside the city, and relief authorities were able to establish an isolation facility out on the lower slopes of Lookout Mountain only under the protection of police bayonets. But as events developed, the infection failed to spread from the city to the country, and within Chattanooga it stayed confined almost entirely to a slum district situated in a low, swampy area in the middle of town. The locale was inhabited mainly by Negroes and poor whites, and sanitary conditions were compromised not only by bad drainage but by the presence of numerous old corrals and filthy privies. In the elevated parts of town surrounding this valley, the fever refused to propagate. To Dr. J. H. Vandeman, the city's registrar of vital statistics, the distribution of yellow fever in Chattanooga only served to confirm the standard theory about the disease's etiology: "The more filth, the more yellow fever; the lower the ground, the poorer the drainage and water

66. Minor, *Yellow Fever in Ohio*, 19–28, 79–102; W. H. Long, "Yellow Fever at Gallipolis, 1878," in U.S. Marine Hospital Service, *Report for 1878 and 1879*, 127–40. On some other notable floating epidemics, see E. M. Eager, *Yellow Fever in France, Italy, Great Britain, and Austria, with Bibliography of Yellow Fever in Europe* (Washington, D.C., 1902).

67. Chicago *Tribune*, September 24, 27, 30, 1878.

supply, there you would find this disease the worst, following in its course the track of the cholera of 1873."[68] Chattanooga was one place where a difference in water supply was clearly indicated as a factor influencing the occurrence of the fever. A report by E. M. Wight observed that the better-class neighborhoods on the heights, which remained free from yellow fever, were supplied with river water "conveyed by iron pipe," while the people of the infected district got their water from a line of shallow wells in the bottom of the valley—a fact significant not because of the unwholesomeness of the source, as Dr. Wight supposed, but because it implied storage of water in the houses, creating opportunities for the breeding of *A. aegypti:*

> The water of the wells, which is much in use by the poorer classes at all times, is all bad. . . . These wells are situated in the main valley of the town, which was the heart of the infected district. This valley receives the drainage of the hills upon which are the residences of most of the well-to-do people, on both sides, which sewerage drains sluggishly out of the soaked soil by one main open drain. . . . Nine-tenths of the people in the infected district used water from the wells in this valley situated along both sides of this drain.[69]

Chattanooga had been accepting refugees from fever stricken cities right along, confident that its higher elevation and cooler night air made it impossible for the infection to spread. When yellow fever erupted in the highland city, it presented another great shock to believers in the "zone theory." "Great excitement" was reported in the mountain counties of northern Georgia, where people, watchful and worried, feared they would be next. The mood in the city of Atlanta was said to remain calm. The disease was breaking out in some of the important railroad towns of northern Alabama, bringing dislocation and paralysis in its wake. On September 26, for example, Decatur reported "business entirely suspended" and that all but 200 of its 1,500 white people had scattered. Decatur was

68. J. H. Vandeman, "Yellow Fever as It Existed in Chattanooga, Tenn., Its Origins, Progress, and the Probable Remedy for Its Abatement in the Future," *Reports and Papers, American Public Health Association,* IV (1878), 210–22.

69. E. M. Wight, "Yellow Fever at Chattanooga in 1878—Topographic, Telluric, Atmospheric, and Other Influences," in *Transactions of the Medical Society of the State of Tennessee, 1879* (Nashville, 1879), 162.

an important transfer point for freight on the Memphis & Charleston Railroad, and shipments of various goods had tended to back up when rigidly quarantined places farther up the line refused to receive them. The fact that the town's first cases had been among railroad employees and people who lived close to the railroad yards made infection from fomites the logical inference, though Dr. Jerome Cochran acknowledged in his final report that "the exact method of the introduction of yellow fever into Decatur admits of some question." There were 35 deaths among Decatur's whites; among the town's 600 black people, nearly all of whom remained through the epidemic, there were just 19 deaths.[70]

At Tuscumbia, Alabama, circumstances pointed to importation, but here again the facts of the matter were unclear and would remain so. The mayor of the town had tried to impose a railroad quarantine early on, but his effort was thwarted by the frank opposition of the merchants and hotelkeepers, and by the noncooperation of many residents who wanted to bring in friends and relatives who were escaping from infected places. Many refugees, it was said, simply hopped off the trains at water stops in the nearby country and walked in unchallenged. By the end of September, several focuses of infection had been established, sources unknown or at least unnamed, and local people who had been maintaining that "in their pure air yellow fever could not live" were now scared and beginning to flee. By October 12, when the town was finally reached by a relief train from Memphis, only 300 of its 1,200 inhabitants remained.[71] At nearby Florence, unrecognized yellow fever had evidently been prevailing since the latter part of August among the Negroes and poor whites living around an undrained flat on the outskirts of town. A certain number of malaria cases occurred in this locality almost every summer, and even as the infection grew more violent and began to penetrate the main part of town, a majority of doctors continued to hold that it was not really yellow fever but just "a malignant type of malarial fever." Advocates of the malaria theory ascribed the unusual sickness to emanations from the slimy bed of a side channel of the Tennessee River that had been diverted earlier that summer so a gravel bar could be removed. On October 3, with the town and surrounding country falling into a panic, the project crew was dis-

70. "The Epidemic in Decatur," Paper 18 in "Report of the Yellow Fever Commission," RG 90, NA.

71. "The Epidemic in Tuscumbia," Paper 16, *ibid.*

charged, the diversion weir was opened, and the slough was reflooded, with no effect whatsoever on the Florence epidemic. Yellow fever eventually claimed 44 lives at Florence, and 30 at Tuscumbia.[72]

The experience of Huntsville, Alabama, during this epidemic illustrated once again the contradictory and unaccountable behavior that had confused and bedeviled yellow fever epidemiology for two hundred years. While Decatur, Tuscumbia, and Florence were ravaged by an infection whose origin remained debatable and obscure, Huntsville played host to a succession of well-marked imported cases without a single house becoming infected. Over the course of the epidemic, the town took in an estimated five hundred to six hundred refugees, mostly from Memphis at first, with many coming later from Tuscumbia. From August 27 down to the end of October, a total of twenty-three known cases of yellow fever occurred among the refugees in Huntsville. They were nursed in its hotels and private homes in all parts of town and eleven yellow fever corpses were buried from its churches. Not one native case ensued, however, with the single exception of "a dissipated young man" who was known to spend his nights in railroad cars. Neither climate, topography, nor the composition of its population differentiated Huntsville from neighboring towns. "We attribute our immunity from yellow fever to our superior sanitary condition," concluded Dr. J. J. Dement, president of the local board of health. "The germ of the disease had every opportunity of being propagated, since we placed no restrictions on the commerce or travel of the country, or upon the intermingling of our fellow citizens with persons from infected places." Among its distinguishing sanitary qualities, it was observed that Huntsville drew its water from a large, pure spring, whose flow was distributed through the town in pipes; accordingly, wells and cisterns were few.[73]

"After having ravaged Memphis, the pestilence is seeking new victims in the interior, and is marching with swift steps even to the healthy cities of North Alabama," the *Avalanche* observed on October 9, adding gloomily: "One week more of the present warm weather will suffice to infect the whole of West Tennessee, and all the horrors of an epidemic will be experienced throughout this whole section of country." The protracted warm spell had caused a recrudescence of the fever at Cairo, Illinois, prompting

72. "The Epidemic in Florence," Paper 17, *ibid.*
73. "The Epidemic in Huntsville," Paper 21, *ibid.*

a renewed exodus and another suspension of business. The death toll at Memphis had been falling pretty steadily since September 18, however, and by the first week of October was running from 30 to 40 a day. This slackening was correctly attributed to the fever's having "gone through all its human material." Wherever it could still locate such material, however, the pestilence refused to relax its ravages. As relief workers extended their rounds out along Poston, Deane, and other fashionable avenues in the better-class suburbs south of the city, it was reported that "many instances are discovered of whole families who are stricken and have lain for days without any attention whatever." "Death was everywhere," reflected the editor of the *Avalanche* after he toured these streets. "They thought they were safe there in those lovely houses. God preserve us. There was never a scourge like this." In a letter published in the *Medical and Surgical Reporter* on the nineteenth, Dr. Greensville Dowell expressed a veteran's dismay at the amazing fatality of this visitation. He said that of the 41 unacclimated physicians originally engaged by the Howard Medical Corps, 22 had perished, along with 300 of the nurses. Dr. Dowell—a Galveston professor recognized as one of the country's leading authorities on yellow fever—also disclosed that he had lost 101 of the 226 cases he had personally treated: "We have tried almost every plan, but all fail, and this is the almost universal report."[74]

Memphis' economic life was still utterly prostrate, and the nation's charity was feeding the city's survivors. The Citizens' Relief Committee was distributing subsistence in the city at a rate of 18,000 rations a day, comprising 10,000 pounds of bacon and 20,000 pounds of flour and cornmeal, besides sundries like salt and soap; this did not include the supplies forwarded to the municipal camp. Normal retail channels in the city were still sluggish and the stocks on hand small and dwindling, partly due to the competition from the rations issues. Nearly all the stores were still closed, but some merchants were beginning to place invoices in anticipation of frost and the return of the city's people. The arrival of the steamer *Goff* with a barge of freight from St. Louis on October 11 at least "made things look a little better" in that regard. In cotton circles, there was a glimmer of activity on October 9 when a steamer dropped off 25 bales, the first received by river this season, and there were also a few arrivals by

74. Memphis *Avalanche*, September 24, 26, October 10, 1878; "The Yellow Fever in Memphis," *Medical and Surgical Reporter*, XXXIX (1878), 349.

wagon. What little was coming in was being stored to await a market. There were no calls and no quotations at the cotton exchange because sellers were so few and reshipments impossible; some small dealing by "guerilla" traders was known to be going on but not at quotable prices. More than 3,000 bales were reported to be piled up at Helena on the Arkansas shore, waiting to be forwarded to Memphis as soon as communication was opened. A few days later, Helena's board of health vacillated, and then in the most careful language admitted the existence of fever in the town: "This Board believes it now becomes a duty to announce to the citizens that, while the prevailing disease may not be strictly yellow fever, it certainly is seemingly quite as fatal, and the citizens are hereby so advised." The businessmen of the place immediately organized an indignation meeting and baldly declared that there was no yellow fever at all in Helena, that the general health of the town was good, and that "all parties can come here with perfect safety." It was not until well into November, safely after frost, and after the fever had racked up 74 victims, that Helena would acknowledge the infection.[75]

Some inclement feelings were being expressed against the blacks in Memphis. "Negroes will not work, will not leave town, but lie about idle and draw rations, and then get sick and become a burden intolerable," the president of the local Howard Association had exclaimed. "The fields are white with cotton, but not a foot will they move. They seem to think they must be nursed in idleness." Patience was evidently growing short, along with supplies, and it was easy for the gentleman to forget that if the blacks had gone out to seek work, they would undoubtedly have been driven straight back into the city by rural quarantine posses, as actually happened in a number of reported instances. Throughout the stressful season, the region's endemic racial tensions had never been very far below the surface. In September, there had been a scuffle and shooting at the main relief commissary on Court Street in Memphis, and scurrilous rumors of a general uprising of the blacks came and went. Two companies of militia were posted outside town, ready to go into the city at a moment's notice if the alarm were given. Actually, most of the police on duty in Memphis were blacks deputized back in August after most of the regular force quit in disgust at the salary situation or fled the city because of yellow fever.

75. Memphis *Avalanche*, October 10–12, November 12, 1878; Chicago *Tribune*, October 15, 1878.

"While they behave very well," the Louisville *Courier-Journal*'s correspondent said of the Negroes, "there is still a lurking fear on the part of the whites of some evil." From Grenada, Brownsville, and other places had come reports of looting and other depredations by blacks—stories that were mostly unfounded, but were enough to pitch up the general mood of "lurking fear." When the sheriff of Shelby County died of yellow fever, the *Avalanche* nervously admonished on the need to find an immediate replacement: "Delays are dangerous. At any moment the chaos of Hell may be upon us." No significant trouble ever developed, and even the editor of the local Democratic monitor was obliged to praise the blacks for their "responsive, patient, forbearant" behavior during the crisis.[76]

Relief trains began running out from Memphis to country towns after October 10, meeting with "sore affliction and dread suspense" all along the line. Clear out to Chattanooga it was reported that "suffering prevails in nearly all the towns," and needy refugees were scattered over the fields and forests. In the immediate orbit of Memphis it seemed that "every station and woodpile" had its tale of woe, involving either disease or privation, or both. The town of Somerville, deserted by two-thirds of its people in September, was without telegraph facilities and had not received any mail at all for three weeks. In the last week of September, the postal superintendent at Atlanta had suspended deliveries along many routes in Alabama, Mississippi, and Tennessee, complaining that mail agents and carriers were being treated "like enemies of mankind," often subjected to heavy fines by local quarantine enforcers and sometimes pulled off the trains by main force and dumped in the woods. In a few places, as around Collierville, public roads had been wrecked and bridges had been burned by terrified farmers and crossroads dwellers opposing the townspeoples' flight to the country. It was expected that the Shelby County grand jury would look into those incidents and issue indictments after frost. Brownsville, reached on October 16, was found in "the most deplorable condition imaginable," with more than 200 dead, only 450 remaining in town, mostly blacks, and hundreds of others, blacks as well as whites, camped around in the nearby

---

76. Memphis *Avalanche*, September 8, 26, 1878; Memphis *Appeal*, September 3, October 16, 1878; Louisville *Courier-Journal*, September 14, 1878. Even though all relief requisitions were supposed to be countersigned by two visitors, there were persistent allegations of widespread rations fraud, and Negroes were accused of hoarding supplies to get through the coming winter without work or to swap for tobacco and whiskey on the black market. There were mutterings against a similar "communistic" spirit on the part of the Irish.

woods in improvised lean-tos and "bush arbors." The town's little relief commissary was down to thirteen barrels of crackers, seven of flour, one of rice, and a single chest of tea. Two carloads of supplies were delivered to the town. Until then, Memphis had been in no condition to extend relief, the frightened country population was in no mood to succor the town, and food and other basics had been available only by means of the occasional train from Louisville, 320 miles away. At Martin's Station, reached on the twenty-first, only 300 people remained out of a community of 600. The place had suffered 136 yellow fever cases and 35 deaths up to that date, and was completely out of everything from quinine to coal oil.[77]

Supplies of all sorts of fresh eatables in Memphis were meanwhile running down "with thrilling celerity." Vegetable gardens on the outskirts of the city had been thoroughly plundered by the campers, and on October 9 the *Appeal* had made the rather startling observation that "chanticleer cannot be heard now," the chicken coops of the suburbs having been cleaned out as well. The daily list of deaths in the city was steadily falling, however, and by the third week of October was down to fewer than twenty a day. A chilly rain had passed over Memphis on October 5, followed by another weather front on the tenth, and mean temperatures had begun dropping into the sixties; *A. aegypti* would have been growing torpid under those conditions. Killing frost finally came on the morning of October 19, when grateful Memphians discovered thin ice on puddles in the suburbs. Refugees immediately started back into the city, although the board of health and newspapers warned against anyone returning for another week at least: "The Great Plague of 1878 is of a more venomous character than any ever known. One black frost will not kill it, nor two." Yet by the twenty-third, the bar at the Peabody Hotel had reopened, and advertisements for Memphis restaurants and saloons began reappearing in the *Avalanche*. A few columns over from those teasers, an incongruous dispatch from one of the relief trains observed that many poor families camped in the immediate vicinity of the city were still subsisting by hunting possums and foraging wild nuts.[78]

By October 25, cotton was reported to be coming in quite steadily in wagons from the surrounding country. So too were many more of the

77. Memphis *Appeal*, October 11–13, 15, 16, 1878; Memphis *Avalanche*, October 22, 1878; Chicago *Tribune*, October 1, 1878.

78. Memphis *Avalanche*, October 20, 24, 1878.

people who had been rusticating in the woods around Memphis, but who now preferred to brave the hazards of food, bed, and wages in a city where infection still lingered rather than endure further exposure to cold and hunger in the spots of refuge they had been occupying for two long months. One returnee remarked that a person could literally feel "the heavy pressure of the poisoned atmosphere the moment he comes in contact with the infected belt or district." On the twenty-fifth, the Citizens' Relief Committee saw fit to terminate distribution of rations in the city. Newspapers advised the city's blacks that the frost had been heavier in the country than in Memphis, that the fields around town were full of cotton to be picked, and that planters would now be pleased to accept their services. Surplus relief funds were entrusted to the mayor's office to be disbursed on an individual case basis. The general mood had lightened to the point that the *Avalanche* could wax facetious on the rations matter: "A week ago the time between drinks around this office was fifteen minutes. That ration has been reduced to ten minutes."[79]

Another heavy frost occurred on the morning of October 28, and the board of health officially declared the epidemic to be over. "Come home," the *Avalanche* advised the absentees. "Those words have a talismanic sound. We thank God the hour has come. The epidemic is at an end." The municipal camp broke up on October 30, and the Memphis & Louisville Railroad was running its trains on double schedule to accommodate the throngs coming back from northern cities. The resiliency that was manifested in all facets of New Orleans' urban life as the pestilence lifted shone forth even more remarkably in the rebound taking place in Memphis. Boats "heavy with freight" and barges "full of cotton" had responded immediately to the liberating news of frost, and on November 5 a commercial reporter at the wharves under the bluff marveled, "To look at the immense piles of freight of every description, no one could imagine the desolation and dread silence that reigned supreme where now is heard the noise of hundreds of wagons and drays." The directors of the cotton exchange met on November 11 for the first time since August, in a trading atmosphere that was said to match the briskness of the weather. Meanwhile, the leather works, iron works, oil presses, and other industries of the city were reporting themselves to be back on their feet and ready for fresh orders. The

79. *Ibid.*, October 25, 26, 1878.

city's refugees were still returning, and the city's newspapers, which two weeks before had honestly advised them to remain away "until the atmosphere becomes thoroughly purified," now turned their efforts to quashing rumors circulating at Knoxville and other places that the fever was still dangerously prevalent in Memphis. Oxford and other Mississippi towns that still had Memphis under rigid quarantine were called "foolish." As heavy rains fell on the 15th, the city's regrouped board of health admitted that scattered cases of yellow fever were still being reported, but declared: "We are satisfied that every case is directly traceable to ill or no ventilation, or to the use of infected bedding."[80]

Just as commerce was regenerating in all its branches, the city's population seemed to be restoring itself in all its former range of character. The *Avalanche* resumed its humorous reporting of "The Matinee," the afternoon sessions of the police court, as well as its frequent editorials on "The Tramp Nuisance," Memphis, like New Orleans, being one of the nation's premier resorts for "the floating class." The *Appeal* quoted the Hartford *Courant* as saying the country's major life insurance companies did not expect to sustain much loss in Memphis after all, since their clientele was mostly among the well-to-do, and the well-to-do had mostly fled ahead of the epidemic. That was reported as encouraging news. The public schools reopened as the season's first snow fell on November 28. Taking it all into account, the *Avalanche* in a December editorial tossed off those pessimists who were suggesting that the yellow fever disaster had effectively blasted Memphis' future as a center of trade and population, and that, like the ancient Memphis on the Nile, it was fated to become a ghost city. The bluff it sat upon commanded the only capacious landing to be found for several hundred miles along the Mississippi, and it looked out over a trade area stretching from Fort Smith to Chattanooga: "This Memphis is a veritable city set upon a hill, and her light is bound to shine."[81] The question of the city's survival was renewed in a more serious way when yellow fever reappeared the following July.

80. *Ibid.*, October 29, November 2, 6, 9, 10, 16, 1878.
81. *Ibid.*, December 15, 1878.

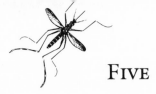

FIVE

The Epidemic of 1879

"There is reason to fear the development of yellow fever at Memphis is but the dirge-like prelude to another appalling tragedy in that most unfortunate of American communities," the Washington *Post* announced in July, 1879. "The germs of disease appear to have been kept alive through the winter and spring, and have burst into fury under the heat of midsummer." The distressing news was that Yellow Jack had surfaced again in Memphis. A cobbler residing on DeSoto Street in the Sixth Ward had died on July 9 with undeniable symptoms. A committee of doctors from the board of health held a conference over the body and decided it was probably a "sporadic" case, caused by germs that had overwintered in old clothing the man had taken from the house of some in-laws, who had perished in the previous summer's epidemic. The city newspapers assured that "the atmosphere was never purer than at present," and doctors offered the hopeful theory that such attenuated "sporads" were unlikely to reproduce to any extent, and that another violent or fast-spreading epidemic could only arise from a fresh importation of virulent germs from the Caribbean.[1]

The following morning, three more cases were reported at a house in the Tenth Ward and another two in the Eighth Ward. Savvy citizens began to evacuate, and the chaotic scene of eleven months before was reenacted in all particulars. Once again Memphis streets "echoed to the roll of baggage wagons" and trains were going out "crowded with fugitives," slip-

1. Memphis *Avalanche*, July 10, 1879.

ping away with all possible haste as rigid quarantines were put into effect in towns and cities from Little Rock to Montgomery. Sixty miles out, at Brownsville, many people were already fleeing, and daily business was paralyzed in anticipation of what was to come. The local quarantine was made so strict that even first class mail was prohibited. All roads around Brownsville were picketed day and night, although the town council repudiated suggestions that the trestles of the Memphis & Louisville Railroad west of town be demolished. Meanwhile, the management of that line notified the public of standby plans to terminate its runs at Milan, Tennessee, one hundred miles northeast of Memphis.[2]

"The medical faculty are as impotent today before such a visitation as they were half a century ago," the *Post* commented. "We do not say it in disparagement, but state it as a lamentable fact, that science has made scarcely any progress in discovering the causes and preventions of yellow fever." The previous fall, the American Public Health Association had voted a small appropriation that, along with contributions from several New York and Washington philanthropists, supplied funds to Surgeon General J. M. Woodworth of the U.S. Marine Hospital Service. Woodworth was to organize a scientific panel charged with visiting towns that had been scourged by the great epidemic, to study the circumstances of how the fever appeared and spread at each locality. This so-called Yellow Fever Commission was also requested to arrive at some general conclusions about "the habitudes of the poison," with a view to curbing future outbreaks. Apparently, the association had in mind something similar to the major report on cholera submitted to Congress by Woodworth, J. C. Peters, and Ely McClellan in 1875.

The experts delivered their preliminary findings in November at the Richmond meeting of the American Public Health Association. They concluded that, while yellow fever clearly depended on a certain set of atmospheric conditions and to some extent was an "air-infecting agent," it did not represent an inorganic malarial toxin but was the product of a specific living germ. At no place, according to everything they had been able to discover, had the disease arisen independently of human traffic and inter-

2. *Ibid.*, July 11–13, 16, 1879; Memphis *Appeal*, 11–13, 16, 1879; Tennessee Board of Health, *First Report, April 1887 to October 1880* (Nashville, 1880), 360–61.

course, and in every instance they believed the infection could be traced to persons from previously infected places (or, more exactly, to the fomites those persons carried). The germ evidently bred and multiplied outside the human body and was only communicated indirectly, through its prior infection of an area, undergoing "some process of maturation" in the environment after its introduction to a new locality. At each town they visited, the doctors of the commission prepared spot maps showing the sequence of the first cases, similar to those worked out earlier in the decade by the New Orleans Board of Health. These charts reconfirmed the tendency of yellow fever to occur in "concentrations of cases," progressing outward from initial centers or focuses of infection that often originated with a single case. The infection's "slow but regular" spread was compared to "the growth of mould on leather," and it was not deemed insignificant that both mold and yellow fever were favored in their development by the same sanitary and meteorological conditions. The experts believed the germ was primarily diffused by means of fomites, but organic debris in a state of putrefaction was judged to be "the fittest soil or hotbed for its maturation" in any particular place.[3] Despite the rather cloudy language, some of the commission's observations on the *modus operandi* of the germ deserve quoting at length:

> The natural history of yellow fever poison affords a certain degree of support to the opinion that under favorable meteorologic and telluric conditions it undergoes some form of change outside the human body which increases its toxic effects. Witness, for example, the singular local attachments of the poison, so often observed during the prevalence of

3. "The American Public Health Association: The Yellow Fever Epidemic of 1878," *Sanitarian*, VII (1879), 3–10. The fullest exposition of the commission's conclusions on the etiology of yellow fever is found in S. M. Bemiss, "Chapters from the Report of Yellow Fever Commission of 1878," *New Orleans Medical and Surgical Journal*, n.s., X (1882), 321–37. A congressional appropriation to publish the complete report was not forthcoming, and Bemiss, who had been chairman of the commission, subsequently published some of its more important sections in the *New Orleans Medical and Surgical Journal*, of which he was editor. On the background of the commission, see "The Yellow Fever Commission and the American Public Health Association," *New Orleans Medical and Surgical Journal*, n.s., VI (1878), 496–504. On its fact-gathering methods, see remarks by E. Lloyd Howard in "Abstract of Discussions," *Reports and Papers, American Public Health Association*, IV (1878), 385–87.

yellow fever. A certain locality or area of a city may be intensely infected by yellow fever, while other parts are entirely free from it. These conditions may exist for one, two, or three months. Under such circumstances the medical observer can often define quite precisely the boundaries of the infected districts and warn unprotected persons of the danger of entering within those limits. It must be admitted, therefore, that under these circumstances the yellow fever poison has a degree of life and permanence of presence not exhibited by it except in infected localities. In other words, it must infect localities either by some quality which causes it to adhere to material substances when accidentally brought in contact with them, or because on the other hand these substances afford it an area for growth, or point d'appui, during certain life cycles which it may be capable of undergoing outside the human body. While it is not known by which of these methods places become infected by yellow fever, there is one very old and often quoted observation which favors the belief that the materies morbi is capable either of multiplying in the open air or of extending its area of prevalence in some manner quite independent of atmospheric currents. This is the slow but regular extension of the boundary of infected localities which marks some epidemics; an extension often apparently uninfluenced by human intercourse. Some observers have endeavored to formulate this rate of progression of yellow fever poison, asserting that infected localities enlarge their boundaries forty feet daily.

The atmosphere is undoubtedly the vehicle for the infection in the communication of the yellow fever poison to exposed persons. There are however certain peculiarities in the behavior of yellow fever infection, which cannot in our present state of knowledge be accounted for. I shall simply state these peculiarities as we and others have recorded them:

Yellow fever is spread with much more certainty through means of infected localities or things than directly from the persons of the sick. Indeed, it is questionable if the poison as primarily developed in the human body is in a marked degree infectious. The fact is indisputable that the unprotected may expose themselves with but little danger around the sick bed of one seized in an uninfected locality, while it is exceptional that an unprotected person shall expose himself in an intensely infected locality and escape an attack.

It must be understood, however, that the arrival of a person sick with yellow fever, or with the disease in its incubative stage, into an uninfected locality, is liable to be followed by a new focus of infection. If we take the ground that this is brought about by first infecting the surroundings of the sick person, we will be in accord with the opinion held by a large number of the oldest and most careful of yellow fever observers.[4]

We still see the term *poison* being used to denote the causative agent of yellow fever, but such usage by this time was merely habitual and concessionary; the context makes it clear that the reference was to some kind of "living germ." The Yellow Fever Commission had disappointingly little to offer on the prophylaxis and control of the disease. While allowing that sulfur smoke had demonstrated "a certain degree of efficacy as a special germicide," chemical disinfectants on the whole had been "signal failures." At Port Gibson, Mississippi, carbolic acid had been poured onto the streets so copiously that the lower branches of the shade trees had wilted, but it had not prevented yellow fever from destroying a quarter of the population. The experts' interviews and investigations had not turned up any breakthroughs in the way of personal prophylaxis, either. In one town, individuals might testify that their escape had been entirely due to charcoal pills, or to chalybeate water, but at another place, the people had suffered frightfully despite heavy doses of those very things. The doctors were disturbed to meet a few poor devils who had fallen back on the "Hunterian doctrine"—an obsolete medical theory maintaining that two different infections could not exist together in the same host—and had deliberately contracted syphilis to elude the greater terror of yellow fever. In fact, the only measure that had proved at all effective in excluding infection was quarantine, in the sense of absolute nonintercourse. "In some instances this fact was illustrated where the quarantined localities were very contiguous to those which were infected."[5]

The Memphis *Avalanche* had predicted that any additional light shed by the Yellow Fever Commission on the topic of yellow fever "would not be visible to the naked eye." The highstanding *British Medical Journal* reviewed the findings and found them to be "not devoid of value," but only because "they agree with those of other observers." A special review committee of the American Public Health Association saw nothing new, either. It considered the conclusions of the Yellow Fever Commission to be

4. Bemiss, "Chapters from the Report," 323–25.
5. *Ibid.*, 345, 350–52.

"satisfactory" and "in accordance with the prevailing views of the medical profession," but thought the investigation should have taken on "a much wider range." Among the various "accompanying phenomena" that should have received more attention were allegations that "certain insects are unusually prevalent" whenever yellow fever raged. It was also noted that "certain analogies between the yellow fever and the Texas or Spanish cattle fever have been pointed out." Those comments had a significance only dimly perceived at the time. The report's failure to establish the exact relationship between filth and the yellow fever germ was seen as its chief shortcoming: "If the current theories about yellow fever are correct, the yellow fever poison may be developed by adding some one or more of the excretions of a person affected with yellow fever to decomposing organic matter under well-known conditions of temperature and moisture. We have then to carry out a process of elimination to find out what constituents of the decaying filth are essential and what non-essential, what secretions or excretions of the body are essential and what non-essential to the production of the poison."[6]

The unhelpful muddle of perspectives and opinions on yellow fever was evident in subsequent discussions among attending members of the association. A Vicksburg doctor said the description of yellow fever's creeping, fungating spread from house to house and street to street agreed with his own observations, and he threw in the suggestion that when gaps appeared in the pattern and no explanation could be given for the disease skipping quite a distance, perhaps the fact that an animal had passed along there with the spores in its fur supplied the missing link. "A dog can carry yellow fever poison just as well as a man can. Every dog in the city carries it about with him." Points generally taken for granted by the profession at the time were severely criticized by some individuals. Greensville Dowell of the Texas Medicial College was one who believed yellow fever spread contagiously, just like smallpox, only under a narrower range of atmospheric conditions, and he questioned the fixed ideas about its transmission by fomites and propagation outside the human body. "Gentlemen say it is in clothing, trunks, steamboats. Do people carry it in their satchels and clothing? No sir. You tell me that the body does not reproduce and

6. "Report upon the Work of the Yellow Fever Commission," *Reports and Papers, American Public Health Association*, IV (1878), 361–62.

develop the disease. Where does it come from? The body does develop the poison. I do not see how it is possible to reason to any other conclusion." Concerning the presumed role of filth in propagating the disease, one of the experts of the commission, E. Lloyd Howard of the Maryland Board of Health, admitted that in many instances it had not been the most filthy sections of towns where the fever originated or was most malignant. A sanitarian from Mobile, Alabama, went so far as to declare: "It has seemed to be assumed that perfect sanitary conditions would check yellow fever. My experience upon this point is to the contrary. Where yellow fever has prevailed worst has been in the cleanest places. . . . The only thing that I consider established is that sanitary conditions have no effect whatever." Facts, however, had a way of proving refractory to countertheories as well as to established beliefs. A Chattanooga doctor hesitated to say his city developed yellow fever in 1878 because it was unusually filthy, but claimed he could nevertheless cite numerous instances of the efficacy of sanitation and disinfection. "When a case was once recognized as yellow fever, the family was removed, the house was quarantined, cleansed, and shut up, and absolutely filled with the fumes of burning sulphur. From such instances we could trace no cases of yellow fever." Dr. A. N. Bell of New York, editor of the *Sanitarian,* sternly warned: "Let it never go abroad that filth is to be indulged because in some one place it did not happen to be heated enough to promote putrefaction and develop disease."[7]

No more cases were reported in Memphis for five consecutive days after July 10, and fears of another widespread epidemic began to wane. "Nothing has occurred so far to show that sporadic cases can spread the disease," the *Avalanche* maintained. "The old theory, based on experience, holds good thus far." The paper published interviews with several respected doctors in private practice, all vouching for the official "sporadic" theory, and printed a special letter from the keeper of the municipal cemetery, formally denying stories that yellow fever corpses were being sneaked into the grounds after dark at the behest of city politicians more concerned with containing panic and preserving trade than with safeguarding the public health. Some towns in the countryside began to declare their willingness to receive Memphis freight and passengers again, and prices in

7. "Abstract of Discussions," *Reports and Papers, American Public Health Association,* IV (1878), 363–88.

local markets "ran wild," as hundreds of wagons came in from the country to quickly load up on supplies and carry them out to the surrounding villages and plantations, which were still wary of a recrudescence of fever in the city and another shutdown in communications.[8]

That interlude did not last long, for a fresh outbreak was reported at a Clay Street tenement on July 16, and by the twenty-first, no less than fifty-one new cases had been brought to the attention of the board of health. "The best thing the citizens of Memphis can do is drop their theories and scatter for the hills," an out-of-town paper advised, and thousands who had not fled in the first wave of panic mobbed the ticket counters at the train stations. The city council of Louisville, Kentucky, which had risked much by keeping the gates wide open in 1878, decided to impose nominal quarantine restrictions against Memphis traffic on July 19. "Business and sentiment are essentially different in all their qualities," the Louisville *Argus* stated editorially, and made it clear which meant most when it demanded even tougher measures. "The yellow fever question has become a practical one, and while it is lamentable that we must shut out our fleeing and distressed fellowmen, we can not do otherwise. The era of flapdoodle and sentiment is past; we must do as other people do or we are losers. Last year we received the refugees with open arms, and what was the result?" The Cincinnati *Enquirer* affirmed that rigid quarantine represented "the right kind of humanity." On the advice of the newly organized state board of health, the governor of Arkansas dispatched mounted patrolmen to the Tennessee crossings.[9] A bulletin from the National Board of Health begged local authorities to endeavor to secure the best possible sanitary condition of the places and people under their charge. Inasmuch as the fever in Memphis seemed to be arising from germs surviving from 1878, sanitation rather than quarantine was given top priority. The board reaffirmed the germ theory in language that indicated it was aware of the publicity directed toward recent theoretical conflicts over the nature of yellow fever:

> It is best to act as if it were a disease due to a specific particulate cause, which is capable of growth and reproduction, and transportable, and may be destroyed by exposure to temperature above 250°F or by chemical

8. Memphis *Avalanche*, July 13, 15, 17, 1878.
9. *Ibid.*, July 18, 20, 22, 24–26, 1879; Tennessee Board of Health, *First Report*, 381–83.

disinfectants of sufficient strength if brought into immediate contact. It is also prudent to assume that the growth and reproduction of this cause are connected with the presence of filth, in the sanitary sense of the word, including decaying organic matter and defective ventilation, as well as of high temperature. . . . A careful sanitary inspection of almost any town or city will show the existence of collections of decaying or offensive matters, previously unknown, and which everyone will admit should be promptly removed and destroyed. Such inspections to be of value must be thorough, and made by persons competent to recognize foul soils, water, and air as well as grosser and more palpable forms of nuisances. They should be made by persons who would report fully and frankly the results of their observations without reference to the wishes of persons or corporations.[10]

Evansville, Indiana, instituted rigid quarantine and began a thorough sanitary inspection of tenements and produce stores, "as would leave no chance for them to offer the slightest inducement for the habitation of infection." New York City officials provided for the impounding of fomites on Staten Island and intensified clean-up activities in Manhattan, which, as the New York *Tribune* apprehensively noted, "abounds in putrescent localities, which only await a few germinating seeds from the South to become the foci of some hideous contagion."

A crash program to eliminate the many fruitful sources of germs in Memphis was again put in operation, with some interesting variations on the campaign of 1878. A new citizens' organization, the Auxiliary Sanitary Association, took particular note of Bayou Gayoso, the turbid natural drainageway that snaked through the north-central part of town, "full of stagnant and offensive pools . . . which are the receptacles for dead animals, exhaling noxious and poisonous vapors hurtful to the public health, not to mention the privies, stables, and private sewers which discharge their deadly contents into it." In one day and at a cost of just $75, the association figured, a wheelbarrow crew could throw up an eleven-foot dirt weir across the bayou below Eliot Street, and a quarter of a million cubic feet of water from city hydrants in the neighborhood could quickly be sluiced into the little reservoir. The weir could then be blown out with explosives and the rush of water would purge the dirty channel clear to its

10. Memphis *Appeal*, July 15, 1879.

confluence with the Mississippi. This dam was constructed and filled on July 17, then washed out fortuitously in a rainstorm that night. High hopes had been pegged on this experiment, but it was soon evident that the sludge and slime had merely been lifted up and spread over the bayou's banks, killing the grass and weeds and adding measurably to the putridity of the air.

Another resolution by the Auxiliary Sanitary Association urged the city to abolish its ubiquitous privy vaults, reasoning that they had been the principal lurking-places of sporads. The deep "cess-pits," according to this theory, had "no doubt been used as receptacles for black vomit and other excreta during the fever of 1878, and being too far from the surface to be influenced by the breezes of winter, have been vitalized by the present heated term sufficiently to endanger life." The association recognized that the city was destitute of both the revenue and the supply of water—not to mention the time—necessary to install water closets and build costly sewers, and recommended immediate substitution of a system of dry-earth latrines as the next best thing. "The excreta quickly becomes incorporated with the earth and loses its identity. . . . Moses, in his wanderings in the wilderness, was taught this principle by the same authority that prepared the tablets of stone," the resolution said, recalling the prescription in Deuteronomy—and in fact, the city's position at that moment was not too much better than that of the Israelites adrift in Sinai. The earth-closet suggestion was emphatically and repeatedly endorsed by Memphis newspapers.[11]

The Cleveland *Herald* severely chided the indifference of Memphis' property holders and civic officials, who had ignored the opportunity to rectify the town's sanitary condition during the cold of winter. "What will be the final result of the terrible lesson which has just begun in Memphis no man can imagine. No one can guess how far or how wide this scourge of unclean cities in the South will extend, but as it goes we can imagine the personal misery and commercial ruin that follow in the dreadful wake of terror, disease, and death." New York City's onward weekly, the *Nation*, saw the recurrence of yellow fever as a fundamental comment on post-Reconstruction southern society and Bourbon political leadership. "The cities of the South will never be guarded from pestilence until they are

11. Memphis *Avalanche*, July 16, 18, 1879.

filled with a new, progressive, and prosperous population, who will make the necessary improvements, take the necessary precautions, and raise the necessary taxes." Other journals began to take an even darker view of the situation, and there was speculation that the yellow fever germ had in fact become "naturalized" in Memphis, established on a permanent basis as it was at Havana and Rio, to flare up every summer and present a recurring threat to the whole surrounding region. The disgusted health officer of Cincinnati declared that he was personally convinced that it was naturalized, "and this trouble of quarantining the city will have to be continued from year to year." [12] "It is hard to say what Memphis can do in such a crisis. She is bankrupt in purse and without means to do anything substantial for her own protection. About the only plan that seems to be left to the Memphis people is to desert the city." That was the pessimistic conclusion of the Cincinnati *Enquirer,* and the faraway Denver *Tribune* agreed: "Memphis is doomed. Yellow fever is there and means to stay there, and there is nothing for the people to do but leave." The *Avalanche* observed "a very general disposition to rule out Memphis from the list of American cities," and bravely tried to counter: "There are few people hereabouts who would not now prefer to live in Colorado rather than Memphis. The river and the cotton trade are the two great points in favor of the 'yellow fever city,' and in good years there are advantages which offset the mines. The boy who in looking over his geography wondered why the large rivers always run past the large cities, struck upon one of those universal coincidences which help to explain why there will always be a Memphis, no matter how many die in the summer time." [13]

By the end of July, 187 cases of yellow fever had been officially reported in Memphis, and 57 deaths had been recorded. The Tennessee State Board of Health, actually established in 1877, had remained entirely in the background during the 1878 epidemic for want of money and authority, but it had been voted more funds and wider powers by the legislature in March and presently stepped in to direct an intensified, house-by-house attack on the yellow fever germ. It could not be denied that Memphis was, as the New York *Herald* bluntly put it, "crammed with fomites." Stables and sheds, not to mention rooms and closets in hotels, houses, and shanties in

12. *Ibid.,* July 26, 1879; Memphis *Appeal,* July 20, August 2, 1879.
13. Memphis *Avalanche,* July 30, 1879.

all parts of the city, were still full of clothes, bedding, curtains, carpets, and other fabrics that had been left behind by refugees the previous summer. It was supposed those articles had received in trust, as it were, the "poisonous germs" that had diffused everywhere and permeated everything in the great epidemic, and they had never been adequately aired out or disinfected. It was even said that in some abandoned houses, boarded up after their inhabitants had been annihilated by the fever, unemptied kettles of black vomit and other excreta could still be found. "Winter arrested the development and activity of these germs but it was a mild winter and did not destroy them. In this respect the city—perhaps others—is in the condition of places in the tropics, where the poison lives through from year to year and resumes its great activity upon the return of the hot season."[14]

A force of 13 wagons and 76 men was organized and sent on a regular circuit through infected neighborhoods. When an infected house was identified, adjoining privies, cesspools, and gutters were treated with a saturated copperas solution, mixed at a ratio of two pounds per gallon of water. All possible fomites were taken from the house, drenched with crude carbolic acid, and put in an express wagon to be carried, covered with a tarpaulin, to a municipal incinerator under the bluff at the foot of McComb Street. After the disappointments of 1878, much less faith was placed in the efficacy of carbolic acid as a squelcher of yellow fever, and it was explained that the chemical was being used in this connection chiefly to make the fomites more flammable, and secondarily to reduce any possibility of dribbling live germs through the streets. Reviewing the official records of this operation, it is interesting to see 33 mosquito nets listed among the hundreds of items taken out and destroyed by fire. Sulfur was burned in the sickroom (but not the whole house, unfortunately), which was then shut up with orders to keep it closed for 24 hours. The next day a squad came to reopen the room and carry out the additional measure of pouring unslaked lime into the house privy. Over the course of the summer, 939 infected houses in Memphis were visited and treated by the sanitary teams. In addition, virtually all privy vaults in the city, in uninfected as well as infected districts, were systematically disinfected, requiring a total expenditure of 56 tons of copperas and 9,343 barrels of lime.[15]

14. *Ibid.*, July 17, 1879.
15. *Ibid.*, August 19, September 28, 1879; Tennessee Board of Health, *First Report*, 391–98.

By August 8, 97 yellow fever deaths had occurred in the city, and the following morning a bulletin from the Memphis Board of Health officially declared that a general epidemic existed. It observed that in July the disease had confined itself mainly to the south part of the city, to the Fifth Ward and parts of the Seventh, Eighth, and Tenth Wards, but in the past week it had "extended generally in so many different localities of the city that it is now impossible to say what portion is not infected." This was two calendar weeks earlier than when a similar declaration had been issued in 1878, and optimism collapsed. "All hope of averting the frightful yellow fever plague has now departed in Memphis," said the Washington *Post*. "It now becomes an anxious question whether the fever, by virtue of the strictest outside quarantine regulations, can be housed up in Memphis, and thus prevented from striking its terror into the surrounding country." In July, the state board of health had restored railroad communication in west Tennessee by introducing a complicated system of train relays and inspections. Outbound travelers were required to check their baggage at a disinfecting station 12 hours before departing Memphis, and all cars and coaches were thoroughly fumigated with sulfur and closed up tight for 6 hours before being loaded and boarded. At a point 5 miles outside the city, there was a complete transfer of passengers and baggage to clean cars, which were never taken any nearer to the infected city. This transfer was repeated at a second point fifty miles out. At each transfer, the trains and their contents were given a general going-over by special sanitary inspectors. One of the instructions was: "No person with fever shall be allowed to proceed but shall return to the point of departure"; yet there was no general detention of city refugees. Freight and baggage were regarded as the chief danger. If the inspectors had reason to believe that a passenger car had become infected, the coach was to be sidetracked and left open to ventilate for 20 days, and its curtains and upholstery were to be taken out for a thorough scrubbing.[16]

The state board of health insisted that its program gave the surrounding region ample security against a spread of yellow fever from Memphis, but "the excitement throughout Tennessee had by this time become very great, and the wildest rumors were freely circulated as to the condition of affairs at Memphis." Many localities began reimposing independent quar-

16. Tennessee Board of Health, *First Report*, 361–66; Memphis *Avalanche*, July 13, August 10, 1879.

antine measures. When the state board refused to defray the cost of hiring extra police for them, some towns seized on the pretext to disclaim allegiance to the board and sever official connections, falling back on the trusty "shotgun" policy of the summer before. By the middle of August, only two of the four railroads serving Memphis and west Tennessee were still in operation, and only on a tri-weekly schedule at that, with the predictable consequences to commerce. According to the Chicago *Commercial Report,* the loss to the Chicago provisions trade already stood at not less than $1.5 million. The worried speculators of the Pit were unloading hog and grain options and depressing prices in anticipation of fever in southern cities, and southern railroad shares were sliding fast in value, "though the total mortality from the disease at Memphis is really less than occurs almost any day through the summer in any of the tenement house wards in this city."

The state board also devised an involved and unwelcome system of internal quarantine for within the city of Memphis. Infected houses were immediately marked with yellow flags, and none but doctors, nurses, and clergymen were allowed to approach them. "Dangerously infected" streets were sealed off with picket guards, debarring not only peddlers and casual visitors but also keeping the milk, meat, wood, and ice wagons from their regular rounds. A general 9 P.M. to 4 A.M. street curfew was imposed. The scheme was theoretically sound, the *Avalanche* gibed, and only needed "the whole available force of the German Empire to make it a success." The *Appeal* groaned, "We wish the mosquitoes could be isolated and quarantined during the remainder of the summer."[17]

Another municipal camp for the poor classes had been set up in the woods south of Memphis, its 1,500 A-tents laid out in good military order, with lines of bonfires kept burning between the rows at night to warm the air and discourage the germ. By day a sanitary force made constant rounds with lime, copperas solution, and mops. A pass system was enforced this year, and at-will excursions into the infected city were prohibited. A special census completed at the end of July had revealed that only 16,110 blacks and 4,283 whites remained in Memphis. Most of the standpatters of both races were believed to be people who had been acclimated in 1878, but the

17. Tennessee Board of Health, *First Report,* 385–86; Memphis *Appeal,* August 15, 1879; Memphis *Avalanche,* August 15, 23, 1879.

superintendent of quarantine continued to plead for total depopulation as "the only knowable barrier to the onward march of the unknowable scourge which now afflicts our city." Despite official urgings, nearly all the blacks of Memphis resisted the inconvenience of moving out to the camps, as explained in a little manifesto by a group of their preachers: "We have but little to fear from yellow fever as compared with the whites. Hence there is no necessity for our leaving the comforts and conveniences of our humble city homes, leaving our personal property exposed to probable destruction, and exposing ourselves to the certainty of contracting those pulmonary diseases which are so very prevalent and fatal among the colored people in this damp and changeable climate."[18]

Apparently, the problem of housebreaking, pilfering, and vandalism during the 1878 epidemic had been worse than city officials or the newspapers had ever admitted. A more theoretical concern was that the presence of any people in Memphis, acclimated or not, would have the effect of keeping the infection from being effectively "starved out." Some talked of using military force to completely evacuate the city, and a semiofficial vigilante organization came into existence, suggestively named the Committee of Safety. One night, a downtown fire whipped up the general sense of anxiety. The New York *Herald* sardonically commented that perhaps "some of the wild creatures left in Memphis would do the country a service by firing the city." The St. Louis *Times-Journal* called the suggestion "simply atrocious" and said: "There is enough business sense in the land, as well as enough humanity in our civilization, to compass the difficulty without resorting to that truculent and barbarous plan." There ensued one of the strangest discussions in the history of American journalism, on the question of whether the best solution to the yellow fever problem in Memphis might not be the wholesale abandonment and destruction of the city by fire.[19]

The Indianapolis *News* thoroughly explored the idea in a long editorial. It reasoned that there were only two conceivable means of purifying a plague-ridden area of such dimensions. If absolutely everything on top of the ground could be simultaneously drenched with some powerful dis-

18. Tennessee Board of Health, *First Report,* 376–77, 398–400; John F. Cameron, "Camps: Depopulation of Memphis, Epidemics of 1878 and 1879," *Reports and Papers, American Public Health Association,* V (1879), 156–63; Memphis *Avalanche,* August 1, 1879.

19. Memphis *Appeal,* July 25, 26, 1879.

infectant, the germ might be killed out. That plan was probably, if not surely, impossible. The other plan was fire. "It was the great fire of London that ended the great plague. Russia stopped the advance of the plague last year by the same means—whole districts were burned." The yellow fever germs in Memphis had just withstood as cold a winter as the city was ever likely to have. As the *News* interpreted the situation, the great concern now was that Memphis, "from her local conditions, has become the habitat of this human destroyer, to be yearly devastated by it, and yearly to be a threat to the whole country." Just so would Memphis be retaining "in the heart of the country, in the very center of the traffic on its largest inland watercourse, a plague that yearly shall paralyze the industries of one of the most important sections of the country." Such recurrent interruptions to commerce more than overbalanced the capital values represented by the city: "Is not Memphis bankrupt already? If this plague goes on this summer as it did last (and it certainly will) will she not be destroyed as a business point? Will not property be worthless where to venture is death during the term of the busy season?"

"Will Memphis willingly be a leper to yearly threaten the lives of all that have intercourse with her, rather than be cleansed, even though by fire?" The *News* argued that the work could be carried out under authority of an executive order from Washington, D.C., with Memphis property holders to be compensated with special federal bonds. "The intense heat of the conflagration will destroy every vestige of the poison germs, in every hollow and on every height. . . . If there is to be a holocaust, let it be one of lifeless material, not human beings." The *Times-Journal* finally acknowledged that perhaps it would be better for Memphis and all its property to be destroyed in a general conflagration than "to permit the yellow fever to get a permanent foothold in the Mississippi Valley. . . . If it should be deemed better to thoroughly purify the place, let that plan be adopted. But it is clearly evident that any work, to be thoroughly effective, must be undertaken by the government." The gears of decision making in a representative government, however, ground slowly on this as on less sensational issues—fortunately, in this case—and Memphis was preserved for a more sparing and precise program of sanitation.[20]

20. Memphis *Avalanche,* July 31, 1879. The following year, 189 houses in Memphis were condemned for sanitary reasons by the state board of health and ordered demolished;

By the end of August, 234 people in Memphis had died from the fever, and a need was perceived for drawing a picket line around the entire city to check ingress and egress by way of the dirt roads. This was established on September 4. Passes were issued only to those who could demonstrate that they were on pressing business, and admissions were made only between the hours of 6 A.M. and noon, with the stipulation that all persons had to be out by 5 P.M. No baggage or personal effects of any kind could be carried either way. The season's first bale of new cotton had been shipped into Memphis on August 30, and the authorities decided to include in the pickets' instructions the rule that neither lint nor seed cotton be allowed into the city. One reason for this was to remove any temptation for refugees to reenter the infected city to seek work in the gins and presses, but the main concern was that the cotton might trap and absorb the pervasive yellow fever infection and later become a means of broadcasting the disease far and wide. The *Appeal* instantly thundered: "No such thing occurred last year when nearly the entire cotton crop of the Mississippi Valley was ginned and baled at a time when the air of nearly every city, town, village, hamlet, and farmhouse was laden to a thickness that could almost be felt with the poison of the most malignant plague that ever visited the American continent." Any kind of trammel on the cotton trade, of course, pinched the very taproot of Memphis' commercial existence. A letter in the *Avalanche* insisted that the whole quarantine scheme was nothing but a conspiracy by a ring of speculators to build up some other shipping point by thoroughly crushing Memphis: "Who is behind the curtain?"[21]

Some rich and influential Memphis cotton processors immediately filed a bill of complaint, and injunction proceedings batted about in chancery until the issue was obviated by cool weather in October. The defensive president of the state board of health, Dr. J. D. Plunkett, who had been hooted and reviled in the Memphis papers and hanged in effigy in front of the Opera House, delivered a paper justifying this particular mea-

---

the owners were allowed no compensation. See G. B. Thornton, "Memphis Sanitation and Quarantine, 1879 and 1880," *Reports and Papers, American Public Health Association,* VI (1880), 196.

21. Tennessee Board of Health, *First Report,* 388–91, 408–45; Memphis *Appeal,* September 6, 11, 23, 1879; Memphis *Avalanche,* September 17, 23, 1879.

sure to the American Public Health Association in the fall. He pointed out that the transmission of disease by fomites was "a fact unquestioned by all intelligent physicians of this age," and if rags, furs, feathers, and sponges could be proscribed in quarantines, it was only reasonable to put similar restrictions on cotton, "which by its peculiarly porous, flocculent nature is particularly adapted to the absorption and imbibation of the infectious or propagating cause of yellow fever." Plunkett acknowledged that the decision had come as an added embarrassment to the commerce of a city that was already badly strapped, and he admitted that no case had ever been documented of anyone catching yellow fever from handling un-wrought cotton; nevertheless, he had thought it best to "err on the safe side." He recalled that cotton imported from the Levant was supposed to have brought the Great Plague of 1665 to England, and as recently as 1835, during an outbreak of plague in Alexandria, the Privy Council had ordered 31,000 bales of Egyptian cotton to be ripped open and exposed to fresh air and sunshine for two weeks on the London docks before being allowed into the city.[22]

Outlying towns and cities in Tennessee had, in fact, warmly supported the state board on this question. The Memphis interests that kicked against the measure were denounced by the Chattanooga *Times* in these terms: "They may fool the surrounding cotton planters into carrying on a two-party barter of seed cotton for yellow fever germs, but they will not be allowed, nor will the fools who mix with them, to go cantering over the world as heretofore, dumping the pestilence here and there as they go." The fomites theory was firmly ensconced in general acceptance, but leaders of commerce and industry in quarantined cities—and their hand-maidens, the local newspapers—were bound by sheer self-interest to cry out against it. The columns of the *Avalanche* and *Appeal* almost every day

---

22. J. D. Plunkett, "Cotton as a Fomite," *Reports and Papers, American Public Health Association,* V (1879), 84–88. In 1908, almost thirty years after this controversy, some sporadic cases of smallpox were found among mill workers at Stockport, England, traced to cotton imported from Ziftah, Egypt, and Memphis, Tennessee. Health officials observed that low-grade variola was endemic at both Ziftah and Memphis, and that at both places field hands were addicted to chewing tobacco. "Raw cotton, on account of its texture and organic nature, would no doubt constitute a suitable nidus for the organism of the disease," the health officer at Stockport commented (H. E. Corbin, "Small-pox from Imported Cotton," *Public Health,* XXIII [1909], 20–23).

contained editorial fulminations against "the quarantine anaconda" and "the murderous clutches of political doctors." It is perhaps a wonder that such protests, loud and importunate as they were, and coming from such influential quarters, did not have more of an effect in getting the medical profession to reexamine the fomites doctrine and its inconsistencies, nudging it along to other ideas about the transmission of yellow fever. New Orleans was also battered by quarantines in 1879, and in August the exasperated New Orleans *Times* made this editorial statement, which must have sounded extremely rash and radical at the time, though it reads today like the plainest good sense:

> Out of this fomite which casts no shadow, and has no more substance than the fabric of a vision, the whole world has put on a madcap and gone crazy. We are told that the germs or spores of fomites travel, that they may be carried about in leather or prunella, in groceries, hardware and dry goods. In consequence, we have unreasonable quarantines, state and national; learned commissioners to sit and visit on the subject; country people stand at arms on the highway—and all this to keep away fomites, which have no existence. Though this theory of fomites may have some material and tangible fact to rest on, it is throwing the moral world off its hinges. . . . Are we common people, who are content to sport on the margin of science, to stand still and say nothing against the empiricism of the age?[23]

As it happened, the worst expectations about yellow fever in 1879 did not come to pass. The infection did not subside until cold weather, but neither did it spread with anything like the speed and ferocity it had displayed the summer before. It was finally halted by frost on the morning of October 24. Over the 100-day crisis, only 1,595 cases had been enumerated in Memphis, with 497 deaths—106 blacks, 391 whites. "If the fever has sprung up from the old germs at Memphis," the Jackson *Sun-Tribune* had asked back in July, "why should it not do so in the other towns visited by the pestilence last year?" This reasonable worry fortunately failed to materialize. The Tennessee State Board of Health subsequently traced the diffusion of infection from Memphis to 23 communities situated from 2 to 25 miles outside the city. At 10 places the disease did not spread at all after

23. Memphis *Appeal,* August 9, 1879.

being introduced; at another 11 the secondary infection was limited to just one or two houses. The most serious situation developed at the settlement of Buntyn's Station 5 miles outside the city, where 9 houses became infected and 36 cases were reported. But altogether only 106 cases were reported in Tennessee outside Memphis in 1879, 43 of which proved to have resulted from personal exposure in the city itself.[24] Scattered cases, mostly Memphis refugees, also appeared at various railroad towns around Mississippi, precipitating panics at Corinth, Starkville, and a number of other places, but nowhere did the infection become epidemic. At Grenada, a boy was taken down with suspicious symptoms on the first of September, whereupon a majority of residents promptly forsook the town. It turned out to be a false alarm, and within a few days most of them were reported to be "slipping home on the back streets." The town of Concordia, on the Mississippi River 100 miles below Memphis, did become seriously infected in September and eventually suffered 29 deaths; the infection was traced to certain fomites brought down from Memphis earlier in the summer.[25]

New Orleans was strangely spared another serious visitation, with only 48 reported cases entailing 19 deaths, all in a wealthy and well-kept neighborhood in the Fourth District between Chestnut Street and the river. Since December, an unacclimated family from Mississippi had been living in a Third Street house, in which there had been several cases in 1878. The place was in good sanitary condition except for the privy vault, "which was foul and had not been cleaned for at least a year previous." With the advent of warm weather, this sink became "horribly offensive," and finally was cleaned out on June 8. A week later, one of the boys of the family was seized with yellow fever, and before long, the disease was appearing in other houses, all clustered within 100 yards of this original focus of infection. It broke out two blocks away in the home of General John

24. Tennessee Board of Health, *First Report*, 402–403, 452–78.

25. Memphis *Avalanche*, September 3, 1879; John B. Pease, "Yellow Fever at Concordia, 1879," in *Transactions of the Mississippi State Medical Association, 1880* (Jackson, 1880), 166–70. Yellow fever was also communicated to Forrest City, Arkansas, a railroad town 40 miles off the river, and took 15 lives despite the fact that most of the community's 1,200 people stampeded (R. G. Jennings, "Quarantine and Its Results in the State of Arkansas in 1879," and Jno. B. Cummings, "The Inefficiency of Quarantine in the State of Arkansas during the Year 1879," both in *Reports and Papers, American Public Health Association*, V [1879], 121–26 and 127–30, respectively). See also John H. Rauch, "Yellow Fever in 1879," in Illinois Board of Health, *Report for 1879–80* (Springfield, 1881), 24–93.

Bell Hood, hero of the defense of Atlanta, and within seven days claimed the lives of the general, his wife, and one of his two daughters. Physicians from the board of health carefully examined the Hood mansion and determined that the place, "although elegant in all of its appointments, was really in a sanitary condition of the worst character, due to the existence of a closed and unventilated privy vault in the basement."[26] That winter the sanitary inspector of the Fourth District would write:

> There is not the slightest evidence upon which could be founded a suspicion that the infection was brought into this locality by importation of any kind; but on the contrary, the whole weight of testimony is in favor of the opinion that it was engendered from local causes. It is a safe assumption to say that it was the offspring of germs held over from last year. . . .
>
> We challenge any man to cite, with corroborative evidence, one single instance to the contrary: that is, of yellow fever occurring and spreading in a community where there did not exist bad hygienic conditions due to the massing of human excrement and other filth is close proximity to habitations. Their streets and premises might look severely clean, but to the scrutinizing eye of a sanitarian, the place would be seen disgustingly filthy.[27]

There were 143 deaths in the parishes west of the city, including 25 at Morgan City. From there it diffused to several nearby settlements and caused another 40-odd deaths. The rest were at various places in the Lafourche country, principally around Napoleonville. Most of the Lafourche outbreaks were also thought to be traceable to Morgan City, where the first case had appeared on July 25—a little boy whose source of exposure could not be exactly determined, but who lived on a street where the infection had been intense in 1878. Although Morgan City had been in constant contact with New Orleans all spring, and had been visited by an infected schooner from Tampico besides, it was concluded that there, as

26. Louisiana Board of Health, *Report for 1879* (New Orleans, 1880), 1–7, 112–15, 181; Joseph Holt, "The Chain of Circumstances Connected with the Appearance of Yellow Fever in New Orleans during the Summer of 1879," *New Orleans Medical and Surgical Journal,* n.s., VII (1879), 375–84.

27. Joseph Holt, "Yellow Fever in New Orleans during the Year 1879," *New Orleans Medical and Surgical Journal,* n.s., VII (1879), 623, 625.

in New Orleans itself, the fever was probably the product of germs held over from the previous summer, stimulated and aggravated by the town's "bad sanitary condition."[28]

New Orleans health officials were satisfied that the metropolis' reprieve in 1879 was attributable to their policy of "persistent sanitation in detail." That spring, a citizens' group had raised $30,000. They outfitted an extra force of rubbish carts and also purchased two big garbage scows, which every day carried the city's refuse several miles below and dumped it in the middle of the Mississippi. (Formerly, it had been thrown, along with night soil, off designated "nuisance wharves" along the waterfront.) Some big steam pumps were purchased and a regular program of gutter flushing was instituted. When yellow fever appeared in July, it was attacked with the most thoroughgoing disinfection. The mattresses, linen, and pajamas of the sick were burned, and the clothing of their families, nurses, and doctors was fumigated. In event of death, the cadaver was immediately wrapped in a sheet soaked with copperas solution and placed in a tightly sealed coffin, packed several inches deep all around with powdered charcoal. Sulfur was burned in the sickroom. The floor of the house was scrubbed with carbolized water, and the walls and ceiling painted with carbolized whitewash. Drains and privies connected with the house were treated with copperas and carbolic acid.

All privies and gutters in the general neighborhood of infected houses were treated with chloride of lime. Eventually, more than 10,000 premises on 376 squares in New Orleans were strewn with lime and generally scrubbed up. "The amount of filth removed from the premises in the way of trash, manure, garbage, etc., was simply appalling, in a sanitary point of view, and enough in itself to breed sickness of almost any description, especially during such hot months. The whitewashing of the trees and fences gave a fresh and healthy appearance to the streets in which it was done." Most interesting was an experimental measure said to have been carried out on the suggestion of W. G. Austin, a former board of health official who had been one of the leading advocates of carbolic acid disinfection a few years before. A solution of "glubo," an alkaline residue obtained from local soap factories, was sprayed over all trees and shrubbery on designated blocks, with "the object of killing all forms of low animal

28. Louisiana Board of Health, *Report for 1879*, 7–16.

life"—insects, in other words—"existing thereon, which *may* have something to do with the spread of yellow fever, possibly carrying the germs on their backs." Unfortunately, sources do not reveal any explicit details on the theoretical background of this plan.[29]

The glubo experiment was never heard of again—one more example of the imaginative but inconsecutive thinking an epidemic crisis tended to inspire. In July, the editor of the *Appeal* took note of the many hungry and bewildered cats and dogs wandering around Memphis, turned loose and left to fend for themselves on the streets when their owners "refugeed" to distant places. Not only was this an inhumanity inflicted on the brutes, the editor scolded, but it was by no means yet known that animals were not harborers and spreaders of the yellow fever germ. Old-style miasmatism was still percolating in the public imagination—a September letter to the *Appeal* considered that the stubbornness of yellow fever in recent years was directly related to the progressive denudation of the natural woods around Memphis: "The forest trees formerly absorbed the malaria we now inhale." Other letters in the daily press showed that, even among doctors, there was still considerable variance and skepticism respecting the subtenets of the established germ theory. One local M.D. contended that "sulphur fumigation is a humbug from a scientific standpoint"; another took the completely heretical position that filth had nothing whatever to do with yellow fever.[30]

Page 2 of the August 8 *Avalanche* carried an inconspicuous item under the heading "Settled at Last," giving a glimpse of how far the sallies of causal theorists could go. Affecting a self-deprecating, semihumorous tone—aware that the speculation it offered was at odds with the fixed views of the medical profession—the note explained: "The office of the Board of Health is an arena where journalistic warriors fight an argumentative battle over the yellow fever question every evening, while waiting for the undertakers' reports. The most impossible theories as to the cause, treatment, and spread of the disease are argued, with all the more persistence because they have not the least foundation in fact, or even probability." Chief among the "results" those insouciant debaters had arrived at were the propositions that "yellow fever is caused by animalculae which

29. *Ibid.*, 120–25.
30. Memphis *Appeal*, July 30, September 9, October 23, 24, 1879.

float around loose in the atmosphere and feed upon germs," and that "the poison is disseminated by mosquitoes and bedbugs, which explains why so many more people are attacked at boarding houses than elsewhere." This was two years before Dr. Carlos Finlay formally proposed the mosquito theory of yellow fever transmission, and two decades before Walter Reed and his associates established it as a scientific fact. The newspaper dash was submitted in a spirit of fun or mock-fun, however, and at the time, it went virtually unnoticed and was certainly unremembered.

In medical circles, a certain amount of conjecture about the possibility of insect transmission of disease was afloat, but it was accorded very little discussion and even less acceptance by the profession. In 1863, Dr. William Budd of England had suggested that biting flies might be an important means of disseminating "malignant pustule," the human manifestation of chronic cutaneous anthrax. He observed that the complaint was most prevalent in summer, when bugs abound, and that the lesions were most frequent on the face and hands, parts of the body most exposed to insect bites. In France, a school of veterinary scientists maintained that anthrax was spread among horses and cattle by bloodsucking flies. One of the scientists was Casimir Davaine, discoverer of the anthrax bacillus. In 1875, a French army veterinarian published a paper that explained the theory and discussed its background. He noted David Livingstone's earlier observations on the association of the tsetse fly with "nagana" cattle sickness along the Zambezi River, and presciently commented that instead of being the product of a venom injected by insects, as the explorer supposed, the disease was probably caused by a germ being carried from animal to animal by the flies. (This was twenty-one years before David Bruce, a British army doctor in Zululand, actually demonstrated the transmission of nagana by tsetse). In an article contributed to Hugo von Ziemssen's wellknown *Cyclopaedia,* an American edition of which appeared in 1875, the German veterinarian Otto Bollinger accepted the fly transmission of anthrax, though he did not agree with Davaine that all cases not explainable by direct contagion were to be attributed to inoculation by flies. Bollinger also thought it quite conceivable that rabies virus could be transferred by fleas and lice, but he acknowledged that this had never been demonstrated and could not be a usual mode of infection.[31]

31. William Budd, "Observations on the Occurrence of Malignant Pustule in England," *British Medical Journal,* March 7, 1863, pp. 239–40; J. P. Mégnin, "Mémoire sur le question

In the fall of 1878, Dr. Patrick Manson of Great Britain published a series of papers on the relation of mosquitoes to filariasis, based on his microscopic and pathological studies at Amoy in south China, where he had been stationed in employment with the Customs Service. Manson had squeezed blood from the stomachs of mosquitoes that had bitten filariasis sufferers, and in it he discovered active filaria parasites. This in itself was a momentous finding; unfortunately, Manson failed to conclude that the insects were spreading the disease by direct inoculation, but instead assumed that they contaminated stores of drinking water with the parasite via their excrement.[32] One of the few American journals to take note of this discovery was the *St. Louis Clinical Record,* in its August, 1879, issue. Its editor, William B. Hazard, commented: "It appears to us that there is a simpler way of communicating the disease from man to man by way of the mosquito than that proposed by Manson." Dr. Hazard proceeded to set forth a remarkably advanced—and remarkably accurate—interpretation of the process:

> When the mosquito or fly bites an animal it first injects a portion of the fluid from its own body into the puncture for the purpose of diluting the blood that it intends to appropriate. . . . Some of this fluid from the insect is left in the puncture; it is rapidly diffused and cannot all be withdrawn. Now, if the fluids of the insect are permeated by the living, active filareae, it is but reasonable to suppose that some of them will be injected and left in the subcutaneous lymph-spaces. . . . Those parts of the body best supplied with lymphatics—the external genitals and extremities— are the seat of those most remarkable changes dependent upon obstructive lesions produced by the filareae. Hence our hypothesis derives the strongest supporting evidence. The way of entrance suggested is certainly more direct than that by means of drinking-water.[33]

---

de transport et de l'inoculation des virus par les mouches," *Journal de l'anatomie et de la physiologie normales et pathologiques de l'homme et des animaux,* XI (1875), 121–33; Otto Bollinger, "Infection by Animal Poisons," in *Ziemssen's Cyclopaedia of the Practice of Medicine,* ed. Albert H. Buck (20 vols.; New York, 1875), III, 383, 409, 440. For an alleged case of smallpox transmission through the bite of a flea, see also, "An Insect Vaccinator," *Lancet,* June 22, 1872, p. 885.

32. "The Development of the Filaria Sanguinis Hominis," *Medical Times and Gazette,* September 7, 1878, pp. 275–76.

33. "The Mosquito in a New Relation," *St. Louis Clinical Record,* VI (1879), 146–47. On the matter of yellow fever, Dr. Hazard remained a firm believer in filth and fomites.

Sanitary science obviously had something more than a labor of Hercules in cleaning up Memphis, but citizens bound to the place by circumstance or sentiment realized that self-preservation was the consideration that most starkly confronted the city in the aftermath of the epidemics. J. M. Keating, editor of the *Appeal* and a leading light in Memphis civic life, delivered a strong editorial on the subject on October 21: "A repetition of this infliction (which I am persuaded is wholly due to filth and dirt and the neglect of the simplest forms of sanitation) would prove the destruction of the city as a great commercial point . . . and she would occupy the singular and anomalous position of a dead American city. . . . To live we must sewer, pave, and enforce other sanitary regulations," Keating emphasized. "To escape death we must become clean in a sense unknown to any other people." Certain "men of property" and other influential Memphians waiting out the epidemic in St. Louis and Nashville hotels were simultaneously holding meetings on the question, and finally memorialized the state and national boards of health to map out an agenda for permanent sanitary reform.[34]

In December, a house-to-house inspection was conducted to obtain an exact inventory of the city's sanitary situation, with particular attention to cellars, sinks, and privies. More than 12,000 business and residential premises were visited, the inspection returns filled 96 folio volumes, and the tabulated results were appalling. They revealed that there was practically no sewer system in Memphis, the few private lines in existence having only 215 connections in all. Of the 5,914 privy vaults that received the vast proportion of the city's excreta, 3,668 were found to be foul or overflowing, and it was judged that there was probably an equal number of disused but unemptied old vaults, merely abandoned when full and covered with a scattering of dirt or ashes. The inspectors found 3,408 of the city's 4,744 cisterns and wells within contaminating distance of privies; in several hundred instances the walls were almost touching. Garbage collection was in a scandalous state. A force of sixteen men, four wagons, and five carts was theoretically supposed to cover more than 100 miles of streets and alleys, but an examination of the dumpkeeper's records showed that only 30 loads a day were really being fetched in—only half the stipulated number. Four of Memphis' ten wards were substantially ignored, and refuse was being

34. Memphis *Appeal*, October 18, 21, 1879; Memphis *Avalanche*, October 29, 1879.

disposed of in every conceivable way: scattered over alleys and vacant lots, dumped into disused wells and cisterns, cast down gullies, and thrown into bayous.[35]

The privy vaults and cesspools of Memphis took on a particularly awful significance after the imagination of sanitarians had filled them with yellow fever germs. Accumulated human excrement—"the animal impurities incidental to crowded populations," as the president of the Memphis Board of Health delicately stated the problem—had long been implicated as an especially potent factor in fostering and propagating yellow fever. And not a few theorists believed that the germs of the disease, released into the soil through the discharges and excreta of its victims, could be disseminated subsequently through drinking water as well as through the air—an idea originally advanced by the influential William Budd, who had proved a similar theory about typhoid fever.[36] In Memphis, privies located in cellar closets and backyard blinds, and their unavoidable proximity to house wells and underground cisterns, made the idea seem more than plausible, and the crisis of a second consecutive epidemic made abolition of this nuisance the first imperative. In 1879, the city papers had pounded away on this point all summer long. "The germ that is eating the heart out of Memphis does not come from the West Indies. The germ lies rotting in the vaults under our feet," the *Avalanche* exhorted in an August editorial, explaining how, unless substantial corrections were made, the city was going to be perennially poisoned by the germs battening on its own waste: "And the people not only breathe the mephitic odors arising from it from year to year, but they drink from it." A few days later: "The whole world looks with dismay upon a civilization that permits the existence of a city upon a bed of ancient privy vaults. Burn the city, is their cry. Burn it down and build a new one in another place." In the fall of 1879, one of the country's foremost civil engineers was engaged to lay out a reticulated system of vitrified sewer pipes, which would be flushed daily from water tanks situated at the head of each submain. Trenching for the pipes began

35. "Report on Sanitary Survey of Memphis, Tennessee," in National Board of Health, *Report for 1880,* 416–34.

36. W. Budd, "On the Contagion of Yellow Fever," *Lancet,* April 6, 1861, pp. 337–38; "Proceedings of the Medical and Surgical Society of Baltimore, October 10th, 1878," *Medical and Surgical Reporter,* XXXIX (1878), 471; B. Brown Williams, "Pure Water vs. Yellow Fever," *Medical Brief,* VII (1879), 5–6.

in January, 1880, and by the end of the year, over 26 miles of sewer line were in operation, and over 2,300 house connections had been completed. By the end of the decade, all but two of the city's wards had been sewered.[37]

Another perceived hotbed of yellow fever infection was the "Nicholson" wood-block pavement that many of the downtown streets had been encumbered with. In 1867, an expenditure of half a million dollars had purchased for the city eleven miles of this questionable improvement, consisting of squared sections of cypress set on end and caulked with tar. At the time, southern cypress was being advertised by lumber dealers as "the wood eternal," but after a few seasons of pounding by hoofs and grinding by wagon wheels, the pavement was reduced to what one observer denounced as "a dark, pulpy mass of decay." A correspondent of the Chicago *Times* described the problem in the summer of 1879: "Every rain has carried into the pores of the wood and between the interstices of the blocks, excrementary matter, and this, upon the recurrence of the great heats, has fermented and given off poisonous fumes in unlimited quantities. . . . The foul organic matter, composed largely of the excrements of animals, is retained in the joints, ruts, and gutters, where it undergoes putrefactive fermentation in warm, damp weather and becomes the fruitful source of noxious effluvia." In fact, removal of the Nicholson pavement and replacement with stone had begun in the spring of that year and continued through the epidemic. By the end of the 1880s, over thirty-five miles of Memphis' streets had been paved.[38]

Sewering and paving between them took an outlay of over a million dollars. Together they were viewed as the core of the sanitary reform program; but, however wholesome and commendable the projects were in other regards, they rendered the city no real protection from Yellow Jack. The contingent benefits from changes made in the city's water-supply ar-

37. Memphis *Avalanche*, August 20, 24, 1879; George E. Waring, *Report on the Social Statistics of Cities* (2 vols.; Washington, D.C., 1887), II, 144–47; John Huber Ellis, "Yellow Fever and the Origins of Modern Public Health in Memphis, Tennessee, 1870–1900" (Ph.D. dissertation, Tulane University, 1962), 181–85.

38. Memphis *Appeal*, July 18, 1879; G. B. Thornton, "The Yellow Fever Epidemic in Memphis, 1879," *Reports and Papers, American Public Health Association*, V (1879), 118–19; Ellis, "Modern Public Health in Memphis," 191–92.

rangements were of infinitely greater effect, though no one at the time could have divined the reason. Tied in with the agitation for removal of the privy vaults had been a concern that subsoil pollution had already extended to the point where the purity of house wells and subterranean cisterns was hopelessly compromised. Two days before frost came to put an end to the epidemic of 1879, an editorial in the *Avalanche* had demanded that "the cisterns must be abolished immediately." The cisterns were not contemplated as a source of mosquitoes; mosquitoes were not suspected as a source of yellow fever. Rather, the fear was that widespread seepage and infiltration from the privy vaults had contaminated the cistern water with poisonous and germ-breeding "fecal substances." At first, an immediate solution was seen in putting water tanks up on stilts alongside the houses, as in New Orleans. But when cold weather came, with more time for considering the problem, officials recognized that longterm requirements for pure water in quantity could only be satisfied by a centralized municipal supply. After a few years of deliberation, consulting engineers and city politicians settled upon artesian water as the best source.

The resistance of a preexisting franchise committed to the pumping of river water was finally overcome in March, 1887, when the state legislature passed an act to permit the issue of $150,000 in new waterworks bonds for the city, and the vested interest was bought out and absorbed. Drilling in the countryside behind Memphis got under way that summer, and by the fall of 1888, over thirty good, flowing wells had been struck, capable of delivering 10 million gallons per day. Within two years, 60 miles of mains had been laid and 5,300 of the city's 11,567 dwellings had taps. The gradual extension of this system over the next ten years no doubt served to eliminate the prime breeding locations of *A. aegypti* in most of the incorporated area of the city. However, in the course of 72,014 house inspections performed in 1900, the Memphis sanitary police reported 4,916 inspections of cisterns, which shows that a significant number of tanks were still in use at the very time Walter Reed was at work demonstrating the agency of the "cistern mosquito" in transmitting yellow fever. The owners of small houses and shanties of the "five-dollar-a-month class" were blamed for the difficulty—people who regarded the water tax as a burden and exercised their right to erect tanks, under specified rules, instead of taking water from the municipal company. The board of health was gradually persuading most of those landlords to give up their individualistic arrangements.[39]

The raised cisterns of New Orleans had also come in for a certain amount of sanitary criticism in the wake of the great epidemic. In 1879, a chemist for the National Board of Health had found them abounding in potential pabulum for germs—"recent vegetable tissues, starch cells, confervoid filaments, zoopores, cotton fibers, fungi, and mineral fragments"—and had determined an ammonia content scarcely better than that of surface water sampled from pools in the nearby swamps. Mosquito larvae, the only significant contaminant as far as yellow fever was concerned, were not considered in the analysis. In fact, one of the popular beliefs yellow fever sanitarians had to overcome in later years was that the wrigglers actually contributed to water purity by consuming algae and bacteria. Water from the shallow street wells, used regularly by the city's bakeries and dairies, as well as by many families in periods of drought, was found to be so vile that its total and immediate interdiction was recommended. In 1886, the municipal board of health banned further use of street wells, but declined to interfere with cisterns. Proposals to supply the city via aqueducts from streams in the "pure pine woods" on the other side of Lake Pontchartrain went by the board. In an 1889 report, the city's chief sanitary inspector concluded that there was really no alternative water supply as safe or healthy as the cistern system, that river water with its sediments was not as wholesome, that indeed the practice of rainwater storage was "a God-send to the people, and doubtless it is due to this fact that typhoid fever is so rare a disease amongst us." By 1905 there would be more than 70,000 house cisterns in New Orleans, double the number that had existed in 1878. It was not until after 1912 that the city's cistern system was substantially replaced by piped water.[40]

39. Memphis *Avalanche,* October 22, 1879; Ellis, "Modern Public Health in Memphis," 185–90; J. M. Safford, "The Water Supply of Memphis," *Sanitarian,* XXIV (1890), 289–307; John S. Billings, *Report on Social Statistics of Cities in the United States at the Eleventh Census* (Washington, D.C., 1895), 73; Memphis Board of Health, *Report for 1900* (Memphis, 1901), 23. In fact, yellow fever did appear sporadically in Memphis in the fall of 1897, with fifty-two cases and fourteen deaths reported. And as late as 1956, a U.S. Public Health Service investigation found *A. aegypti* in 4 percent of the premises surveyed in the city. See George R. Hayes, Jr., and Milton E. Tinker, "The 1956–1957 Status of *Aedes aegypti* in the United States," *Mosquito News,* XVIII (1958), 254.

40. Charles Smart, "Report on the Water Supply of New Orleans and Mobile," in

It was easy, in the summer and fall of 1879, for rival cities to come up with words and music for Memphis' funeral dirge. With its commerce apparently shattered, its people scattered, and the ineluctable fear that every spring the city would be on the verge of another calamitous encore of yellow fever, it was easy for commentators to conclude that a pall of uncertainty and depression had been permanently draped over Memphis' future. In July, the Cairo *Bulletin* had summed up the situation:

> Memphis is today the leper among American cities, shunned and avoided by its own people, held as a thing of horror, not to be seen or touched, a dreaded spot, fenced out by the surrounding world, to be ravaged by its own pestilence. . . . Property values are destroyed, citizens by the thousands are flying from their businesses and homes, leaving all to the mercy of burglars and thieves or the more dreaded hunger-driven mob—all that from an ordeal that but few who can avoid it will pass through for the third time. . . . For years to come, though yellow fever gain no hold anywhere in the South, the city will be and remain but a mere shadow, a skeleton of its former self—shorn of its business, its life, its wealth, its air of thrift, of all that rendered it the second city of the lower valley.[41]

U.S. Census figures give a good measure of Memphis' longterm forfeiture to the three sieges of Yellow Jack in the 1870s. Whereas Shelby County had posted a gain in population of nearly 59 percent in the war decade of the 1860s, from 1870 to 1880 the increase was less than 3 percent (from 76,378 to 78,430). In the same period, the increase in the only other Tennessee county of comparable rank was 26 percent (Davidson County, centering on the city of Nashville, which was unaffected by yellow fever). In Tennessee as a whole, the increase was 23 percent. If it was not exactly thrown backward by yellow fever, overall population growth in Shelby County was certainly stalled by the epidemics. That the problem was centered in Memphis and its suburbs and outlying towns is evident in the fact that the acreage of improved land in Shelby County farms increased 24 percent during the 1870s, exactly matching the increase in the state of Tennessee as a whole. It is perhaps significant that the percentage of blacks

National Board of Health, *Report for 1880*, 441–45; Louisiana Board of Health, *Report for 1888–89* (Baton Rouge, 1890), 116.

41. Memphis *Appeal,* July 26, 1879.

in Shelby County increased from 48 percent to 56 percent during these years, while the black population in Davidson County and the state of Tennessee as a whole remained steady at 40 percent and 26 percent, respectively.[42]

Manufacturing statistics showed a marked decline during the yellow fever decade. In 1870, Shelby County housed 20 percent of the total capital invested in manufacturing in the state of Tennessee. By the 1880 census, capital values reported in the county had fallen by 22 percent and accounted for only 12 percent of the Tennessee total, which, indeed, had risen 29 percent since 1870. The number of hands employed in manufacturing in Shelby County had fallen by 30 percent. The number of boilerworks, foundries, and machine shops declined from 14 to 9 during the decade. The number of manufacturers of sawn and planed lumber dropped from 30 to 13; of carriages and wagons, from 27 to 6. The slump seems to have affected the lesser categories of industry just as much; the number of saddleries fell from 18 to 5, and brickyards from 9 to 3. Nor does it appear that local-supply enterprises were exempt from the downward pressure: bakeries declined from 18 to 7, confectioneries from 14 to 5, and Shelby County lost one of its two breweries. A few lines of business thrived: marble works and tombstone-cutters' establishments, alas, increased from 5 to 6.[43]

We should be cautious about interpreting the apparent flight of capital and enterprise with reference to the epidemics alone, for Memphis in the late 1870s was laboring under a complication of grave civic problems, of which yellow fever was merely the most sensational. A municipal debt crisis of terminal proportions had been building steadily since 1866 and was coming to a head in the summer of 1878 when the fever struck. By then a demoralized city government had piled up a bonded debt of over $5 million and had saddled real estate and commercial inventories in Memphis with an *ad valorem* property tax of 5-$\frac{1}{2}$ percent. The debt situation had been gravely impacted by constricted financial conditions prevailing nationwide in the wake of the 1873 Wall Street crash. The city's credit position, never very solid, was progressively hammered down, until after a few years Memphis found itself largely unable to sell new bonds, even at the

42. *Tenth Census, 1880: Population,* 407–408.
43. *Ninth Census, 1870: Wealth and Industry,* 570, 734; *Tenth Census, 1880: Manufactures,* 175, 358.

outrageous discounts from par value that had served to float its issues previously. Taxes were going delinquent, creditors were being stalled and put off, and municipal employees, including many of the police, were quitting. So when yellow fever burst upon the scene, the city's elected government virtually blew away in the chaos.[44]

The anomalous situation lasted until January, 1879, when the state legislature intervened, revoked the city's charter, threw its finances into receivership, and replaced the mayor and council with an appointed commission. The general state of affairs, compounded by the reappearance of the fever that summer, did not bode well for commerce and industry in Memphis, and talk of an extra $2\frac{1}{2}$ percent levy on property for sanitary purposes could not have made future prospects any more inviting for businessmen. This unstable period turned out to be the low point in the city's fortunes, however, and after a few years of strict management, Memphis' cash flow was restored, its streets were cleansed, and its privy vaults done away with. Yellow fever failed to mount another attack. Capital invested in manufacturing in Shelby County rebounded dramatically, increasing 300 percent from 1880 to 1890 to account for 19 percent of the Tennessee total, and the county's population also resumed a healthy upward trend, rising nearly 44 percent to 112,740 by 1890. The state saw fit to restore the city's charter in 1893. Even when Memphis was in the slough of pestilence and depression, a few optimists had predicted its reascendancy. In 1879, the Huntsville *Alabamian* called the idea of permanently abandoning Memphis "simply ridiculous." It said the history of the great cities of Europe and India, repeatedly scourged by cholera and black plague, or indeed the example of places like Havana and Veracruz, where yellow fever was endemic, "contradict the presumption that such visitations inflict any lasting injury upon the regular trade and business of a commanding point." "Memphis is not a doomed city," the Humboldt *Argus* had insisted: "An earthquake will have to sink all the rich cotton lands for 200 miles around for Memphis to be ruined."[45] The prophecy of the St. Louis *Globe-Democrat* furnished a conclusion for historians: "The reaction in Memphis will be greater than her decline. . . . She will pay off all her debts and become a bonafide city again before the headboards of her graveyards

---

44. Ellis, "Modern Public Health in Memphis," 126–42.
45. Memphis *Avalanche,* August 10, October 28, 1879.

become old. The suggestions to burn and forever abandon the city are more sarcastic than reasonable. The fever is as likely to depart suddenly as to remain another year. . . . She occupies a controlling situation in a business point of view, and this cannot be changed. Misfortune is always emphatic, but its opposite is more so."[46]

46. *Ibid.*, August 31, 1879.

SIX

The Final Rounds with Yellow Fever

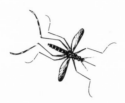

The confused debate over the mystery of yellow fever resumed again at the Nashville meetings of the American Public Health Association in November, 1879. Dr. A. A. Woodhull of the U.S. Army presented an etiological study of the 1876 epidemic at Savannah, Georgia, particulars of which (as Woodhull reconstructed them) seemed to rule out any importation of foreign germs, establishing local causes as the source of the fever. His "most careful scrutiny" had failed to determine "the faintest clue" of any derivation from abroad. Six vessels from Cuba had visited Savannah prior to the outbreak of the fever, but Woodhull was satisfied that all of them had been "entirely free from sickness." Nor was he able to establish evidence of any personal communication between the first local cases. The only connecting link seemed to be their proximity to an abandoned rice canal that was receiving the discharge from numerous local sewer lines. "It was in effect a huge, uncovered, shallow sewer charged with the excremental discharge of a large portion of the city, and fully exposed to atmospheric influences." Woodhull challenged the assumption that the emergence of the first yellow fever germ was a one-of-a-kind biological accident, "with no chance of repetition," and he saw no reason why in this instance it could not have been developed *de novo* by the right combination of heat, humidity, and "fermenting foecal matter in excess." Here was a bid to revive the idea of yellow fever's local causation and spontaneous origin, not in terms of the old miasmatism, but along the new-fashioned lines of evolutionary theory.

With more confidence we may imagine an infinite variety of self-propagating germs, each set of which may gradually yield to adjacent influence, as is conspicuous in the cultivation of vegetation, and is shadowed in animal life; and then suppose that with the metamorphosis induced by the surrounding conditions the yellow fever cause is gradually evolved. Those presumed changes, although perhaps involving many generations of germ life, may easily be accomplished within the period of a single season, and would be developed with a rapidity proportional to the propitiousness of the season. If such a modification has occurred once it may occur a thousand times.[1]

A paper read by one of Memphis' sanitary inspectors maintained that it was entirely probable that the recent epidemic there had been of *de novo* origin, and emphasized that the thousands of foul privy vaults underlying the city made excellent places for the infection's spontaneous generation. Taking the opposite extreme was Dr. Jerome Cochran, a former member of the Yellow Fever Commission who had represented the National Board of Health in Tennessee during the recent epidemic. Cochran declared that he had thought over various inconsistencies in the occurrence of yellow fever, and he had come to agree with the small minority who believed the disease was not in any way the product of ordinary filth and had no necessary connection with filth as such. "If it has any connection with filth, it is with some element of filth that is not manifest to any of the senses, that does not offend the eyes or the nose." "As he had sat here from day to day and had heard almost every theory that had been advanced by one learned member of the body controverted by others, and a general chaos of opinion upon almost every important question, he had been surprised to find how small a modicum of accepted truth there is in medical science, and how much is left to conjecture," a Memphis judge who was sitting in on these sessions was quoted as saying. "Impressed as we have been by the ravages made by this King of Terrors, it is admitted that we know but little if any more today than was known centuries ago as to its origin, its mode of propagation, its prevention, or its cure." He said the current portrayals of Memphis' sanitary degradation were mainly caricatures, and

1. Alfred A. Woodhull, "May Not Yellow Fever Originate in the United States? An Etiological Study of the Epidemic at Savannah in 1876," *Reports and Papers, American Public Health Association*, V (1879), 89–107.

insisted the city was really no worse in that regard than most others in the country, north or south (which was probably true).[2]

At the urging of the American Public Health Association, the newly created National Board of Health had dispatched a group of medical scientists to Havana, Cuba, in the summer of 1879 to collect and analyze all available facts about the occurrence and persistence of yellow fever in that tropical city. Havana—where yellow fever had been recorded every single year since 1761, claiming over 11,000 lives in the nine years since 1870—was appropriately denounced as "the greatest nursery and camping ground of one of man's most ruthless destroyers." The officials reasoned that a study of the disease at an endemic center on its supposed native soil would yield more useful information than any haphazard observations that could be made during its epidemic invasions of the United States mainland. The Havana Yellow Fever Commission published its ponderous final report in the annual report of the National Board of Health for 1880. It concluded that the prevalence of yellow fever at Havana was due "not to any mysterious exceptional cause, but to an exceptional intensity of usual causes. . . . Hence, there are no remedies for this condition other than those which are well known and which have proved successful wherever properly applied."

The commission had encountered the same unspeakable sanitary conditions that had amazed Baron von Humboldt seventy-five years before, and its detailed description of those conditions made the reasons for the perpetuation of yellow fever in the Cuban capital self-evident to any partisan of the conventional germ theory. The low-lying section behind the bay, where most of the poor, immigrant, fever-prone classes lived, was an uncertain landfill built up from rubble, dirt, garbage, and street refuse. Privies rose and fell with the tide; many were overflowing and unusable, and chamber pots were often simply emptied into holes scooped out in the dirt streets. "Nothing more stinking, nasty, and unwholesome than the privy system of Havana can be conceived." The peoples' hovels were damp and ill-ventilated; crooked alleys were thick with kitchen garbage, and prosperous turkey vultures perched on the roofs; and, where not choked up with filth, the foul, open sewers from higher suburbs drained

2. T. J. Tyner, "Etiology of Yellow Fever, with Remarks on Quarantine," *Reports and Papers, American Public Health Association,* V (1879), 147–51; "Proceedings and Discussions," *ibid.,* 213–30.

into the polluted harbor, where ships that would soon be headed for United States ports rested at anchor. The list of abominations singled out for condemnation by the Americans extended even to the decayed paper money kept in circulation by the impoverished colonial government, "so dirty that it stinks," and as dangerous a fomite as rags. It seemed obvious to the investigators that, under such extreme conditions of filth and unsanitary living, the planting and harvesting of the yellow fever germ could go on in the city concurrently and perpetually—in a frost-free climate, with a constant inflow of unacclimated subjects to feed the disease, and with uninterrupted communication between infected neighborhoods.[3]

To the extent that it merely cataloged stenches and unpleasant sights, the report of the Havana Yellow Fever Commission would have gone down as just another documentary relic of the germ theory, but it also contained a certain amount of material that would be of permanent importance in the evolution of scientific thought on yellow fever. The secretary of the commission was a U.S. Army pathologist, who prepared a collection of photomicrographs of blood and tissues from yellow fever victims that is still admired for its quality. This pathologist, Dr. George Sternberg, would serve as Surgeon General of the Army twenty-two years later, when the momentous investigations of Major Walter Reed were undertaken in Cuba. Dr. Stanford Chaillé, chairman of the commission and professor of pathology at the University of Louisiana, attached a series of brilliant critical essays: "The Origin and Some Properties of the Poison of Yellow Fever, and of Other Specific Spreading Diseases," "The Alleged Spontaneous Origin of Yellow Fever on Ships," and "Acclimatization, or Acquisition of Immunity from Yellow Fever." These served to put all atmospheric or "malarial" theories to final rest and reconfirmed, on a deductive basis, the character of yellow fever as a specific, infectious, germ-caused disease. Excerpts from the first of those essays illustrate the tenor of his argument and the clarity of his reasoning:

> It is less than thirty years since Budd denied the spontaneous origin of typhoid fever, an origin still contended for by some. Modern research

3. "Report of the Havana Yellow Fever Commission," in National Board of Health, *Report for 1880*, 95–106, 299–308.

has tended constantly to prove that diseases, above all migratory epidemic diseases, have no such origin; and the spontaneous-generation experiments and the whole tendency of modern science are opposed to any such belief. None the less, "indigenous," "spontaneous," "de novo" origin and development are words incessantly repeated in the present literature of yellow fever, and express the ideas firmly entertained by many. . . .

There are three chief causes for the belief in the spontaneous origin of yellow fever. Some, more deeply impressed by past than by recent knowledge, are not able to understand that a disease may not be personally contagious, in the manner of smallpox, measles, etc., and yet may be portable and communicable, as are trichina, tape-worm, typhoid fever, and cholera. A second cause is the very old one of mistaking those causes which favor the propagation of a poison for those which originate it. Finally, disbelief in the duration of the dormant vitality of disease-poison is a constant source of error. . . .

The poison of yellow fever must be on the one hand either an inorganic or dead organic something, or on the other hand a living organism. Very few if any, even of those who credit its spontaneous origin, deny that this poison has reproductive power. The function of reproduction is limited to living organisms, and such must be the nature of the poison of yellow fever. . . .

The poisons of cholera and typhoid fever are the most important, and to yellow fever the most closely allied, of those disease-poisons which are non-inoculable yet transmissible, and are now classified as miasmatic-contagious poisons, being characterized, apparently, by the peculiarity that while they come from a sick person, yet they require outside of the body favorable conditions for further change or development before acquiring any infective poisonous power. . . .

It is manifest that the failure of the microscope to prove that the causes of yellow fever, as also of typhoid fever, cholera, etc., are living organisms no more disproves this than the failure of all the appliances of science to prove that the cause is an inorganic or a dead substance disproves this conclusion; and the mystery as to what is in truth the poison is increased by supposing it an unknown inorganic something rather than an unknown extra-microscopic organism. . . .

These poisons are markedly characterized by one of the most striking differences between living organisms and inorganic or dead matter, viz., by the fact that their growth and reproduction occur only under special circumstances. They have either climatic limits, or are greatly influenced by climate; they are at one time narrowly localized, at another widely radiated; and they repeatedly refuse to propagate under circumstances apparently identical with those under which they have on other occasions best flourished. All the spreading disease-poisons seem to grow best in decaying, putrefying substances, one of the most noted traits of the fungi; and in the peculiarity of the circumstances required for the propagation of these is also found the best analogy to the often inexplicable appearance and disappearance of disease-poisons.

Dr. Chaillé drew extensively on the literature of biology to show how the various species of microscopically visible fungi each germinated and flourished only in a particular medium and only under certain narrow conditions of light and temperature. "Such facts enable us to understand, among other things, why the poison of yellow fever should much more frequently fail than it succeeds to propagate when imported, the success or failure depending on some perhaps most trifling, though disastrous, contingency." The way some of them would vegetate on one strain of a particular host species and not on another suggested similar peculiarities in yellow fever. "Since this is true of the parasites which attack animals as well as vegetables, it is possible that a special parasite might be, as is yellow fever, more partial to man than to inferior animals, and more partial to a white man than a black man." In all this, Chaillé was not trying to demonstrate that the cause of yellow fever was a fungus, but—much the way Dr. Josiah Nott had once sought analogies in "the habits and movements of the larger insects"—to show how "some of the mysterious phenomena of the unknown and invisible poison of yellow fever have their counterparts in similar phenomena of known and visible living organisms." As an illustration of the prolonged duration of the "dormant vitality of disease-poison," Chaillé could cite recent demonstrations by Pasteur and Koch of the remarkable resistance of anthrax spores to extremes of heat, cold, and drying. This feature of dormant vitality suggested an explanation for yellow fever's long-range transmission via fomites, as well as for its endemic persistence in certain places in spite of the best sanitary efforts. In discussing some of the hidden pathways of transmission that might be available to the yellow fever germ, Chaillé even intimated the possibility of an intermediate host, though he never specifically accused the mosquito:

It is worthy of note that a number of animal parasites are now known which pass through several stages of development, each stage requiring its own special and peculiar favorable conditions, and that in only one of these stages does it cause disease. . . . The egg of the thorn-headed worm of the hog develops in a crab; this must be eaten by a fish, and this by a hog, to gain the stage of maturity. The "rot" in sheep is due to the fluke-worm, the eggs of which require for their first stage of development that they should be eaten by a fresh water snail. In all instances the undeveloped eggs are harmless.[4]

As a means of securing local cooperation, twelve Cuban scientists had been connected to the Havana Yellow Fever Commission as "auxiliary experts." One of them was a Havana physician, Dr. Carlos Finlay, who had earlier impressed his colleagues on the island with a paper that purported to show a relationship between yellow fever and "excessive alkalinity of the atmosphere." He believed he had determined that there was a measurably higher ammonia content in the air where yellow fever prevailed, and he noted a number of similarities between the symptoms of yellow fever and those of ammonia poisoning. One of the tasks assigned to Dr. Finlay as assistant to the commission was that of interviewing the bosses of night-scavenging operations in the city. Finlay found a preponderance of unacclimated Spanish immigrants employed in these excavating crews, but the incidence of yellow fever among them was actually much less than among the general population. "From these facts it would seem that yellow fever is not a faecal disease." Another consideration that weighed on Finlay's mind was that Dr. George Sternberg had failed to find in the air of infected localities in Havana "any gross and conspicuous germ or organism . . . which by its peculiar appearance or abundant presence might arrest the attention of the microscopist and cause suspicion that it is the germ of yellow fever." Finlay began to doubt that there was any connection at all between this disease and "filth," and gave up his search for a special toxic element or pathogenic organism in the soil or air. But he still had the problem of accounting for the mass of evidence that indicated yellow fever was caught from places, not persons—that its "poison" was somehow matured and multiplied in outer nature by certain conditions of the locality. He was impressed by the germ theory advocated by Chaillé,

4. *Ibid.*, 117–28.

but even supposing that certain unsanitary conditions might provide a medium for the extrinsic development of the germ, the theory supplied no clear explanation of just how the infection invaded the body. Most doctors were content to assume that the germs wafted up from the ground and were inhaled, but this seemed to Finlay to be an unsatisfactory explanation, inasmuch as it implied diffusibility of the infection through the air, in contradiction of the acknowledged fact that breezes had little or no effect on the spread of epidemics.[5]

Sternberg's photomicrographs had failed to turn up the specific germ of yellow fever but had displayed one very intriguing pathological change in its victims—the desquamation of the capillaries, which was the source of the hemorrhagic tendency in the disease. Studying the pictures, Finlay conceived the idea that yellow fever was essentially an eruptive infection of the inner lining of the blood vessels. And if the seat of infection were inside the blood vessels, he reasoned, it followed that the infectious element had to be extracted and deposited by some means of inoculation. Finlay postulated that the infection of yellow fever could only be propagated through the agency of some "natural inoculating agent" present in the environment. Some blood-sucking insect seemed the obvious candidate for this role—more particularly, a stinging insect whose environmental conditions were identical with those that were known to favor reproduction of the disease:

> I have had reason to become convinced of the untenable nature of any theory which may attribute the origin or propagation of yellow fever to atmospheric, miasmatic, or meteorological influences, or of its equally weak character if it appeals to filth or neglected hygienic principles. I have thus been obliged to abandon my primitive beliefs. . . .
>
> I must state, however, that the subject of this paper has no relation whatsoever with the nature or form in which the morbigenic factor in yellow fever exists; in this regard I will limit my opinions to the following statement: that I admit the existence of a material or transportable cause, which may be either an amorphous virus, an animal or vegetable germ,

5. *Ibid.*, 162, 165–66; George M. Sternberg, "The Microscopical Investigations of the Havana Yellow Fever Commission," *New Orleans Medical and Surgical Journal*, n.s., VII (1880), 1019; Charles Finlay, "Summary of the Progress Made in the Nineteenth Century in the Study of the Propagation of Yellow Fever," *Medical Record*, LIX (1901), 201–203.

bacterium, etc., etc., but which consists in all cases of a tangible something which has to be communicated from the sick to the healthy in order that the disease may be propagated. What I propose studying is the medium or agent by which the pathogenic material of yellow fever is carried from the bodies of the infected to be implanted in the bodies of the non-infected.

The necessity of admitting the intervention of an element foreign to the disease in order that it may be transmitted follows as a result of numerous observations formulated in the early part of this century and confirmed by latter-day experience. Thus, yellow fever sometimes traverses the ocean and is propagated in very distant cities whose conditions are widely different from those of the focus in which the infection originated; while at other times the same disease does not transgress the boundaries of a very limited epidemic zone, notwithstanding the fact that the meteorology and topography of neighboring localities reveal no differences which would explain so different a behavior of the same disease in two apparently similar places. Admitting the necessary presence of an agent whose behavior would explain the above anomalies, it is evident that the conditions now recognized as affecting the propagation of the yellow fever poison would also be applicable to this agent. In searching for this agent it was not probable that it would be found in the microzoa or zoophytes, for these minute forms of animated nature are little, if at all, influenced by the meteorological variations which most frequently affect the development of yellow fever. In order to meet the exigencies of this question it was found necessary to ascend as high up in the animal scale as the insect class, and keeping in mind at the same time that yellow fever is characterized clinically, and according to most recent labors, histologically, by vascular lesions and physicochemical alterations of the blood, it seems natural that this agent could be found in that class of insects which, by penetrating into the interior of the blood vessels, could suck up the blood together with any infecting particles contained therein, and carry the same from the diseased to the healthy. Finally, I asked myself if it was not the mosquito that transmitted the yellow fever poison.

Finlay recalled the frequent mention of mosquitoes in accounts of earlier epidemics—he had studied the 1854 report of the Sanitary Commission of New Orleans—but instead of regarding them as mere incidentals of a vitiated atmosphere, he guessed that they might in fact be the "natural inoculating agents" he was searching for. He reasoned that the species whose natural history best matched the seasonal peculiarities and locational anomalies of yellow fever was the gray-colored, house-haunting "day mosquito" well known all around the Gulf and Caribbean. He described the mosquito's proboscis and its operation in some detail, supposing that it became encrusted with the germs of the disease when it pierced the blood vessel of an infected subject, thereby spreading the virulent particles like a contaminated needle in subsequent feeds. Finlay was satisfied that his theory of mosquito transmission could finally reconcile "the anomalies, so obscure and difficult of explanation otherwise, which have been observed in the distribution of yellow fever." The disease's inability to spread at higher elevations, for example, was due to the inordinately small wings of this mosquito, which made it less able to get about in a rare atmosphere. The "partial immunity enjoyed by the African," so much in contrast with the malady's "especially active persecution of the members of the Northern races," was explained by the Negro's thicker skin, which made it less attractive to the mosquito. Finlay modestly concluded that "the truth of my suspicions and conceptions be left to the decisive evidence furnished by direct experimentation."[6]

In February, 1882, the *New Orleans Medical and Surgical Journal* published an English translation of Finlay's article submitted by a young New Orleans doctor, Rudolf Matas, who later gained prominence as a professor of surgery at the Tulane Medical School. There is no evidence that, at the time, the publication elicited significant comment or debate either way. In a long lecture before the Orleans Parish Medical Society fifteen years later (1897), Matas reviewed the evolution of the germ theory of yellow fever, dwelling at some length on the mystery of the infection's apparent "maturation" outside the human body, without making any mention whatever of Finlay's proposition. Like most physicians of his generation, Matas preferred to think that the germ penetrated the body through the respiratory passages.[7] Finlay's theory made excellent sense to at least one American layman, and in an 1882 letter to *Science* magazine, Mr. Harry Hammond drew on his own recollections to discuss the association of railroads, cis-

6. Charles Finlay, "The Mosquito Hypothetically Considered as an Agent in the Transmission of Yellow Fever Poison," *New Orleans Medical and Surgical Journal*, n.s., IX (1882), 601–16.

7. R. Matas, "Discussion of the Etiology and Pathology of Yellow Fever," *New Orleans Medical and Surgical Journal*, L (1898), 210–37.

terns, mosquitoes, and yellow fever at various places in South Carolina and Georgia. Finlay, meanwhile, from time to time wrote more about his idea; in 1886, a Memphis medical journal briefly noted one of his publications.[8]

In 1883, a remarkable essay was published in *Popular Science Monthly* by A. F. A. King, a Washington, D.C., physician, on the novel proposition that malaria was transmitted by mosquitoes. King examined nineteen recognized etiological characteristics of malaria and showed how each one could be explained with reference to mosquito activity. The association of malaria and mosquitoes with warm weather and with low, poorly drained localities was notorious. The fact that yellow fever and malaria tended to prevail at the same time of year and shared some of the same "atmospheric peculiarities," as well as some of the same symptoms, was an old observation, and earlier in the century had fed speculation that yellow fever was nothing but an intensified, malignant phase of the common "bilious fever." King took note of Finlay's recent publication on mosquitoes and yellow fever and approvingly commented:

> When it is remembered that disease-producing bacteric germs are so minute that a million may rest on the head of a pin, and that the smallest puncture may be sufficient to infect the body with the septic matter, it scarcely seems possible to ignore any longer the punctures of mosquitoes and other proboscidian insects as possible sources of infection. With our present knowledge of the "germ theory" one would hardly dare, even once, to plunge an inoculating needle into the blood of a yellow fever patient and then plunge it into his own blood or the blood of other persons, yet this is exactly what the mosquito is doing in every yellow fever epidemic. In yellow fever it is to be noted also that the spread of the disease ceases with frost; so also do the perigrinations of the mosquito.[9]

Unfortunately, King's essay went for naught as far as any practical influence on contemporary medical opinion was concerned and, like Fin-

8. Harry Hammond, "For What Purpose Were Mosquitoes Created," *Science,* VIII (1882), 436; *Mississippi Valley Medical Monthly,* VI (1886), 541–42.
9. A. F. A. King, "Insects and Disease—Mosquitoes and Malaria," *Popular Science Monthly,* XXIII (1883), 645.

lay's, is remembered today only as a curious example of scientific clairvoyance. Two reports on malaria that were submitted to the Surgeon General of the Army thirteen years later (1896) show how resolutely—and how long—the mosquito idea would be ignored. Major Charles Smart, assigned to investigate a recent increase in the disease at West Point, believed malaria was engendered by "the presence in the air of some product of fermentation in the soil." Major Walter Reed studied the problem at Washington Barracks, in the District of Columbia, and attributed the prevalence of malarial fevers at that post to its proximity to the flats and marshes of the Potomac bottoms. "I conclude that the source can be referred to the development of the specific cause partly in the soil upon which the post is located, and to a still greater degree, in the extensive marsh lands lying along the river." Neither Smart nor Reed was so backward as to think that malaria was produced by some impalpable gaseous influence: both investigators found plasmodia in the blood of affected individuals and recognized those microscopic parasites as the specific cause. Both of them, however, still supposed that this cause was telluric in origin and miasmatic in operation—that the germs were bred in the muck of low, damp places and exhaled from the soil into the air, a premise that was much closer to the theory propounded by Lancisi two centuries before than it was to the discovery advanced by Ronald Ross just two years later.[10]

Whatever small window the insect theory might have opened in medical thinking about yellow fever was quickly closed by the established germ theory. Investigators continued to focus the keenest attention on the danger of transmission by fomites, and costly and cumbersome quarantines were shaped around that principle. When a coffee ship from Rio de Janeiro landed three cases of yellow fever at New Orleans in July, 1880, the Tennessee State Board of Health promptly banned from the state a long list of articles, including all clothing and baggage of travelers; the whole class of goods known as "junk stores," such as rags, paper stock, old rope, and secondhand clothing, bedding, and furniture; excelsior, moss, jute, and bagging of any kind; hides, pelts, feathers, hair, and all other remains of animals; and coffee, rice, sugar, molasses, and tropical fruits of every description. "Nor," it was added, "shall any other freights which may have

---

10. "Malarial Diseases," in U.S. Secretary of War, *Report for Fiscal 1896* (3 vols.), I, 453–71.

been carried in contact with such articles be allowed to enter." The one-year-old National Board of Health, operating under the federal government's constitutional authority to regulate interstate commerce, stepped in and instituted a system of quadruple inspection for steamboat traffic on the Mississippi, with one station at New Orleans, another below Vicksburg, another below Memphis, and another below Cairo. All boats ascending the river were to be scrutinized from stem to stern with reference to their sanitary condition. Foul bilges were to be thoroughly pumped out and purified; decayed timbers were to be scraped clean and painted with turpentine; copperas solution and whitewash were to be "freely used" wherever necessary. The loading of boats was strictly supervised. Inspectors were to inquire into the history of every article of cargo and baggage, and nothing "known or suspected to be infected" was to be taken on board. They were to focus particular suspicion on shipments of rags and other used fabrics, and on tropical fruits.

Passengers who presented any indications of "dangerous sickness" were to be held back five days for observation. Among the 118 so detained, there were, according to final diagnosis, 98 cases of malaria, 10 of dysentery, 7 of dengue, 2 of hives, and 1 of "senile debility"—not a single case of yellow fever, or at least none recognized as such. Over the course of the season, the river stations inspected and certified a total of 1,514 vessels having an aggregate capacity of over 1.2 million tons of freight and carrying over 81,000 passengers. The inspectors at New Orleans also certified 551 outbound freight and passenger trains that summer, under similar rules of procedure. The measures could not have been of any real service in curbing the spread of yellow fever, but the mental comfort they provided was considerable. A resolution passed by the Memphis Cotton Exchange the following winter said the inspection system had merited "the unqualified approbation of every merchant, taxpayer, and citizen of the valley," and the general superintendent of the Mississippi & Tennessee Railroad reported a 98 percent increase in freight earnings and a 68 percent increase in passenger earnings over 1879, thanks to the board's action, which forestalled the proliferation of local "shotgun" quarantines.[11]

There were tremors again in the summer of 1882 when a few yellow fever cases turned up on St. Peter Street in New Orleans, and again the

11. National Board of Health, *Report for 1880*, 28–41, 617–35.

laborious and expensive freight inspection arrangements of the National Board of Health were put into operation. As the yellow fever menace appeared to recede in subsequent years, however, questions about states' rights and interference with commerce arose. Southern interests had always been extremely suspicious of the idea of a national quarantine against yellow fever, figuring, not unreasonably, that it would be too subject to corrupt manipulation aimed at directing extra trade to northern ports— "perverted by designing men into a gigantic system of commercial oppression," in the words of Joseph Jones. The National Board of Health failed to get its appropriation renewed by Congress and was phased out of existence after 1883. Most of its advisory functions were thereafter assumed by the U.S. Marine Hospital Service, and its field operations were replaced by the quarantine and disinfection programs of the separate state authorities.

The Louisiana Board of Health radically overhauled its maritime quarantine procedures in 1885. All passengers from tropical ports known to be infected were uniformly subject to five days' detainment (a special hotel was built for their accommodation at the Buras Station, eighty miles below New Orleans), and a giant sulfur furnace with a steam-powered blower, mounted on a barge, was introduced for fumigating the holds of inbound ships. Quarantine stations were established on the Rigolets and Atchafalaya channels, capping off entry points that had, unaccountably, been left unguarded up until then. The state of Texas promulgated standby regulations that required, on the first report or intimation of yellow fever, all railroad freight from Louisiana to be offloaded at a special warehouse compound on the Sabine River and fumigated for twenty-four hours, then reloaded onto fresh cars. Similarly, Mississippi required the detainment of freight at the state line for fumigation or two weeks' ventilation, whichever was considered more appropriate for the material in question.[12]

12. Joseph Holt, "The Quarantine System of Louisiana—Methods of Disinfection Practised," *Reports and Papers, American Public Health Association,* XIII (1887), 161–78; Louisiana Board of Health, *Report for 1888–89* (Baton Rouge, 1890), 51–60; Quitman Kohnke, "History of Maritime Quarantine in Louisiana against Yellow Fever," *New Orleans Medical and Surgical Journal,* LVI (1903), 167–80; Robert Rutherford, "History of Quarantine in the State of Texas from 1878 to 1888," *Reports and Papers, American Public Health Association,* XIV (1888), 125–33. For a full history of the National Board of Health, see Peter William Bruton, "The National Board of Health" (Ph.D. dissertation, University of Maryland, 1974).

The uniform detention of travelers at quarantine and the fumigation of ships and railroad cars with sulfur might, as Quitman Kohnke believed, have had some real effect in hindering the ingress of infection, but undoubtedly the Mississippi Valley's chief protection against yellow fever during these years was the widespread immunity produced by the 1878 epidemic. Louisiana, and more particularly New Orleans, had long since been convicted of being the region's primary distributing center for yellow fever. We can hardly expect it to have been recognized that, with the improved means of transportation available by this time, a traveler could have been bitten by an infected mosquito in Havana, taken passage on a steamship to almost any East Coast port, then have gone by railroad to virtually any infectible point in the Mississippi Valley, all within the incubation period of the disease. The infection stole into the region in precisely this fashion in the summer of 1888, when yellow fever broke out rather violently at Decatur, Alabama, and sporadically at Jackson, Mississippi, traceable at both places to railroad contact with Jacksonville, Florida. The disease appeared nowhere else in the valley, but the news of those two outbreaks was enough to "throw the whole Southern country into a panic. . . . In the vast majority of instances local boards of health did nothing to quell the agitation, but on the contrary led the panic and excitedly quarantined against the world." Vicksburg and Memphis, as well as Meridian and Chattanooga, shut off all communication and completely tied up the major inland railroads and their branches. New Orleans was automatically embargoed by most places in its tributary area, although the first and only case there was not reported until late October. "Throughout the breadth of the land there were outrages perpetrated, and cruelties shown, and brief authority arbitrarily and shamefully exercised," the board of health of Louisiana ruefully said in its biennial report, "and all this continued until the chilling frosts of late October, in the opinion of the masses, destroyed danger from the dreaded disease."[13]

The King of Terrors certainly lost none of its inspirational power in the period after 1878, but fresh interpretations of the etiology of yellow

13. New York *Times,* September 21–23, 25, 1888; W. E. Forest, "The Cost of Yellow Fever Epidemics—The Epidemic at Decatur, Ala., in 1888," *Medical Record,* XXXV (1889), 620–26; Wirt Johnson, "The Outbreak of Yellow Fever at Jackson, Mississippi, in September, 1888," *Reports and Papers, American Public Health Association,* XIV (1888), 51–54; Louisiana Board of Health, *Report for 1888–89,* 30–31.

fever were not encouraged by the long recess taken by the disease during these years. The most serious outbreak of the period occurred in Florida in 1888, and may be taken as an illustration of what little progress had been made in practical methods of combating the disease since the great epidemic ten years earlier. When the true character of the unusual "society fever" that had been spreading in Jacksonville for a number of weeks was finally identified and proclaimed on August 10, there ensued a disorderly *sauve-qui-peut* evacuation from the infected city, with much that was reminiscent of events at Memphis in 1878 and 1879. Tar fires were burned in the streets, a battery of artillery was brought in by the state militia to worry the germ with nighttime cannonading, and for a while the movements of Yellow Jack in Florida vied in the national headlines with the dervish crisis in the Sudan and the presidential campaign at home. State authorities accepted the assurances of Jacksonville health officials that cases were being promptly identified and isolated and that houses were being efficiently disinfected, but shotgun quarantines of perfect rigidity were soon in effect in most surrounding towns. These local actions were extremely disruptive to commerce and communication in the region, but politically they were impossible to suppress; when cargoes of creosoted lumber, or fish packed in ice, were intercepted, dumped on the ground, and burned, state doctors could only protest at the absurdity.

On August 17, at Florida's invitation, the U.S. Marine Hospital Service tried to assert some degree of control over the situation by establishing stations for the systematic inspection and disinfection of outbound trains, and a week later a "probation," or detention, camp for Jacksonville refugees was opened under federal auspices on the south bank of the St. Mary's River. More than 1,200 refugees were processed through this camp over the course of the season, each being detained ten days at government expense and then allowed to proceed. Thirty-six cases of yellow fever were intercepted and the experiment was deemed a success—which perhaps it was, as far as it went, but Jacksonville was a city of 25,000 people, perhaps 20,000 of whom had already stampeded away, many of them with the virus already in their blood. Towns all over the state had begun to sprinkle their streets with lime and creosote, but the fever was soon in evidence at Fernandina, Gainesville, and other places. Yellow fever had already been on the increase for several weeks at Macclenny, a railroad town 50 miles west of Jacksonville, while local practitioners persisted in calling it "bilious fever." Commercial interests still demanded that local doctors be slow as well as sure about disclosing yellow fever, and the one who had the temerity to make the first pronouncement could usually count on attracting a shower of contradiction, ridicule, and outright obloquy, and at many places might be liable to a heavy fine if it turned out to be a false alarm. Florida at this time was in the midst of its first big real estate boom, so the mood was especially touchy. An experienced Marine Hospital Service doctor arrived for an inspection on September 9, and the very first case of "bilious fever" he examined presented a particularly repulsive example of undoubtable yellow fever:

> The face was of dusky bronze color, the brow and lower portions of the neck were deep lemon hue, the muscles of the face and mouth quivering with convulsive twitchings, the eyes rotated inward and were deeply injected, the sclerotic stained with the familiar icteroid color, the lips dry and fissured, teeth thickly coated with bloody sordes, the gums and nasal apertures showing signs of recent hemorrhage. The pillows and bed-linen were spotted with the dark coffee-ground vomit, and the atmosphere of the small and tightly-closed room was saturated with the peculiarly sickening emanations from the subjects of this disease.

The doctor condemned the "wretched sanitary condition" of Macclenny's streets and singled out a heap of rotting sawdust dumped beside a stagnant lagoon near the center of town. He explained that under conditions of continuous heat and humidity, those telluric factors had "combined to produce a miasmatic atmosphere, which became a congenial nidus for the propagation of the infection matter already introduced." Roused from apathy, Macclenny people began a vigorous effort to set things right, even burning several infected houses to the ground. The government doctor counseled a more moderate course of action, instructing the people to burn suspected fomites and scrub houses with bichloride of mercury solution. Similar sanitary campaigns were organized in other Florida towns where the yellow fever germ was considered to be active or latent, and "a general and systematic riddance of all supposable fomites, retained air, and niduses" was officially urged. At Plant City, the residents cleared off and burned surrounding tracts of brush and deadwood, thoroughly fumigated every house in town, and liberally sprinkled the streets with lime and copperas. The official report from Plant City emphasized the prevailing conviction that the localizing causes of yellow fever had consisted in "accumulations of filth, especially animal matter and human excreta." One of the first undertakings after the fever subsided at Jacksonville was a detailed survey of the condition of the city's sewers.[14]

Yellow Jack's first serious invasion of the Mississippi Valley in 18 years came in the fall of 1897. At least 42 communities in Louisiana, Mississippi, and Alabama were affected and at least 388 lives were lost, 290 of them in New Orleans. The virus strain was apparently not very pronounced or malignant, and when it first appeared at Ocean Springs on the Mississippi coast in August, it was mistakenly written off as "dengue," one of its favorite symptomological disguises. By September 3, the sickness at Ocean Springs was prevalent enough to cause concern, and the Mobile Board of Health requested the U.S. Marine Hospital Service to investigate. When the team of experts arrived a few days later to study the situation, they found the town depopulating and estimated that there were at least 400 cases on hand. Autopsies confirmed the presence of yellow fever. Within a week, cases had been reported at four other towns in south Mississippi, and at least a dozen suspicious cases had been identified on and around St. Claude Street in New Orleans.

Apprehensions mounted that there was going to be a repetition of the terrible experience of 1878, and determined efforts to spike the menace went into motion at all levels. The Tennessee State Board of Health effected rigid quarantine along the whole southern boundary of the state on September 20, and the city authorities at Memphis as well as at Cairo, Illinois, placed river traffic under the strictest surveillance. The U.S. government forwarded camp gear to the area, and the Marine Hospital Service prepared to establish refugee detention facilities on all railroad lines leading out of New Orleans and Mobile, modeled on the plan implemented at Jacksonville in 1888. In New Orleans, the municipal board of health was bichloriding houses and encouraging the orderly evacuation

14. U.S. Marine Hospital Service, *Report for Fiscal 1888*, 24–47; U.S. Marine Hospital Service, *Report for Fiscal 1889*, 49–99.

of infected neighborhoods. Towns and counties around the state, meanwhile, were throwing up a confusion of quarantines in a virtual replay of 1878.

There was no uniformity in this matter; every state, parish, and town having their own rules of quarantine, which varied from that of places like the parish of Plaquemines, which allowed direct daylight communication with New Orleans, to places like Baton Rouge, which was surrounded by an armed guard and allowed entrance to no one, or even as the parishes in western Louisiana, forbidding the passage of trains through them bound to points beyond. Very generally the places quarantined not only against the infected places but against everywhere, and would not allow persons or things from any place outside of its own limits to enter it. Mails were very generally refused; freight, independently of its character, from New Orleans or through New Orleans, almost universally so, and not a few refused freight from anywhere. A few places in Louisiana forbid the passage of trains, freight or passenger, made up in New Orleans, through them, as did the state of Texas.

In this State (Louisiana) commerce was paralyzed; that from and through New Orleans ceased to exist, and local traffic between points outside of the city very seriously interfered with.

On September 17, disinfection of the mails began at New Orleans. All letter mail was perforated with a spiked paddle and fumigated for three hours with a 6-percent concentration of formaldehyde gas. Newspaper bundles were shipped only after being roasted one hour at 212° F. These measures were well publicized and led to a fairly general, but by no means universal, acceptance of the mails. The Marine Hospital Service simultaneously put into operation a carefully planned system of train relays and inspections on the railroads serving New Orleans. Refugees from infected neighborhoods in the city were required to go to a special detention camp for ten days before being allowed to leave the parish. Other outbound travelers were subjected to a series of stops, inspections, and train changes along the route. Passengers on the Illinois Central line, for example, were required to get off at Kenner, about 10 miles outside New Orleans, to be examined by medical officers and have their baggage disinfected with formaldehyde gas. Afterward, they boarded fresh, disinfected coaches to continue on their trip. They were put through the procedure again at McComb, Mississippi, 110 miles north of New Orleans. Any suspicious cases discovered by the doctors were sent to an outcamp governed by an extremely strict policy of disinfection: all privies were treated twice a day with lime and copperas; detainees when released were subjected to a disinfecting bath, regardless of the final diagnosis of their illness; the ticks they had slept on were burned; their tents and blankets were washed with bichloride solution; and the ground where their tents had stood was seared with blowtorches. The program was highly involved and quite expensive for the government, but it was considered the only way to obviate the dodging, smuggling, and illicit communication that would have resulted from a total nonintercourse quarantine and it ensured a modicum of sanitary supervision over the movement of people and freight.[15]

In the wake of the 1897 outbreak, the surgeon general of the Marine Hospital Service published a collection of articles on the etiology and control of yellow fever written by twelve prominent experts. These essays spanned 165 pages in the annual report for 1898 and are interesting for what they show about the stagnant state of yellow fever epidemiology on the very eve of the momentous discovery of the mosquito vector. Of special interest are two articles by Dr. H. R. Carter, who just two years later would play the lead role in prompting the experiments that led to the mosquito breakthrough. At this time, Carter considered the causative agent of yellow fever to be "unquestionably a saprophytic facultative parasite," in other words, a free-living germ whose primary habitat was outside the human body in sources of dampness and decay. He declared that "the infection is heavy and hangs near the ground," and that the most suitable "culture medium" for its propagation and dissemination was "along sewers, about the dumping places of refuse, etc."

Carter thought experience indicated that the germ was most active at night, and that the infection was least apt to be contracted out-of-doors on clear, breezy days. He decided the practice of daylight communication was "not safe, but it is little dangerous." Locations most secure from yellow fever were elevated places kept free from decaying vegetable and animal refuse. The matter of disinfection was heavily emphasized. All absorbent materials from an infected place were to be regarded as fomites capable

15. U.S. Marine Hospital Service, *Report for Fiscal 1897*, 580–677.

of carrying the germ and establishing new focuses of infection, and should be disinfected or burned. The contaminated bedding of patients should be burned in all cases. Leaves, sawdust, and similar litter around houses should be cleaned up. Rotten wood, Carter believed, was "an especially bad nidus of infection," a fact that in his mind explained the special persistence of infection in ships and houses. The floors of infected houses, and the yards and ditches around them, should be thoroughly treated with germicidal solutions, the best of these being bichloride of mercury. Formaldehyde gas was recommended for fumigating enclosed spaces, though sulfur smoke was still considered adequate "if properly used."[16]

Carter's advice agreed with that of the other contributors to the annual report, and indeed represented all that was responsibly held and professionally maintained about the disease at that time. Practically nothing was offered that could not have been expressed as well in 1888 or in 1878. H. D. Geddings, a respected bacteriologist in the Marine Hospital Service, also regarded yellow fever as an "extrinsic infection," and likewise emphasized hygienic surroundings. Regarding the *modus operandi* of its "epidemic influence," he could only say: "The question has puzzled me greatly, and I can offer no other explanation than that of an intoxication caused by the absorption or ingestion of toxines liberated by the yellow fever organism in the process of its growth, under favorable conditions, outside of the human body." A colleague, Eugene Wasdin, considered yellow fever "an almost inexplicable poison, so insidious in its approach and entrance that no trace is left behind." Wasdin and Geddings were the principal investigators in a study commissioned one year later by the U.S. Treasury Department, which wrongly confirmed that a microorganism recently discovered by a celebrated Italian bacteriologist was the causative germ of yellow fever. They exposed cultures of this so-called *bacillus icteroides* to formaldehyde, carbolic acid, and bichloride of mercury, and concluded that it was "very susceptible to the influences injurious to bacterial life, and its ready control by the processes of disinfection, chemical and mechanical, is assured."[17]

16. H. R. Carter, "Hygiene of Persons Living within an Area of Yellow Fever Infection," in U.S. Marine Hospital Service, *Report for Fiscal 1898,* 319–24; "A Précis on Hygienic Measures to Be Taken in a Town Infected with Yellow Fever," *ibid.,* 339–57.

17. *Ibid.,* 330, 333; "The Aetiology of Yellow Fever: Abstract of the Report of the Commission of Medical Officers, M.H.S.," *Philadelphia Medical Journal,* VI (1899), 326.

There was another extensive diffusion of yellow fever in the region in 1898. The disease touched 21 communities in Louisiana and 28 in Mississippi, but once again the strain of virus was relatively mild and only 114 deaths were recorded. Disinfection efforts of the most strenuous kind were brought to bear, and the Marine Hospital Service was invited by local authorities to superintend the work. At McHenry, Mississippi, all possible fomites were ferreted out and carefully subjected to sulfur smoke, dry steam, or formaldehyde gas, whichever was deemed most effective on the material in question. "Trash and every kind of organic matter" was taken from houses and yards and burned, and the ashes were soaked with a solution of bichloride of mercury in water before they had time to cool. Privy structures adjoining infected houses were burned to the ground, and the pits were then filled with dry sawdust and set on fire, after which the site was drenched with bichloride solution. Five badly infected residences were ordered put to the torch. It is interesting to note that the government doctor detailed to supervise sanitary operations at McHenry was H. R. Carter. Carter contracted the fever while engaged in his work there, but survived the attack and later distinguished himself as the twentieth century's foremost yellow fever scholar.[18]

In terms of sickness and destruction of life, the outbreak of 1898 was not a major epidemic, but it was significant by virtue of one of those odd chains of circumstance that from time to time have figured so importantly in scientific history. It so happened that at Taylor, an unimportant railroad town in northern Mississippi, a local doctor who had not been away from the community all summer came down with yellow fever and died on August 9. Subsequently, others in his house and elsewhere in town were attacked. The doctor had supplemented the income from his practice by running a grocery store. When two members of the Mississippi State Board of Health came to investigate the Taylor outbreak, they decided that, in the apparent absence of any infecting case from the outside world, a bunch of bananas received at the store from New Orleans in May must have been the original source of infection. This comported with the accepted doctrine of transmission by fomites and was considered by them to be a sufficient explanation.

18. U.S. Marine Hospital Service, *Report for Fiscal 1898*, 544–78.

Drs. J. O. Cobb and H. R. Carter of the Marine Hospital Service visited the place later in the season and probed the matter further, and a little more skeptically. They were ready to admit that a banana "might be the means of carrying the organism of yellow fever," if the weather were warm and the fruit decayed, or its peel split. However, the fifty-one days intervening between the receipt of the bananas and the doctor's illness seemed "too long to be probable," and the fact that a young man living on the other side of town had sickened and died just a day after the doctor made that source of infection seem even less likely. They questioned surviving members of the doctor's household and were assured that all mashed and decayed bananas had immediately been picked off and disposed of, the balance of good fruit had peels intact, and the consignment had been quickly sold out and presumably consumed. The doctors concluded that accordingly, there was "no further chance for them to act as culture media."

The Marine Hospital Service investigators determined that there had, in fact, been several importations of possible fomites into Taylor about the time the fever broke out—a box of clothing, a mattress, and so forth. But what interested them most was the information that somewhat earlier in the summer, about mid-July, there had been sickness of an undetermined character among a Negro railroad gang quartered in a set of shanty cars sidetracked alongside the Taylor depot. Most of this gang had hailed from Jackson, and although yellow fever existed there at the time, this fact was unknown to Taylor people. It stood to reason that virtually everybody in the community would have visited the neighborhood of the depot for one reason or another over the course of the season. Cobb wrote up the findings in a short article published in the annual report of the Marine Hospital Service for 1898, forming an interesting discussion of the question of infection from fomites versus personal exposure via inapparent or missed cases. The terms *primary* and *secondary* infection and *extrinsic incubation* were used for the first time in this article.[19]

On several occasions in earlier epidemics, a vaguely defined "elapse of time" or "period of incubation" had been observed between the arrival of infected sojourners at an uninfected place and the eruption of yellow fever

19. J. O. Cobb, "Source of Yellow Fever Infection in Mississippi in 1898," *ibid.*, 570–78.

among residents there. The remarkable article published by Dr. A. P. Jones of Mississippi in 1854 had reflected on this phenomenon. In 1882, a member of the Louisiana State Board of Health had noted: "The length of time intervening between the breaking out in a locality of yellow fever and the appearance of the cases which may be called 'cases of second category' has often been observed. This interval is sometimes of two, three weeks, sometimes more. May not this phenomenon be explained by admitting that the first cases were the product of a germ in active life, when imported, and that a longer time was required for the ripening of a second crop?" H. R. Carter had been contemplating this problem since the early 1890s when, as a quarantine officer at various Gulf Coast stations, he had occasion to study the records of sickness on ships making the long voyage north from infected ports in Brazil. He had not arrived at any conclusions, however, and had not published his notes.[20]

While helping Cobb in his investigations at Taylor in 1898, Carter's attention was diverted to the occurrence of yellow fever at Orwood, a shoestring country settlement linked to Taylor by a few miles of dirt road. It occurred to Carter that conditions at Orwood furnished a nearly ideal laboratory for a precise study and measurement of the phenomena relating to the spread of infection in houses and extrinsic incubation. Here he had a group of twenty widely separated farmhouses, well removed from any river, railroad, or turnpike. The people were all whites and nonimmunes, sedentary in habit and few in number, so their movements could be easily retraced. Above all, they were intelligent and cooperative and furnished information openly—without any professional axes to grind or commercial interests to protect. Carter secured a history of cases and began interrelating and analyzing them in detail. He determined that at each place, the yellow fever infection had required not less than twelve days to be communicated from a sick visitor to the residents, with the average "period of extrinsic incubation" being about seventeen days. Carter published his findings the following May in the *New Orleans Medical and Surgical Journal*, where eventually they would be studied with much interest by Walter Reed. In this rather twisted and improbable way, a box of bananas shipped to an obscure Mississippi town in the spring of 1898 served to

20. Louisiana Board of Health, *Quarantine and Sanitary Operations during 1880, 1881, 1882, and 1883* (Baton Rouge, 1884), 491; Henry R. Carter, "Are Vessels Infected with Yellow Fever? Some Personal Observations," *Medical Record*, LXI (1902), 441–44.

point the way to one of the greatest breakthroughs in medical history. Carter had an opportunity to gather further practical verification of his thesis at Port Tampa, Florida, in the fall of 1899. His report on the Port Tampa outbreak, however, makes it clear that he still considered fomites an important source of infection.[21]

Carter himself did not infer that the intervention of an insect had anything to do with the long interval between infecting and secondary cases in yellow fever. He had been schooled in the germ theory, and his initial assumption was that the "period of extrinsic incubation" represented the time required for the "saprophytic microorganism" that he assumed to be the cause of the disease to multiply and ripen in the environment so as to impart infection to the human system. However, some highly suggestive discoveries had recently come about in related areas of epidemiological research. At an experiment farm in Maryland in 1889, the Bureau of Animal Industry of the U.S. Department of Agriculture had opened a series of fresh investigations into the etiology of bovine piroplasmosis, the southern, or Texas, cattle fever that had scourged American beef herds since colonial times, and had become especially troublesome with the great "long drives" out of Texas after the Civil War. Proceeding on no other basis than an old cattlemen's theory that the sickness was conveyed by ticks, Theobald Smith and F. L. Kilbourne carried out a series of beautifully planned and carefully controlled experiments. Healthy cattle were pastured with infected animals from which all ticks had been removed, and the fever was never communicated. Clean pastures were sown with ticks that had sucked the blood of infected animals, and the disease broke out destructively when healthy animals were turned in. An extrinsic incubation of about fifty days was determined, directly referable to the life cycle of the tick. The results were published in 1892 and confirmed the investigators' original hunch, and science had its first solid demonstration of the transmission of an animal disease by arthropods.[22]

A few writers had remarked earlier on certain broad similarities be-

21. H. R. Carter, "A Note on the Interval between Infecting and Secondary Cases of Yellow Fever," *New Orleans Medical and Surgical Journal*, LII (1900), 617–36; U.S. Marine Hospital Service, *Report for Fiscal 1899*, 744–47.

22. Theobald Smith and F. L. Kilbourne, "Investigations into the Nature, Causation, and Prevention of Texas or Southern Cattle Fever," in U.S. Bureau of Animal Industry, *Report for Fiscal 1892*, 177–304.

tween the etiological characteristics of Texas fever and yellow fever. Both diseases were mysteriously controlled by climate and temperature, and ceased to spread after a hard frost. In both diseases the infection seemed to be retained and apparently even multiplied by something in the environment—localities somehow remained infected long after the death or removal of the infecting case. And for reasons that could only be guessed at, in both diseases the sphere of infection often tended to be rigidly localized. In the same way that yellow fever was often confined to a single house or to one side of a boulevard and not the other, Texas fever could not cross a running stream (provided, of course, that cattle could not ford it), and often a simple wire fence was enough to check its spread to adjoining pastures. Some experts theorized that pasture grass became contaminated by the saliva of infected animals; others maintained that the germ was harbored in the dung dropped by the cattle. Prominent in the latter camp was a Nebraska veterinary pathologist, Frank Billings, who in 1888 published a long monograph in which he justified his position on bacteriological, pathological, and etiological grounds.

In developing his argument, Billings carried the parallel with yellow fever further than anyone had before, even to the point of declaring that the diseases were virtually identical. Billings discussed his autopsies of cattle dead from Texas fever and noted the same hemorrhagic tendency and the same congestion, discoloration, and fatty infiltration of internal organs that were reported in yellow fever in humans. He had obtained, courtesy of his friend George Sternberg, a sample of liver tissue from a yellow fever victim, had sectioned and stained it and studied it under his microscope, and insisted that he had seen the same or very similar "belted ovoid germs" he claimed to have discovered in the blood, dung, and organ tissue of animals infected with Texas fever. Billings reviewed the etiological similarities of the two fevers and reasoned that both were "extraorganismal" infections, having their primary development outside the animal organism, nourished by similar climatic and telluric conditions. To the objection that the diseases must be fundamentally different in nature because one was a malady of pastures and ranges and the other one of congested cities, he had a ready answer:

> In view of the fact that my own work has conclusively shown that the foeces of southern cattle are the chief means by which they infect our

northern pastures . . . and as they are held in immense droves on their native plains, it is safe to assert that the same materials are the means by which the continued infection of the land and extension and support of the disease is supported in the South, which in reality places those infected and pestiferous plains in the same condition as those densely populated and filthy portions of the cities where the yellow fever finds it permanent home in the South.

Dr. Billings took it for granted that in southern cities "the population take little or no care of their refuse material and hence are continually supplying the means themselves for the continued pestilential infection oftheir surroundings." He concluded in his amusingly assertive manner: "I think that I may be pardoned the egotism of claiming this to be the first occasion in the history of American medicine that not only one but two germ diseases of animal life have been traced out and their origin placed upon an impregnable scientific basis. . . . The sun of original research, in disease, seems to be rising in the west instead of the east! . . . This honor does not belong to me alone," he added, "but the credit of it is equally to be shared by the State Board of Agriculture of Nebraska" (which had sponsored his research).[23] Dr. Billings argued further for his fecal theory in a long article published in the *Journal of Comparative Medicine* in 1892, but by then his ideas had been thoroughly discredited by the careful field and laboratory work of Smith and Kilbourne. In their final report, the two scoffed at Billings and called the parallel with yellow fever "unwarranted." Unfortunately, the useful part of Billings' argument—which, considered in light of Smith and Kilbourne's discovery, might have prompted some investigator toward the possible role of insects in yellow fever—was cast out with the bathwater and forgotten.

The parallels with other arthropod-borne diseases were not immediately recognized, either. The long legacy of miasmatism was not easily shaken, even by the most progressive scientists, and the handful who were beginning to think that the mosquito played some role in malaria transmission still found it difficult to see the process of infection as one of simple inoculation by the insect. In a series of lectures published in March of 1896, Ronald Ross's great mentor, Dr. Patrick Manson, correctly argued

23. Frank S. Billings, *Southern Cattle Plague and Yellow Fever, from the Etiological and Practical Standpoints* (Lincoln, Nebr., 1888), 83–87, 119–34.

that the malaria parasite was not excreted naturally by the human host and thus could only be extracted by some external agent, probably the mosquito. But Manson did not thereby conclude that the germ was introduced to the next victim when the mosquito took its next blood meal. He supposed, rather, that the parasite entered a "resting stage" after it was extracted by the mosquito and that it returned to the earth when the mosquito died and decomposed, to be eventually "swallowed by man in water," "inhaled in dust," or "shaken out by man when he disturbs the soil."[24]

The potential role of insects as direct communicators of disease germs and parasites nevertheless became an increasingly alluring theme for speculation in medical writing during these years. Indeed, by the end of the decade Nuttall could catalog over three hundred publications on the subject. If it did not gain anything in hard proof, the idea of insect agency in the transmission of disease could not have suffered any in prestige when, in an 1893 note to the *British Medical Journal*, Sir William Moore, surgeon general of the Royal Army and author of a pioneer textbook on tropical medicine, submitted his opinion that flies were important conveyors of cholera infection. Moore went on to suggest that a whole range of other diseases were probably carried by flies as well, among them typhoid fever, anthrax, ophthalmia, and leprosy. "That syphilis is not frequently communicated by flies is explainable from the parts affected being less exposed."[25] By 1897 the transmission of cholera and typhoid by flies was virtually a given in sanitary circles. The surgeon general of the U.S. Army, George Sternberg, was of the opinion that they were also carriers of yellow fever. The fact that yellow fever, like cholera and typhoid, found "a favorable nidus in filthy localities," and produced its severest effects on organs connected with the digestive tract, indicated to Sternberg that the infec-

24. Patrick Manson, "The Goulstonian Lectures on the Life-History of the Malaria Germ Outside the Human Body," *British Medical Journal*, March 14, 1896, pp. 641–46, March 21, 1896, pp. 712–17, March 28, 1896, pp. 774–79. See also Amico Bignami, "Hypotheses as to the Life-History of the Malarial Parasite Outside the Human Body," *Lancet*, November 14, 1896, pp. 1363–67, November 21, pp. 1441–44.

25. George H. F. Nuttall, "On the Role of Insects, Arachnids, and Myriapods, as Carriers in the Spread of Bacterial and Parasitic Diseases of Man and Animals," *Johns Hopkins Hospital Reports*, VIII (1900), 1–152; William Moore, "Diseases Probably Carried by Flies," *British Medical Journal*, June 3, 1893, p. 1154.

tion was concentrated in excrement, and analogy made it "extremely probable" that flies, passing constantly between privies and houses, were its main distributors.[26]

In June, 1898, United States forces invaded Cuba, and within a month completed their conquest of the island. The army had been troubled by typhoid fever at its staging camps in Florida, and to head off more serious problems with the disease during the occupation, Surgeon General Sternberg organized and dispatched a special Typhoid Board under the leadership of Major Walter Reed, head of the Bacteriological Laboratory of the Army Medical Department. Yellow fever had always been known as a major scourge of unacclimated Spanish troops in the colony, and the American command prudently kept its men bivouaced outside Havana and the other towns known to be haunted by the germ. Meanwhile, with the Typhoid Board advising, the occupation government exerted itself in a vigorous campaign of sanitation along traditional lines, and in Havana programs of street sweeping, garbage collection, and night soil disposal were put into effect with military severity. For a season this campaign had superficially beneficial effects, as the incidence of yellow fever dropped off markedly. In 1899, only 103 deaths from yellow fever were recorded in Havana, contrasting with average annual losses of 500 to 600 during the later years of Spanish rule. As it was later recognized, the real cause underlying this sudden decline resided in the fact that the inflow of susceptible Spanish immigrants had been temporarily choked off by the war and unsettled conditions on the island. The stream of immigration from the old country struck up again with the return of peace, and with this fresh nourishment the infection began reasserting itself. By the summer of 1900, yellow fever was once again a serious worry in Cuba, flaring up not only in the cities but also in many of the garrisons, forcing the abandonment of Cabana Fortress as well as the barracks at Guanajay, Pinar del Río, and Santiago. The disease caused over 300 civilian deaths in the city of Havana that year and also claimed over 200 American soldiers, including some casualties among the general staff.[27]

26. For Sternberg's view on flies and yellow fever, see "Discussion," *Reports and Papers, American Public Health Association,* XXIII (1897), 438; U.S. Secretary of War, *Report for Fiscal 1899* (3 vols.), I, 504.

27. U.S. Secretary of War, *Report for Fiscal 1899* (3 vols.), I, 490–507, 602–17; U.S. Secretary of War, *Report for Fiscal 1900* (3 vols.), I, 678–82, 737–38.

"Our increased experience with yellow fever has shown us that there is much about the nature, development, and communicability of the contagium of which we are ignorant," one of the chief division surgeons in Cuba remarked in 1900. "It continues to strike when and where it listeth, regardless of our most reasonable expectations and best hygienic measures." That spring the War Department published regulations forbidding the shipment of yellow fever dead to the mainland for burial during the summer months. The danger posed to the United States by increased contact with areas of endemic infection had been made apparent by an outbreak at the National Soldiers' Home at Hampton, Virginia, in 1899, the infection evidently having been introduced by Cuban returnees. The facility recorded 44 cases and 12 deaths, and half of its 3,200 inmates had to be evacuated to tents. Yellow fever also appeared at Key West, Miami, New Orleans, and several towns in Mississippi that fall, causing a total of 116 deaths, and for the third year in a row the Gulf States were paralyzed by official and unofficial quarantines.[28]

The army's Typhoid Board was reconstituted as the Yellow Fever Commission, still under the direction of Walter Reed. Dr. Carlos Finlay, by then an old man, approached the medical authorities several times with his mosquito theory, and encountered a changed climate of opinion. At the annual meeting of the British Medical Association at Edinburgh in July, 1898, Dr. Patrick Manson had announced recent discoveries by his protégé Major Ronald Ross on the subject of malaria transmission. After three years of sedulous experimentation in makeshift laboratories at Sunderabad and Calcutta, Ross had managed to completely describe the development of the malarial parasite in the *Anopheles* mosquito, and had effected transmission of the disease by mosquitoes under controlled circumstances. Ross had used birds in his experiments, because of local objections to employment of human subjects, but what his results implied about the malaria cycle in humans were quite obvious. Later that year, corroboratory evidence was supplied by a group of Italian doctors who had discovered plasmodia in wild *Anopheles* collected in the Maccarese, a notoriously malarious district on the Tyrrhenian coastal plain. They also produced test cases of malaria in human volunteers under controlled con-

28. U.S. Marine Hospital Service, *Report for Fiscal 1899*, 643–748; U.S. Marine Hospital Service, *Report for Fiscal 1900*, 344–45.

ditions at a clinic in downtown Rome, using mosquitoes imported from the Maccarese.[29]

Dr. H. R. Carter was soon cognizant of the breakthrough in malaria research and recognized its significance for his recent observations on house infection and extrinsic incubation in yellow fever; he began to reorient his inferences. In 1899, he contacted Dr. Finlay and suggested that, as a partial test of his theory, he check for the presence or absence of his mosquito at places known to be infectible or noninfectible. Detailed to Havana by the Marine Hospital Service in the spring of 1900, he talked further with Finlay and forwarded a copy of his publication on extrinsic incubation to Reed's group with the remark that the a priori argument for the mosquito theory had much in its favor and to him was quite plausible. In July, a pair of epidemiologists from the Liverpool School of Tropical Medicine stopped off at Havana on their way to perform field studies of yellow fever in Brazil. They met with Finlay and Carter and declared their own opinion that the mosquito theory "hardly appears so fanciful" in view of recent developments in malariology. They agreed that it supplied a more than likely explanation for many of the most perplexing points about yellow fever's behavior: the limiting influence of cold; the spread of infection in neighborhoods where neither fomites nor personal communication could be implicated; and the appearance and persistence of infection in places like hospitals, whose evident sanitary condition was unimpeachable. In a communication to the *British Medical Journal* they said: "Some means of transmission by the aid of an intermediate host—a town-loving host for this town-loving disease—is to some extent more plausible than might be anticipated. Whether that host is of the nature of a gnat remains unknown."[30]

In August, the Yellow Fever Commission secured a batch of mosquito eggs from Finlay and arranged for experiments with volunteers from the Hospital Corps. A field hospital and experiment station was established at Quemados, a fever-free location in the open hills about six miles outside

29. Patrick Manson, "The Mosquito and the Malarial Parasite," *British Medical Journal*, September 24, 1898, pp. 849–53.

30. Henry Rose Carter, *Yellow Fever: An Historical and Epidemiological Study of Its Place of Origin* (Baltimore, 1931), 44; Herbert E. Durham and Walter Myers, "Liverpool School of Tropical Medicine—Yellow Fever Expedition—Some Preliminary Notes," *British Medical Journal*, September 8, 1900, pp. 656–57.

Havana. To nine nonimmune subjects, mosquitoes were applied that had bitten yellow fever cases from two to ten days before, all with negative results. Positive results were finally obtained with two 16-day mosquitoes; thereafter, the army doctors obtained twelve successful mosquito inoculations producing well-marked cases. A memorable series of counterexperiments was devised and carried out. A snugly framed house was built with specially tongued and grooved lumber that had been brought around from the other side of the island, to preclude any possibility of picking up germs in passing through Havana. The structure was carefully disinfected on-site, and its interior surfaces and corners were lined with clean cloth. This house was partitioned by a screen of a mesh small enough to exclude mosquitoes while allowing perfectly free passage to any conceivable miasm, emanation, or germ floating in the air. On one side, a succession of yellow fever cases was hospitalized, while a group of nonimmune volunteers occupied the other. After thirty days of exposure, no cases appeared among the volunteers, after which infected mosquitoes were introduced with immediate results. The house was subsequently ridded of its mosquitoes and then reoccupied harmlessly by other volunteers.

Another, more dramatic test served to demolish the fomites bogy once and for all. A small, tight, practically airless cabin was constructed at Quemados, with the idea of duplicating conditions in "the hold of a ship in the tropics," as Dr. James Carroll, one of the protagonists, later recalled. A small stove was installed to keep temperature and humidity constantly high. From the army's yellow fever hospital at Las Animas, boxfuls of dirty laundry—smeared and spattered bed clothes, and sheets and blankets stiff with the black vomit, blood, and excreta of fatal yellow fever cases—were brought to the cabin and piled in the corners and festooned from the walls and ceiling. In this human sweatbox of ineffable putridity, three volunteers spent twenty days and nights without developing the least symptom of yellow fever. Reed read the preliminary findings at the annual meeting of the American Public Health Association in Indianapolis in October, and published the report later that month in the *Philadelphia Medical Journal,* concluding: "The mosquito serves as the intermediate host of the parasite of yellow fever, and it is highly probable that the disease is only propagated through the bite of this insect."[31]

31. Walter Reed, James Carroll, A. Agramonte, and Jesse W. Lazear, "Etiology of Yellow Fever: A Preliminary Note," *Philadelphia Medical Journal,* VI (1900), 790–96.

The demonstrations by Reed's group in Cuba were not immediately endorsed by the profession back home. Dr. J. O. Cobb, then stationed at an army post in New Mexico, wrote a skeptical commentary that was published in the *Philadelphia Medical Journal* less than a month after Reed's first article appeared there. Aware of the key role that Dr. Carter's observations at Taylor and Orwood had played in ushering in the mosquito experiments, Cobb reviewed some of his own recollections from the fall of 1898. He confessed that he had been "a partial though weak-kneed convert to Finlay's mosquito theory" back then, but admitted that he had been "careless" about making special observations with reference to it because he, along with the whole medical fraternity, had been substantially wedded to the germ theory at that time. Cobb said he had stayed in several houses and finally in a tent at Taylor for a good part of the season, but he did not remember the mosquitoes to have been bothersome or even noticeable. Based on his own experience, he thought fleas or bedbugs should be likelier suspects as vectors. He pointed out that mosquitoes were notoriously bad at Nashville, but yellow fever was unknown there; they had been a plague at the railroad detention camps outside New Orleans in 1897, but the camps had remained secure from yellow fever. In any case, Cobb could not understand how the theory of man-to-man transmission of yellow fever through the single agency of insect bites could adequately account for all leaps and somersaults of the disease. He recalled a farmhouse outside Taylor, four miles from the nearest infected habitation, where two cases cropped up after the family had quarantined itself against the outside world for three full weeks. Surely fomites would have been a more probable means of introducing the germ in that instance, or perhaps the mosquitoes had imbibed the infection from some intermediate source close by, like the cesspool.[32]

There was really nothing captious about these objections—they stemmed from proper scientific doubts arising from excusable ignorance or confusion about the natural history of *A. aegypti*, about the phenomenon of extrinsic incubation, and about the role of inapparent cases in spreading yellow fever. In a 1901 article, also in the *Philadelphia Medical Journal*, one of the officers of the Mississippi State Board of Health de-

---

32. J. O. Cobb, "Conveyance of Yellow Fever Infection," *Philadelphia Medical Journal*, VI (1900), 993–94.

clared that it was mathematically impossible to explain the explosive epidemic spread of yellow fever in terms of the bites of individual mosquitoes, each of which had stung a case two weeks before. He pointed to places like Memphis, where yellow fever had not recurred despite the fact that the mosquitoes had never been molested by sanitarians. Concerning the fomites dogma, he acknowledged that on many occasions materials from an infected center had failed to spread the fever, but he insisted the principle was not invalidated by such instances. Surely the scores of cases of fomites transmission reported in the medical literature had enough in them that was "sufficiently authentic," and the profession could not afford to ignore them.[33]

The Louisiana State Board of Health initially called Reed's announcement "captivating" and declared itself "willing to be convinced," but noted that "officers charged by the law with the grave responsibility of excluding infection are not warranted by theoretical beliefs in neglecting known and proved methods of safety." In a critical essay on the fomites principle and quarantine reform, the president of the board, Dr. Edmond Souchon, gleaned from the medical literature twenty-seven cases where mosquito transmission seemed to be "impossible or superfluous." How, for example, could anything but fomites exposure account for the fact that the only cases at Summit, Mississippi, in 1878 were five persons who had been present at the unpacking of a trunk from New Orleans?[34] Dr. Stanford Chaillé, who had been writing on the disease since the 1850s, hailed Reed's demonstrations and freely acknowledged that the attention he had formerly devoted to fomites had been a waste of time. He insisted that closer analysis of alleged cases of fomites infection would always show such reports stemmed from mere failure to recognize the infection's presence in the community early on. This was due partly to the inherent difficulties in diagnosing yellow fever and, more often than not, to the deliberate nonreport of early cases—by poor people who could not afford to call in a doctor, by doctors afraid of being denounced as alarmists, or by citizens anxious to suppress the news to avoid quarantine and related problems:

33. John H. Purnell, "The Mosquito an Insignificant Factor in the Propagation of Yellow Fever," *Philadelphia Medical Journal,* VIII (1901), 189–93.

34. Louisiana Board of Health, *Report for 1900–1901* (2 vols.; Baton Rouge, 1902), I, 78–79, 81–102.

The history of the remarkable change of view in New Orleans as to belief in fomites is instructive. A great majority of its physicians, myself included, firmly believed that yellow fever originated in this city as was then universally claimed as to other habitually infected cities, and all of this great majority unhesitatingly testified that they had never observed a single case either of direct contagion or of infection by fomites. As steamboats and railroads multiplied and many adjacent places on the routes of travel became infected after outbreaks of the disease in New Orleans, the conviction gradually gained ground that yellow fever did follow the routes of travel and was an infectious disease. Then followed numerous reports that some places on these routes had not had any case of yellow fever introduced therein, certainly the usual precursor of an outbreak, but that fomites had been introduced. Our imaginations failed to invent any explanation for these credited reports except infection by fomites. However, this concession to fomites was made very grudgingly because New Orleans physicians could not ignore their innumerable experiences of the failure of fomites to infect. Hence the hypothesis invented to explain these credited reports was that, while fomites were usually innocuous yet under the rare influence of some unknown mysterious condition fomites did become infectious. . . .

I, like others, have advocated fomites, always, however, citing authority. For my part, I have never secured satisfactory proof of a single case of infection by fomites. I have investigated reported cases of infection by fomites, and I have known several cases, supported by very strong evidence, which, after laborious investigation, were conclusively traced to a usual cause, viz., to infected houses wherein were women of easy virtue. These had received night visits, carefully concealed and denied by men who, living in uninfected country places, had contracted the disease in said infected houses, and not by fomites in their uninfected country places.[35]

Dr. Chaillé admitted that "time is required to convert these probabilities into certainties," and he declared that Louisiana was justified in continuing to disinfect fomites "as long as public opinion may favor this measure." There was, after all, a very reasonable concern on the part of many officials that the manifest sanitary gains of the previous twenty years were

35. Stanford E. Chaillé, "The Stegomyia and Fomites," *Journal of the American Medical Association*, XL (1903), 1433–40.

about to be flung away because of a specious theory. T. C. Minor, a retired health officer of Cincinnati and another veteran of 1878, commented in the *Cincinnati Lancet:* "Does anyone imagine that the destruction of the entire mosquito tribe would result in the disappearance of malaria and yellow fever? . . . As long as filth and weather exist and eternal decomposition goes on, as long as ordinary filth conditions are unremedied, so long will Nature spread abroad the poisonous toxines that have existed since the world has been known, no matter whether they be carried by rats, cats, flies, or mosquitoes." In an editorial in the *Sanitarian,* A. N. Bell similarly questioned the "exclusive instrumentality of the mosquito." The *Texas Medical Journal,* official organ of the Texas State Association of Health Officers, came out unreservedly against the mosquito theory.[36] In Havana, meanwhile, U.S. Army personnel under the direction of Major W. C. Gorgas pressed ahead with a reformed program of sanitation based solely on the mosquito principle. Beginning in March, 1901, more than 26,000 breeding places in the city were identified and systematically eliminated. Twenty-three cases and six deaths from yellow fever were reported that summer, but by October the 140-year-old cycle of infection had been broken and Yellow Jack had virtually vanished from the Cuban capital.[37]

On United States soil, the first object lesson in the control of yellow fever through control of the mosquito vector came to pass in 1903 at the somewhat unlikely place of Laredo, a dusty railroad town on the southern border of Texas, more than one hundred miles from the sea. The fever had appeared far to the south at Veracruz in early spring and was gradually disseminated northward along the Mexican railroads, and by summer quite a number of communities in northeast Mexico were infected. On September 13, it was confirmed that the city of Monterrey was seriously infected, and "epidemic dengue" was reported to be raging at Nuevo Laredo just across the border from Laredo. The state of Texas reflexively ordered the disinfection of the mails, quarantined railroad communication

36. T. C. M., "The Mosquito in Yellow Fever," *Cincinnati Lancet,* XLVII (1901), 231–34; A. N. Bell, "Fomites and Yellow Fever," *Sanitarian,* XLVII (1901), 302–10; "That Mosquito Fallacy" and "Yellow Fever and the Mosquito," both in *Texas Medical Journal,* XVII (1902), 221–23 and 245–48, respectively.

37. W. C. Gorgas, "Disappearance of Yellow Fever from Havana, Cuba," *Medical News,* LXXXII (1903), 1–7.

with the neighboring country, and deployed Texas Rangers along the Rio Grande to guard the shallow crossings. The key cities of Corpus Christi and San Antonio shut down the railroads and imposed rigid and unconditional nonintercourse quarantines against Laredo and the rest of the border area. Soon the presence of yellow fever in Laredo itself was ascertained, and the state government requested the U.S. Public Health Service to step in and direct the effort to stamp it out. Dr. John Guiteras, who had been Gorgas' adjutant in the final campaign against Yellow Jack in Havana, was dispatched to the city and quantities of mosquito netting and pyrethrum were forwarded from New Orleans.

When he arrived in Laredo, on September 25, Guiteras was informed that two people had died and numerous suspicious cases were being watched. He was distressed to find *A. aegypti* "in enormous numbers and widely distributed." Laredo was in semiarid country, and most drinking water was delivered from the river by street vendors and stored in crocks and casks in the houses. What little was supplied through pipes by the small local waterworks was objectionably muddy, and had to be turned into settling barrels for clarifying before it could be used. Needless to say, as breeding places for the yellow fever mosquito, those arrangements left little to improve on. Workers were hired and instructed, and under conditions less than favorable, the necessary operations were organized. Officials had every reason to believe the infection had a head start of at least three weeks, and the people were unfamiliar with yellow fever and wholly ignorant of the mosquito theory of transmission. The Mexicans, who comprised the majority of the local population, had an ingrained distrust of gringo doctors and their methods, and many families took to concealing their sick. There was an almost superstitious resistance to the oiling of the water barrels, and "serious and menacing opposition" to this vital part of the work had to be overcome. "This was certainly an amazing condition of affairs," the cultivated Guiteras remarked, "and it was difficult to believe that such perversion and crass ignorance could exist within the confines of the Republic."

The *jacales* most of the people lived in were rude shacks clapped together with loose boards and sheet iron, and the screening and fumigating squads had to be accompanied by carpenters to make alterations preparatory to disinfection. There was still some uncertainty about the exact habitat of *A. aegypti,* so the streets of Laredo had to be thoroughly oiled to clean up countless puddles, ruts, and potholes, and oil was also sprayed along all the arroyos surrounding the city. The autumn was protracted, and warm, sultry weather lasted into mid-November. At the end of October, hundreds of seasonal laborers had started drifting back to town from cotton picking in the north, and the Texas attorney general declared that he had no law to prevent them. Steady headway was being made against the mosquito, nevertheless, and 2,952 habitations were disinfected by the end of the season. The epidemic in Laredo was limited to 1,050 known cases and 103 deaths, which was regarded as a satisfactory outcome in view of the peculiar drawbacks presented by the situation, and in consideration of the fact that Laredo's 18,000 people were virtually all nonimmune Mexicans, with a minority of equally susceptible whites.[38]

New Orleans sanitarians had not ignored or resisted the principle of mosquito transmission, but neither had they publicized the idea forcefully enough to stimulate adequate preventive measures in the community. In 1901, immediately after the findings of the Reed Commission were published and confirmed, a group of expert entomologists commissioned by the Orleans Parish Medical Society made a spot check of 200 cisterns in different parts of the city and found mosquitoes breeding in 198 of them. In July, the board of health issued a circular urging citizens to oil and screen their cisterns and also to get rid of disused tubs, pots, and similar water receptacles around their yards. There followed a desultory effort to back this advice with practical action, but the campaign fizzled out by September. The official report said that just enough indifference and antagonism had been encountered in the community to "vitiate the experiment." In 1903, the board reviewed the corpus of sanitary ordinances directed against yellow fever that had accumulated over the previous half-century and eliminated most of them as irrelevant or ineffective. The long-standing rule that forbade the tearing up of streets, dredging of ditches, or excavations of any other kind from May to September was struck out as "innocuous." Statutes relating to fomites were likewise weeded from the books, with suitable reflections on the terrible waste of time and money they had entailed over the years. From a practical standpoint, how-

38. U.S. Public Health Service, *Report for Fiscal 1904,* 230–325.

ever, these actions had only the marginal effect of propaganda, and no compulsory measures to eliminate the breeding places of *A. aegypti* were promulgated.[39]

It required another epidemic crisis, in 1905, to finally galvanize an effective program against the mosquito and conclusively banish yellow fever from New Orleans and the region to which it was the main portal of infection. New Orleans officials had no better luck pinpointing the origin of this outbreak than they had in past invasions, but the infection was known to have been prevalent at Belize and Colón earlier that year. It was also known that an amorphous "roman fever" had been circulating for some time among immigrant Italians of the Second District, but they were regarded as a furtive and suspicious lot who did not trust accredited doctors and were disinclined to seek help outside their own ethnic circle. The Italians blamed their sickness on putrid miasms from the dirty gutters, which the authorities neglected to clean up despite repeated protests. On July 12, 13, and 14, a number of probable cases on Decatur Street were reported by doctors in private practice. By July 18, the situation was serious enough to attract outside notice, and the U.S. Public Health Service sent two experts to "quietly investigate" matters. The next day, a visiting delegation from the board of health of Alabama concluded that "cases presenting the symptoms of yellow fever" had indeed been uncovered, and the port of Mobile, taking no chances, promptly declared rigid quarantine against New Orleans. The Public Health Service representatives proceeded with their investigation, and on July 25 verified that there had been at least fifty-four cases and twelve deaths from yellow fever in the city, and estimated that an area of forty to fifty blocks was infected. Weather conditions were "the worst possible . . . unusually hot and close," and by August 1, fifty-six deaths from yellow fever had been recorded in the Crescent City.[40]

Steps were taken immediately to meet the emergency in New Orleans. On July 24, a proclamation by the mayor and printed appeals from the Orleans Parish Medical Society explained the mosquito transmission of yellow fever and outlined the program that had to be put in motion. Vol-

39. Louisiana Board of Health, *Report for 1900–1901*, II, 46–56; Louisiana Board of Health, *Report for 1902–1903* (2 vols.; Baton Rouge, 1904), I, 91–92; Rubert W. Boyce, *Yellow Fever Prophylaxis in New Orleans, 1905* (Liverpool, 1906), 8–9.

40. *Public Health Reports*, XX (1905), 1505–10.

unteer directing committees were organized in each of the city's 17 wards, and screening and fumigating crews were hired, outfitted, and given instructions. Within a week, more than 2,000 cisterns had been oiled and screened, but the infection had improved its lead and new cases were on the increase, running at more than 40 a day by August 1. Mosquito destruction was cast into hard law on August 2, when the city council passed an order requiring householders to oil their cisterns and cover them with screen or cheesecloth within 48 hours; horse troughs and backyard ponds were to be immediately stocked with mosquito fish. There were at least 70,000 house cisterns in New Orleans, besides countless other breeding places, and it was forecast that "it is not improbable that the fight may be a long one." A citizens' committee quickly raised $150,000 in a series of subscription drives to fund the necessary work.[41]

In the interest of a better-coordinated campaign, local authorities formally requested the U.S. Public Health Service to assume supervision of operations on August 5. In promising the full support of the federal government, President Roosevelt remarked: "No one who has not been through an epidemic of that kind can appreciate the full horror that it brings." Detention camps were set up and a system of train inspection was instituted on all lines going out of the city. More detailed directives on fumigation and mosquito sanitation were issued, as were admonitions about promptly reporting cases, with special warnings about the danger presented by mild and juvenile cases. The influence of churches, public schools, and daily newspapers was tapped for a large-scale public education effort that attempted to reach all classes of the community and overcome any pockets of indifference or skepticism. Informational fliers and posters were printed in several languages and distributed by the thousands, and almost every evening there were neighborhood lectures and lantern shows on the mosquito problem, explaining how the puny pests were indeed "as dangerous as so many rattlesnakes." Saturdays and Sundays were designated "General Fumigation Days," and the people were requested to burn sulfur in their houses more or less simultaneously in the forenoon hours to better smoke the mosquito from all possible hiding places. Out of a misplaced concern that significant numbers of *A. aegypti*

41. Louisiana Board of Health, *Report for 1904–1905* (2 vols.; Baton Rouge, 1906), I, 11–45, II, 56–69; Boyce, *Yellow Fever Prophylaxis,* 16–34.

might be breeding in the gutters, an extensive campaign was launched to clean, oil, and salt all the gutters and street ditches.[42] New Orleans in 1905 was a city of 325,000 inhabitants, and the gutters were more than 700 miles in extent, but betterments in drainage and sewage disposal had not kept pace despite 50 years of exhortations from the board of health. The prominent British sanitarian Sir Rubert Boyce was a witness to these events and described the condition of the streets in language that might have been used in 1878:

> The paving of the streets was exceedingly bad and irregular and allowed for the formation of numerous pools after rains. An open drain on each side of the roadway contained for the most part very slowly moving or stagnant and putrescent water. The sewage fungus, *Sphoerotilus natans,* and the red worm (*Chironomus*) were present everywhere there was the least current. An abundance of decomposing refuse partially blocked them up at frequent intervals. Every now and then drains were "cleaned out" and the sludge was deposited on the roadway, there to be allowed to remain on the street till it had been completely scattered, or had found its way back to the drain again. The results of the absence of a proper system of garbage and sewage disposal was the production of an all-pervading odour of sewage, impossible to dissipate in the close and intensely hot summer months.[43]

There was still a deeply rooted dread of the conveyance of infection by fomites, and just as in 1878, 1888, and 1897, New Orleans found itself faced with an array of inland quarantines "so numerous and complicated as to defy description, causing many needless hardships, and almost total suspension of travel." Such curious items as candy and sheet music were among the things being turned back at some places. On August 8, the Louisiana State Board of Health published a proclamation that denied the legal or scientific right of parishes, towns, and villages to block the passage of trains or boats or to refuse to receive mail or freight. Officials threatened to call upon the governor to order out the state militia to restore the rule of reason at places that persisted in such interference. There were numer-

---

42. U.S. Public Health Service, *Report for Fiscal 1906,* 128–38, 143–46; Boyce, *Yellow Fever Prophylaxis,* 35–59.
43. Boyce, *Yellow Fever Prophylaxis,* 4.

ous appeals to Washington from local post offices for loan of the old form-aldehyde gas disinfecting apparatuses that had been used in 1897, but those requests were turned down by the Public Health Service as "unnecessary, and likely to confuse the public mind as to the real necessities in dealing with yellow fever."

The overwhelming public sentiment had to be accommodated to some degree, however. After July 25, outbound mail and freight cars were fumigated with sulfur immediately before leaving New Orleans, and sent out officially sealed and placarded by the Public Health Service. This measure was quite superfluous as far as any real probability of conveying infected mosquitoes was concerned, but it was nevertheless performed to allay local fears and satisfy the most rigid restrictions that might be met along the line. Over the course of the season, exactly 33,565 railroad cars were processed this way and sent forth. On August 9, the secretary of the Illinois State Board of Health complained that mosquitoes had been found in some of the banana cars crossing into the state at Cairo, and he reported serious protests on the part of the public against admitting any more fruit cars. The health officer of Los Angeles, California, made a similar declaration. Bananas could not be exposed to sulfur smoke because they became discolored. Later in the month, the United Fruit Company was constrained to shift its operations to Chalmette, seven miles below New Orleans, for discharge of cargoes. Fruit was loaded there into screened refrigerator cars that detoured around the infected city on a terminal line connecting to the Illinois Central.[44]

The infection had already become more or less diffused before its presence was recognized in New Orleans, and undoubtedly it continued to spread even after quarantine and mosquito-control measures were put into effect. A case had been discovered at Montgomery, Alabama, as early as July 28; the victim was promptly removed to the country and the state of Alabama banned all Louisiana travelers from its limits. Another case turned up at Morgan City, Louisiana, on July 31, in the person of a small boy with no apparent connection to New Orleans. On the second of August, Natchez, Mississippi, stated that several suspicious cases were being "closely watched" ; meanwhile, standing water around the town was being

44. *Public Health Reports,* XX (1905), 1679–81; U.S. Public Health Service, *Report for Fiscal 1906,* 139–41.

oiled, and lime was being scattered over the streets. By mid-August, cases had been reported in 23 towns in 15 parishes in Louisiana. Shotgun quarantines were thrown up all along the Red River in Louisiana and along the highways leading out of Vicksburg and other Mississippi landings, and Illinois began to require passenger trains from the south to keep moving at a designated speed, with all doors securely padlocked, until past Salem, 110 miles north of Cairo.[45]

To head off chaos, the Public Health Service sent its most reputable and persuasive experts through the main towns of the region, to explain rational measures of yellow fever prophylaxis and control based on the principle of mosquito transmission. Most places had not waited for official directions and had initiated their own hasty and somewhat confused campaigns against the pestilence, and many were still beset with antiquated notions about the propagation of the disease. Dr. Guiteras arrived at Vicksburg on August 2, where extra garbage squads had been deployed, the fire department had been set to work hosing out gutters, and special crews were busy scattering lime over the streets and disinfecting privies with carbolic acid. He observed: "Unfortunately, little if any attention has been given to the destruction of the mosquitoes and their breeding places." Despite the existence of a water company, barrels and cisterns were everywhere. Guiteras found *A. aegypti* abundant in the larval and pupal stages, and warned that conditions were ripe for a violent epidemic if an infecting case found its way into the city. He summoned the mayor, aldermen, and city health officer to a morning lecture and enlightened them on the role of the mosquito in transmitting the fever, sketching its natural history and explaining the approved means of destroying the insect. "It seems incredible," Guiteras reflected in his report to the surgeon general, "that so little should have been done on scientific lines to make impossible the spread of yellow fever in our southern cities." With few exceptions, however, medical and civic leaders at Vicksburg and elsewhere proved quite open in their thinking and gladly accepted the official advice. An energetic campaign was soon under way throughout the region, promoting screened cisterns and house fumigation.[46]

By the end of August, it was apparent that the worst outbreak of

45. *Public Health Reports*, XX (1905), 1559–60, 1618–19, 1675; Louisiana Board of Health, *Report for 1904–1905*, I, 45–67.

46. U.S. Public Health Service, *Report for Fiscal 1906*, 148–55.

yellow fever anywhere since 1878 was shaping up, and the proponents of the new mosquito doctrine were being put to their sorest test. Local authorities and the Public Health Service were having to play a desperate game of catch-up in both educational and sanitary efforts, and the week-by-week accounts published in the *Public Health Reports* series during this period make quite dramatic reading. Whole blocks were cordoned off and disinfected in Mobile after several Greek fruit peddlers were discovered convalescing from evident yellow fever. Pensacola had become seriously infected, and camp gear was forwarded to the vicinity in the expectation that the city would have to be depopulated. No cases had come to light in Memphis, but the president of the board of health observed that "the country around us is panicky," and requested Public Health Service help in clearing railroad traffic. Business in Natchez and the territory dependent on it for supplies was reported "paralyzed" after the confirmation of yellow fever in that city, and merchants were imploring the federal officials to take charge of train inspection and other matters.

Reports and rumors of fever came in from all corners of the region and, whether ultimately grounded in fact or not, had to be responsibly investigated by the Public Health Service. On September 1, a fatal case was reported at Maysville in the Chickasaw Nation of Indian Territory, and a government doctor was immediately dispatched from Galveston. When the physician arrived, he found evacuation of the settlement under way and the body in question too decomposed for a postmortem, but he began screening and fumigating houses and maintained a close scrutiny on things. He stayed in Maysville through the middle of the month and finally decided the case must have been one of malignant malaria. The surgeon general's office in Washington received numerous cables asking for reassurance about the truth of the mosquito doctrine and confirmation that former beliefs about yellow fever were defunct. On August 16, the president of the New Orleans Board of Trade related that "merchants of competitive cities are telling our customers that our goods are unsafe," and asked: "Is it not a fact that goods of any kind per se cannot carry infection?" He was informed that they could only be dangerous if they somehow harbored infected mosquitoes. People in Ellis County, in the heart of Texas, wondered if their elevation of 540 feet above sea level made them secure from yellow fever, and learned that no place no matter how high

was safe if mosquitoes bred there. On September 20, quarantine preparations by the state of Michigan were deemed "absolutely unnecessary."[47]

Quarantine lines were still tightly drawn around most areas at the end
of September, but nighttime temperatures were dipping into the fifties by
then, and frosts were falling by mid-October. The last case in New Orleans
was reported on November 22. There had been, in all, 452 deaths from
yellow fever in the city and another 536 in the parishes, yet this was considered a satisfactory showing in view of the exceptionally wide diffusion of
infection, the many conditions favoring an epidemic, and the peculiar set
of handicaps the sanitarians had to overcome. The expenditure necessary
to achieve this measure of success had been considerable. In New Orleans
alone, 68,000 cisterns had been screened and oiled and more than 55,000
apartments had been fumigated, requiring 448,000 pounds of sulfur and
5,000 pounds of pyrethrum. The season had been costly in terms of labor
and material, but the savings in human life were incalculable. In 1853, Yellow Jack had killed 165 of the 1,000 inhabitants of Lake Providence, Louisiana; Lake Providence was now a community of over 2,000, but a vigorous and timely antimosquito program had limited the death list to just 23.
In 1878, there had been 250 deaths in and around Port Gibson, Mississippi,
then a town of little more than 1,000 people; the losses in 1905 were held
to just 4. Vicksburg had been horribly ravaged by the fever in both 1853
and 1878, but this year the deaths in that city of 15,000 stopped at 26.

The mosquito doctrine had been thoroughly vindicated in professional circles, and even more importantly, it had found a broad foundation of popular acceptance. The report of the surgeon general of the U.S.
Public Health Service called the campaign of 1905 a "great triumph,"
which had finally "established confidence in human mastery of the yellow
scourge." This was a bold declaration, and statements like it had been
made before, but this time the pronouncement was based on truly verifi-
able results. That fall the New Orleans City Council enacted permanent
ordinances relating to screening of cisterns and mosquito suppression generally. Residual centers of endemicity around the Caribbean were gradually cleaned up. Belize and West Indian ports were freed from yellow fever

---

47. *Public Health Reports,* XX (1905), 1741–52, 1803–17, 1871–83, 1923–35, 1983–93,
2061–67; U.S. Public Health Service, *Report for Fiscal 1906,* 147–94.

by British authorities within a few years, and the Isthmian cities were made secure soon after construction of the Panama Canal began in 1907. Mexico and the Central American republics completed their sanitation programs by 1924. The last serious urban outbreak in the Americas was suppressed at Rio de Janeiro in 1928. The last direct threat to North American was during the years from 1948 to 1956, when jungle yellow fever swept around the margins of the Caribbean in a major epizootic wave, decimating howler monkey populations from Venezuela to Guatemala. Although a few rural settlements in Panama and Costa Rica became infected, the situation was closely watched and the fever failed to invade any sizeable community.[48]

48. On early mosquito control efforts around the Caribbean, see Rubert W. Boyce, *Health Progress and Administration in the West Indies* (New York, 1911). On later yellow fever sanitation in South America, see John Duffy, ed., *Ventures in World Health: The Memoirs of Fred Lowe Soper* (New York, 1977), 326–43. For a good firsthand account of one early campaign, see H. R. Carter, "Yellow Fever in Peru—Epidemic of 1919 and 1920," *American Journal of Tropical Medicine*, II (1922), 87–106. On recent problems, see Robert T. Tonn, Rafael Figueredo, and Luis J. Uribe, "*Aedes aegypti,* Yellow Fever, and Dengue in the Americas," *Mosquito News,* XLII (1982), 497–501. For a general history of yellow fever since 1900, see A. W. A. Brown, "Yellow Fever, Dengue, and Dengue Haemorrhagic Fever," in *A World Geography of Human Diseases,* ed. G. Melvyn Howe (London, 1977), 293–302. On a major 1950s epizootic and the discussion it evoked, see "Yellow Fever Conference," *American Journal of Tropical Medicine and Hygiene,* IV (1955), 571–661. On *A. aegypti* control in the United States, see Duffy, ed., *Ventures in World Health,* 344–57; Harvey B. Marlon and Milton E. Tinker, "Distribution of *Aedes aegypti* Infestations in the United States," *American Journal of Tropical Medicine and Hygiene,* XIV (1965), 892–99; Asa C. Chandler, "History of *Aedes aegypti* Control Work in Texas," *Mosquito News,* XVI (1956), 58–63. Some recent discussions of the yellow fever problem are "Yellow Fever: Cause for Concern?" *British Medical Journal,* 282 (1981), 1735–36; Hernando Groot, "*Aedes aegypti:* A Sword of Damocles Hanging over Tropical America," *Bulletin of the Pan American Health Organization,* XV (1981), 267–70.

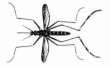

SEVEN

The 1878 Epidemic in Summary and Perspective

All in all, the year 1878 had been a satisfactory one for the United States, as President Hayes reviewed it in his annual message to Congress that December. The nation was at peace. Crops had been good in most sections of the country, and manufacturing and commerce were showing welcome signs of recovery after five years of depression. The administration had continued to make progress on the public debt and was able to report a $20 million revenue surplus for the current year. But the otherwise happy state of the Union had been seriously marred by the appearance that summer of "a fatal pestilence, the yellow fever." The whole nation had been disconcerted by the yellow fever invasion; several states had been completely overwhelmed by it. More than 100,000 cases were believed to have occurred, and estimates put the number of dead as high as 20,000. "It is impossible to estimate with any approach to accuracy the loss to the country occasioned by this epidemic," said Hayes. "It is to be reckoned by the hundred millions of dollars."

As a matter of fact, $100 million was the very lowest estimate of what yellow fever had cost the country, and while economists might disagree about the specific figure, no one could deny the enormous expense of the epidemic. It was conservatively stated that the city of New Orleans had suffered direct losses of $15 million, involving huge commercial forfeitures due to suspension of industry and diversion of trade, with additional millions in lost wages, and the heavy cost of medical attendance and relief for thousands of sick and unemployed. Some claimed that a full calculation of the city's losses, covering the capitalized value of lives lost and long-term depreciation of property values, would add at least $15 million more. For the nation as a whole, estimates of the damage wrought by the great epidemic ran as high as $200 million. What $200 million represented at that time was put in perspective by J. M. Keating of Memphis, who called it "a sum nearly equal to the annual expenditures of the United States Government for all purposes, including interest payment, which in 1877, was $238,000,000; a total that, if levied in one year as an addition to existing public burdens, would create a revolution and endanger the stability of our government; a sum nearly equal to the total of our annual exports of cotton, and nearly equal to one-third of the total of all our annual exports."

The exceptional malignancy of the infection was a signal feature of the 1878 epidemic. At least 4,000 and probably more than 5,000 lives were claimed by the fever at New Orleans, at least 5,000 and possibly more than 6,000 at Memphis. Authorities settled on the round number of 18,000 as the best estimate of the epidemic's total cost in American life. At New Orleans, long familiarity with yellow fever had evolved a community that was fairly hardened to the disease, immunologically and psychologically. The actual losses there were proportionately much lighter than elsewhere and the situation was borne by the people with comparative equipoise. But at many inland communities, where yellow fever had never been experienced, the epidemic fell as a dreadful exotic scourge; the ravages were terrible and the reaction was hysterical, highlighted by shotgun quarantines, the abandonment of towns, miasmatists who demanded fires and gunpowder explosions, and pietists who called for fasting and prayer. At some places the reported fatality rate among white inhabitants approached or exceeded 50 percent, and absolute losses were kept down only by the pell-mell scattering of the people. A mortality experience like this was unmatched in American medical history. Imagination sought parallels in the plagues of ancient and medieval times; the destroyer was apostrophized in biblical terms, as the "King of Terrors."

The fact that the fever appeared at many new and surprising places in 1878 was a feature of the epidemic that contributed much to its virulence, and also to subsequent interest in it. The spread of the disease revealed the wide though irregular extent to which the yellow fever mosquito had established itself in the region since it was first introduced a century earlier.

Louisville and St. Louis marked the northern limits of the epidemic, with small but serious outbreaks confirmed in both cities. Neither city had ever seen yellow fever before, and neither would ever experience it again. The unusual weather was apparently the controlling variable everywhere; the region had just passed through a freakishly mild winter, which presumably allowed high survival of fall-laid eggs, succeeded by a long, warm spring that favored extended breeding. Up until 1878, places like Grenada and Holly Springs had always considered themselves to be noninfectible, and there is good evidence that they really were so as late as 1873. But the rapid and severe spread of infection in those towns in 1878 presupposed a heavy infestation of mosquitoes, which indicates that breeding, if not permanent, was at least abundant and generally distributed at that time. At borderline places like Bowling Green, where the infected area was quite circumscribed and developed only late in the season after repeated exposures, the mosquitoes were likely the progeny of ones introduced earlier that same year. It seems clear that the remarkable outbreak at Gallipolis, away up the Ohio River, was produced by infected mosquitoes brought directly to the place on one pestiferous riverboat.

A century of observation had fostered a general belief that the yellow fever menace was confined to fairly well-defined geographical limits, an essentially tropical and deep-southern problem that the rest of the country could afford to look upon with indifference, or at least with charitable detachment. The comfortable notion of a "yellow fever zone" was shaken by the severe epidemic at Memphis in 1873; it was completely upset by the occurrence of epidemics hundreds of miles beyond Memphis in 1878. The recurrence of the fever in 1879 only emphasized the fact that it had suddenly become, "in its mysterious strides into the interior, a great national scourge, afflicting to the hearts of the people, and interrupting great avenues of trade and commerce essential to the wholesome development of important industries and the material wealth of the country." Important river cities and railroad towns drew their vital nourishment from the very lines of transportation with which yellow fever was so peculiarly associated, making the question of quarantine against this disease a peculiarly anxious one. The old doctrine of local origin still had some adherents, but their ranks were dwindling and their arguments were steadily less persuasive. Many localities in the heart of the fever region were congratulating themselves on having shut out the pestilence with shotguns, and while

those spontaneous arrangements might be decried as barbaric, their osten-
sible success served to stimulate feeling that a regulated system of quarantine for the whole region was feasible. The National Board of Health attempted such a system in the 1880s, emphasizing sanitation of riverboats
and interception of fomites. State authorities provided for the breaking
and disinfection of railroad freights at their borders. All such arrangements
would have offered no resistance whatever to yellow fever had it attempted
another assault.

Depopulation—the defusing of yellow fever epidemics by deliberately
evacuating infected communities—was a time-tested idea brought into
wider practice in the 1870s. It was undertaken rather helplessly by local
authorities at Memphis in 1878, but a little more methodically by the Tennessee State Board of Health the following year. In subsequent years, the
U.S. Marine Hospital Service attempted to reduce depopulation to an
exact system. People originally assumed that yellow fever was fundamentally noncontagious—the germs locally saprophytic, adhering to places
and things, and only facultatively infectious to human beings—and that
persons fleeing an infected center presented little or no danger of infection
to the places they fled to. The problem of depopulation merged into that
of quarantine with the dawning recognition that refugees themselves,
apart from any fomites they carried, might be dangerous sources of infection after all. At the camps it administered outside Jacksonville in 1888 and
New Orleans in 1897, the Marine Hospital Service enforced a ten-day
"probation" for refugees before allowing them to leave the area. This
would have encompassed the actual incubation period of yellow fever in
humans and, on paper at least, should have constituted an effective check
on the spread of yellow fever. But given the realities of enforcement, it is
doubtful that even the most theoretically correct quarantine against yellow
fever could, in practice, have succeeded in establishing anything but a
more sophisticated system of leaks.

Sanitarians correctly recognized that the ultimate answer in yellow
fever prevention would have to consist in altering or abolishing the local
conditions on which it manifestly depended for its propagation. Unfortunately, the one notable development in yellow fever prophylaxis to come
out of the 1878 epidemic was a negative one—the debacle of carbolic acid
disinfection that earlier experience had made to appear so promising. But
it was the particular chemical used and not the principle of disinfection

that seemed to be discredited. The epidemiological observations and etio-logical statements that emerged from the epidemic were not particularly brilliant or insightful, but they did tend to confirm the infectious character of the disease and thus its germ origin—and an inferential belief in germs could only invite continued efforts to kill them off by artificial means. Clear to the end of the century, sanitarians maintained their fascination with the possibility of neutralizing the yellow fever germ with antiseptic compounds applied to drains, floors, and pavements. Bichloride of mer-cury was the fad in the 1880s, and formaldehyde in the 1890s. Some per-ceived a special disinfecting power in sulfur smoke—coincidentally an ef-fective mosquito-killer—but fumigations were usually imperfect, so the evidence remained unclear and its continued use was only in a subsidiary manner.

"The lesson that good sanitary conditions are the prime protection for a community, is the main lesson," the New Orleans *Times* editorialized in 1879. "The fever-breeding alley will avenge itself on the avenue sooner or later, and the tenement house will send its infection to the mansion in time." The circular logic that associated yellow fever with cities, and cities with filth, and therefore filth with yellow fever, had survived the decline of the local-causation doctrine with which it had originated, and indeed seemed unshakable. Only a few of the more penetrating observers doubted it. The grand schemes of municipal cleansing and sanitary improvement proposed after 1878—the schemes proposed were grander than any actu-ally implemented—were all based on that illusory premise, and any good they could have done was only incidental. Street paving and garbage dis-posal would have had even less potential effect on the yellow fever mos-quito than burning pine tar. But at many cities, the push for thorough municipal hygiene included the demand for pure drinking water; at Mem-phis and elsewhere, this meant that vats and barrels were replaced with a piped water supply, which as a matter of fact would have greatly reduced mosquito infestation and thus the liability to yellow fever.

The practice was right even if the theory was off the mark. By the 1870s, American sanitarians generally recognized that foul water was a ma-jor vehicle for typhoid and cholera infection, and there was a feeling that some of the other "zymotic" diseases might have a similar etiology. The town of Huntsville claimed that its exemption from yellow fever in 1878 was largely owing to the piped water supply it had installed after suffering an epidemic of cholera in 1873. Some interesting observations along the same lines were made at Chattanooga, where yellow fever in 1878 was seen to follow the same pattern cholera had in 1873: neighborhoods served with piped water remained uninfected, while the epidemic raged in an adjoining district where the people still drew their water from shallow wells. But here again the body of evidence was conflicting. When National Board of Health chemists examined the well water at Grenada, they concluded that it was pure and wholesome, and had not been a factor in the pestilence there. No one suggested any connection with mosquitoes, but that would have required a leap of imagination considerably greater than John Snow contemplating the Broad Street pump.

Whatever the reason, Yellow Jack's prowlings in the Mississippi Valley later in the century never again approached the wide scope of the 1878 epidemic. Nor did its depredations ever again attain the same dreadful magnitude. But the King of Terrors was firmly planted in the memories of that generation, and even at a distance of twenty years, the very rumor of the fever's reappearance was enough to derange the region's daily life and addle its communities with panic. A series of disruptive outbreaks at the end of the 1890s suggested that the situation was beginning to deteriorate again, but the fortunate discovery of the mosquito vector in 1900 uncovered the secret of effective control and redefined the sanitation of yellow fever. What might have been a very malignant epidemic in the summer of 1905 was cut short by the hasty implementation of mosquito abatement measures worked out by army sanitarians in Cuba a few years before. Yellow fever retreated over the southern horizon, never to reappear in epidemic form on United States soil.

The yellow fever virus still lurks among the monkeys of South America's tropical forests, and in that vast wild reservoir, its ultimate lair, it is considered ineradicable. And it is a lamentable fact that the policy of complete elimination of the domestic vector in this hemisphere, so hopeful a prospect at the beginning of this century, was permitted to lapse in most countries in later decades. Indeed, the United States has been one of the worst delinquents in developing and maintaining a consistent program against *A. aegypti*. In 1964, the U.S. Public Health Service surveyed 5,257 communities in eleven southeastern states and found *A. aegypti* infestations in 566 of them. Large cities showed a particularly high frequency of infestation, with the mosquito found in 23 of 41 cities with populations over 50,000. But while sanitarians continue to warn of the danger to infectible towns and cities from chance importations of yellow fever from jungle sources, the present consensus seems to be that any urban outbreak of the disease would quickly be recognized and brought under heel, aborted by largescale spraying, before it attained serious proportions. For now, it seems safe to hazard the statement that the King of Terrors is deposed as a matter of fact, and if its final execution has been impossible to arrange, it has at least been effectively exiled.

INDEX